Patient and Family Education

Tools, Techniques, and Theory

Patient and Family Education

Tools, Techniques, and Theory

Edited by

Rose-Marie Duda McCormick, RN, BS

Tamar Gilson-Parkevich, RN, MS

A Wiley Medical Publication

JOHN WILEY & SONS

New York · Chichester · Brisbane · Toronto

The proceeds derived from the sale of this publication have been designated for the advancement of patient care and education for children and families of The Children's Hospital, Columbus, Ohio.

The information contained in this book, especially the Helping Hands, should be viewed as a guide. It is recommended by the authors that the reader obtain the necessary and appropriate administrative and/or medical guidance before implementing the systems or using the teaching aids provided. The authors and publisher cannot be held responsible for any consequences resulting from the use or misuse of information contained in this book.

Cover design and illustrations by Jenene DeMars Warmbier.

"Whatever Your Gift" from HOLD TO YOUR DREAM by Helen Lowrie Marshall. Copyright 1965 by Helen Lowrie Marshall. Reprinted by permission of Doubleday & Company, Inc.

Library of Congress Cataloging in Publication Data

McCormick, Rose-Marie.
  Patient and family education.

  (A Wiley medical publication)
  Includes index.
  1. Patient education. I. Parkevich, Tamar
J., joint author. II. Title.

RA440.5.M28   615'.5   79–10014
ISBN 0-471-04269-2

Printed in the United States of America

10 9 8 7 6 5 4 3 2 1

To the children, families, and staff
of Children's Hospital

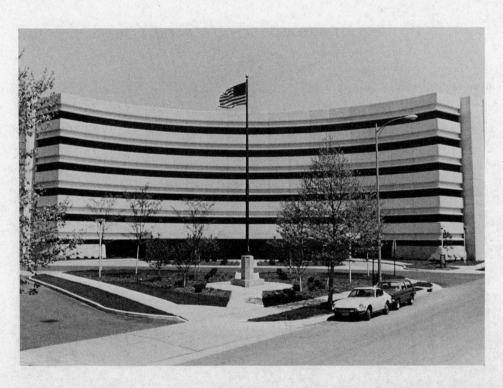

Contributors

JANE HARMAN HOOKER, RN, MS, is the Associate Director of Nursing Education at Children's Hospital. She received her bachelor's degree in nursing and her master's degree in nursing education from Ohio State University. She has held a variety of positions at Children's Hospital, including Assistant Head Nurse and Clinical Instructor for affiliating students. Presently, she is responsible for administering staff development programs for the Nursing Department and for coordinating pediatric experiences for eight schools of nursing.

BARBARA TURNER HORD, RN, is the Nursing Quality Assurance Director at Children's Hospital. She is a graduate of the St. Francis School of Nursing, Columbus, Ohio. Her career in pediatric nursing has included supervision, education, program planning, and editing of the Nursing Department newsletter, *Caring*. Ms. Hord's concern for maintaining consistently high standards of patient care has led to her involvement in quality assurance and the H.E.L.P. program. With a focus on evaluation, her responsibilities include coordinating nursing and medical audits of patient records, communicating audit findings, and collaborating with staff for improvements in patient care.

EVALEE KECK LEEPER, RN, is the Homegoing Education and Literature Program Coordinator at Children's Hospital. A graduate of White Cross School of Nursing, Columbus, Ohio, she has thirty years of experience in pediatrics, including operating room and emergency room nursing and the initiation and organization of the Poison Control Center in Columbus. Interested in improving patient care through education, she has been involved in developing and coordinating the Continuity of Patient Care program and teaching students and health professionals.

ROSE-MARIE DUDA McCORMICK, RN, BS, is the Director of the Homegoing Education and Literature Program at Children's Hospital. She received her bachelor's degree in nursing from the University of Cincinnati. She developed an interest in improving health care in the home as a result of her experience in community health nursing. Before developing H.E.L.P., she was involved in organizing the Continuity of Patient Care and Diabetes Education programs at Children's Hospital and in coordinating the pediatric clinical experiences of nursing students.

TAMAR GILSON-PARKEVICH, RN, MS, is Director of Nursing at Children's Hospital and a member of the hospital's upper management team. She received her baccalaureate degree in nursing and master's degree in nursing administration and pediatric clinical specialty from the Ohio State University. Her professional experience includes staff nursing, clinical instruction, and various nursing management roles. With a sense of commitment to the highest standards of patient care and nursing, Ms. Parkevich strives to stimulate and generate innovative programs through participative management aimed at holistic nursing service. She supported and guided the initiation and development of the H.E.L.P. program at Children's Hospital.

DAVID S. STEIN, PhD, is the Educational Consultant for Children's Hospital. He is also Assistant Professor of Medical Communications at the Ohio State University School of Allied Medical Professions. He received his bachelor's degree from the State University of New York, his master's degree in education from the University of Rochester, and his doctorate in education from the University of Michigan. He is responsible for planning and coordinating continuing medical education programs and inservice education for hospital personnel. Dr. Stein has developed a number of audiovisual patient education programs for children which are being used throughout the state of Ohio.

LAUREL RATCLIFF TALABERE, RN, MS, is a pulmonary clinical specialist at Children's Hospital. She received her bachelor's degree in nursing from the University of Connecticut and her master's degree from Ohio State University. Her previous experience includes staff nursing, in-service education, and faculty positions in pediatric and community health nursing. In her present position, she provides family teaching and counseling and serves as a consultant to the staff for the nursing management of chronically ill children with respiratory problems. She is also involved in research and has published several articles.

JENENE DeMARS WARMBIER is the Homegoing Education and Literature Program illustrator. She studied fine arts and communications at the University of Toledo and is currently pursuing a bachelor's degree in medical communications at Ohio State University. Her background includes experience in business administration, advertising, and graphics. She created and illustrated an educational coloring book for children with cancer and helped to organize the Pediatric Oncology Helpers, a parent support group. These experiences led to a personal commitment to family health education and involvement with the H.E.L.P. program.

Preface

*"Education is man's best friend
in his struggle with the unknown . . .
an enlightened and prepared man is
a better master of himself
than one kept in the dark."*

L.E. Celestin

This book is designed for today's health professionals and students who, by virtue of their involvement in patient/client care, are committed to patient education and have assumed responsibility for providing it. Without this commitment, a successful program of patient education cannot be accomplished. *Patient and Family Education: Tools, Techniques, and Theory* aids in creating a successful program by helping the health professional or student review patient education theory, develop a system for creating teaching aids, write and illustrate teaching aids, document the components of teaching, evaluate teaching aids and the effectiveness of instruction, and plan a patient education conference.

We not only review patient education theory but also show how to apply this theory in creating and implementing an instructional program. The concepts, systems, tools, and techniques provide a practical approach readily applicable to any pediatric or adult care setting. In addition, more than seventy patient education aids on a variety of health topics are included for immediate use or adaptation.

This publication is an outgrowth of the Homegoing Education and Literature Program (H.E.L.P.) of Children's Hospital in Columbus, Ohio. The H.E.L.P. program evolved as a result of our belief in the patient's and family's right to know and our dissatisfaction with the teaching aids that were currently available. Hence, we decided to prepare our own teaching aids for use in our institution. Now, after creating a substantial number of "Helping Hands" and a workable system of patient instruction, we wish to share this information with you.

We are witnessing a change in the attitude of the health professional and the consumer toward patient education. The consumer rights movement, the requirements of governmental and accrediting agencies, and today's emphasis on prevention of health problems attest to this change. With this change comes the challenge of providing accumulated knowledge with a fresh approach. This easy-to-use, practical handbook is designed to help you meet this challenge.

Patient and Family Education brings together the expertise of many knowledgeable and dedicated persons without whose contributions our efforts would have fallen short of our goal. Our medical and nursing staffs, as well as our physical, occupational, and respiratory therapists, pharmacists, laboratory personnel, dietitians, social workers, patient activities staff, and patients and families have generously shared their time and experience in developing the Helping Hands teaching aids. Other significant contributions were made by people in numerous administrative departments and in the departments of education and nursing education. In addition, our printing department was instrumental in helping us devise systems for paper flow, printing, ordering, and storage. We wish to thank the many photographers who contributed pictures to the book. We owe a special word of thanks to Linda Rugh, our very dedicated and capable secretary/typist, and others who assisted in preparing the teaching materials and the manuscript. We wish to express our appreciation to all those who so ably and willingly contributed their knowledge and experience in the development of the H.E.L.P. program.

Rose-Marie Duda McCormick, RN, BS
Tamar Gilson-Parkevich, RN, MS

Contents

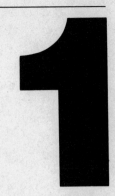

Theory
and Techniques

They Heard . . . But Did Not Remember

In the beginning—there was life.
  The life of a child and parent—
Both "patients"
  In our vast medical system.

Far be it from us to think these
  Patients capable of understanding
Complex medical information. So . . .
  They were not told.

Then came
  The patient's right to know.
So we told . . .
  And they "listened."

Listening
  Through their preoccupations and fears,
They heard—
  But did not remember.

Dismayed, we asked ourselves,
  Why won't these people follow our guidance?
Why do they jeopardize
  The life of this child?

Then—I was "the patient."
  They told me and I listened.
I heard . . . but did not remember.
  I now understand.

Rose-Marie McCormick

chapter 1
Focus
on Patient Education

Tamar Gilson-Parkevich

"To be what we are, and to become what we are capable of becoming, is the only end of life."

Robert Louis Stevenson

Patient education has come of age. The *patient's right to know* and *informed consent* are discussed everywhere from the halls of Congress to television and magazines. To some patient education is a blessing, to others a headache—but to all it's a reality which is here to stay.

Daily we are reminded that patients and their families are more aware of their needs as health care consumers. Newspaper headlines depict legal claims of inadequate care. Consumers' dinner table conversations include shocked statements, and sometimes protestations, over the high cost of health care. Television and communications media graphically reflect society's concern over moral issues—such as the right to life, the right to die—and the impact of these issues on health institutions. Consumer movements have encouraged participation of the public in the decision-making processes of health insurance companies, hospital boards, and other health agencies. Increasingly, clients are developing much of the necessary sense of individual responsibility for acquiring and maintaining optimum health status. And, as consumers of health care services, our patients are developing expectations, educating themselves about their needs and rights, and demanding quality health care services at reasonable costs.

Many health care professionals recognize patients' needs for health education but, for a variety of reasons, are not adequately providing for these needs. One reason may be that relatively few instructional resources are available to assist in this effort. There are many books and articles that expound the *importance* of patient education but few that explain the "how to's" in a realistic, usable manner.

So, we have H.E.L.P. for you. We want to HELP you to provide and to promote patient education. We want to HELP you to gain the security and confidence to teach. We want to HELP you to achieve the satisfaction of knowing your patients' educational needs are being met.

How can we help? By sharing with you our Homegoing Education and Literature Program (H.E.L.P.). The health care professionals of Children's Hospital, Columbus, Ohio, have undertaken the exciting and thoroughly challenging project of developing health education tools for patients, parents, and staff. The H.E.L.P. concept is designed to provide pertinent, high quality, cost-effective instructional aids, which we call "Helping Hands." This program was developed by members of our Nursing Department in response to the deficiencies of many of the available patient education materials. After 3 years' time and much

3

effort, we are eager to share our Homegoing Education and Literature Program with you.

HEALTH EDUCATION: WHAT IS IT?

Health care is undergoing rapid change. Many needs, issues, and problems are being identified and pursued. Technology and treatment modes are developing and are becoming more sophisticated and complex. At the same time, the heretofore "sacred" health care professions are receiving scrutiny from the federal government, third party payors, peer review organizations, and the public. Many committed health care workers are themselves evaluating the needs of their patients and the quality and effectiveness of their care. The goal of these many efforts is to develop and insure high standards of care for all consumers.

As a result of these forces, health education is gaining greater importance. The responsibility for providing health education is being recognized as fundamental to the health care delivery system. Obviously, health education is not new. Patients have always had a need to know and to understand health alterations and preventive health care measures, as well as the health care delivery system itself. These needs, however, have been sorely overlooked or neglected in the past. Now, *finally*, the patient's need and right to know are being fully recognized.

DEFINITION OF HEALTH EDUCATION

What exactly is health education? Health education is the process by which individuals and groups learn to promote, to maintain, and to restore health. According to Somers, the objectives of health education are:

1. To improve health by (a) communication of information to prevent illness and disability and (b) facilitation of necessary modification in behavior or life style if indicated

2. To restrain inflation of health care costs through preventive health care, thereby relieving some of the demand for more costly curative health services

3. To involve the patient constructively in his own health maintenance and in his effective use of the health care system

In short, health education is guiding people in perceiving healthful actions as consistent with their own values and goals (Somers, p. 15).

Health education is an emerging career field "drawing upon knowledge of biomedical, biostatistical, and behavioral sciences as well as various administrative, planning, and research skills" (Somers, p. xxvi). Health education also incorporates communication skills and concepts, including audiovisual media, graphics, and verbal dialogue.

Patient education, that component of health education directed toward persons already accessing the health care system, requires the use of similar skills and knowledge. Patient education can take a variety of forms—from a videotape acquainting patients with the hospital to a one-on-one counseling session for a diabetic patient. It may involve instruction about chronic, acute, or preventive care or the most effective and efficient use of the health care system. Patient education is conducted in a variety of settings, with different emotional climates, different types of teachers, and different types of learners. The only link which can tie it all together, however, is the written word, and our Helping Hands provide that vital link.

WHO IS RESPONSIBLE FOR PATIENT EDUCATION?

We all are. All of us associated with health care delivery are in some way involved in patient education. In our present system, the responsibility for health education does not rest solely on the shoulders of a single group of health professionals. Health education cannot be separated from the total health care delivery system. Each organization within the system faces educational challenges and opportunities relative to clients' needs, prevalent diseases, population demographics, and so on. Therefore, we are all responsible for the education and preparation of the patients we serve. The patient educator is *you,* the hospital administrator, and *you,* the physician or nurse. And also *you,* the x-ray or laboratory technician, and *you,* the student health professional.

What is the impact of this responsibility on health care professionals? We know that the provision of health education requires trained personnel, knowledgeable in both the health topic and the teaching-learning process. We have also learned that effective patient education requires the resources of time and materials to support the educational endeavor.

Many health care workers may be threatened by this type of responsibility, feeling inadequate or unqualified to teach. Many, while recognizing the need, may not have time to teach and as a result may feel frustrated. Still others, while attempting to meet their patient's educational needs, may lack appropriate teaching materials and a sophisticated system to support their educational effort. In many settings, patient education rates a low priority, and when efforts are made to provide education on a routine basis, a team approach is seldom used.

What is your perspective on patient education? Are your patients receiving appropriate instruction? Is your health care facility meeting the information needs of patients and families? Do you have teaching materials available? Do you reap the personal satisfaction of having taught your patients to achieve and to maintain their optimum health status? Do you sense the challenge and delight of meeting individual patient education needs with creativity and sensitivity? If you cannot respond affirmatively to each question, do not feel dismayed. You are *not* alone.

With the increasing recognition of patient education needs, hospitals and other health care organizations are developing various approaches to the design and implementation of patient education programs. In some settings, patient education committees have been appointed to develop and to coordinate patient education programs. Other institutions have developed a decentralized model in which each functional area or unit develops its own programs in conjunction with a hospital education department. This department assumes responsibility for coordination, consultation, staff education, and "change agent" functions. A new breed of health care worker, the patient education coordinator, is also being developed to promote and to assist in patient education. The role of this health educator is being defined in various ways, typically including responsibility for the planning, coordination and/or provision of patient education. Creation of this kind of role appears to be a popular means of implementing formal programs of patient education in hospitals. The coordinator provides a resource for knowledge and teaching materials and supports staff members through role model activities and group classes on teaching.

Each program model emphasizes the primary importance of involving the total staff in the provision of patient education. Each institution and organization must define its own approach to patient education first by developing objectives and content and then by deciding how and by whom these objectives will be accomplished.

According to Somers, it is not possible at this point to say which health care discipline will emerge as dominant in the field of patient education. Today nurses are providing more health education than any other group. This is explained by the large number of nurses, their general knowledge of health and illness, and their direct contact with patients (Somers, p. 42). Historically, nurses have willingly accepted the responsibility for planning and coordinating many elements of patient care (short of diagnosis and prescription of medical care) and in general have acted as patient advocates. It thus seems appropriate that nurses lead the way in promoting, developing, and executing formal programs to meet the educational needs of patients.

COMPONENTS OF A HEALTH EDUCATION SYSTEM

The approach to health education must be organized, deliberate, and specifically designed to meet the needs of the consumer. There are six components to an effective system of patient education:

Organizational structure. Patient education, as an integral part of health care organizations, requires the support of administration, health care workers, and the consumer. The patient education system must be able to relate effectively to the organization, its workers, and its clients.

Philosophy and objectives. The organization, and the individuals within it, must recognize and believe in the integral relationship between patient education and other health care services. Educational needs must be identified and given priorities, and alternative approaches must be evaluated and decisions made.

Allocation of resources. Staff, materials, and thoughtful support must be provided to develop, to refine, and to evaluate patient education programs. "A significant corporate commitment, including staff and financial resources, is essential if hospitals and other health care institutions are to fulfill their leadership role in health education" (American Hospital Association, p. 2).

System design. The health education system must be designed to meet the consumer's needs in the most economic and efficient manner, with awareness of and sensitivity to the problems of those responsible for client education. The system must have the flexibility to change and to improve.

Caregiver involvement. Caregivers must have the direction, knowledge, skills, and time to fulfill health education responsibilities.

Patient involvement. Direct patient and family involvement must occur if learning is to take place. Education is an active process involving the mutual exchange of information between the teacher and the learner.

DEVELOPMENTS AND INFLUENCES IN PATIENT EDUCATION

While patient education is not a new development, it has only been given formal recognition in the last 2 decades. In 1964 the American Medical Association sponsored the First National Conference on Health Education Goals. This conference identified two primary objectives for health education: (1) to educate the individual to assume responsibility for maintaining personal health and (2) to develop responsibility for participation in community health programs. Methods envisioned to meet these goals included individual motivation, school health education, and educational activities in a variety of health agencies and associations (Holder, p. 2308).

The President's Committee on Health Education, created in 1971, released a report 2 years later that recommended, among other things, the establishment of independent focal points within both the public and private sectors to coordinate the various health education-related activities of each respective sector and to foster research in effective methods of health education. The year 1973 also witnessed the passage of the Health Maintenance Organization Act (P.L. 93-222), which assigned HMO's the responsibility of providing health education to their subscribers. The National Health Planning and Resources Development Act of 1974 (P.L. 93-641) further identified public education in preventive health care and in effective use of health services as one of ten national health planning goals.

In response to the recommendations of the 1973 report of the President's Committee, the federal government in 1974 established the Bureau of Health Education within the Center for Disease Control. The private sector counterpart was realized the following year with the awarding of an HEW contract to the National Center for Health Education, an initiative of private industry.

In a 1974 position statement, the American Hospital Association identified the role of hospitals in patient

---

A PATIENT'S BILL OF RIGHTS

AMERICAN HOSPITAL ASSOCIATION

The American Hospital Association presents a Patient's Bill of Rights with the expectation that observance of these rights will contribute to more effective patient care and greater satisfaction for the patient, his physician, and the hospital organization. Further, the Association presents these rights in the expectation that they will be supported by the hospital on behalf of its patients as an integral part of the healing process. It is recognized that a personal relationship between the physician and the patient is essential for the provision of proper medical care.

The traditional physician-patient relationship takes on a new dimension when care is rendered within an organizational structure. Legal precedent has established that the institution itself also has a responsibility to the patient. It is in recognition of these factors that these rights are affirmed.

1. The patient has the right to considerate and respectful care.

2. The patient has the right to obtain from his physician complete current information concerning his diagnosis, treatment, and prognosis in terms the patient can be reasonably expected to understand. When it is not medically advisable to give such information to the patient, the information should be made available to an appropriate person in his behalf. He has the right to know by name, the physician responsible for coordinating his care.

3. The patient has the right to receive from his physician information necessary to give informed consent prior to the start of any procedure and/or treatment. Except in emergencies, such information for informed consent, should include but not necessarily be limited to the specific procedure and/or treatment, the medically significant risks involved, and the probable duration of incapacitation. Where medically significant alternatives for care or treatment exist, or when the patient requests information concerning medical alternatives, the patient has the right to such information. The patient also has the right to know the name of the person responsible for the procedures and/or treatment.

4. The patient has the right to refuse treatment to the extent permitted by law, and to be informed of the medical consequences of his action.

5. The patient has the right to every consideration of his privacy concerning his own medical care program. Case discussion, consultation, examination, and treatment are confidential and should be conducted discreetly. Those not directly involved in his care must have the permission of the patient to be present.

6. The patient has the right to expect that all communications and records pertaining to his care should be treated as confidential.

7. The patient has the right to expect that within its capacity a hospital must make reasonable response to the request of a patient for services. The hospital must provide evaluation, service, and/or referral as indicated by the urgency of the case. When medically permissible a patient may be transferred to another facility only after he has received complete information and explanation concerning the needs for and alternatives to such a transfer. The institution to which the patient is to be transferred must first have accepted the patient for transfer.

8. The patient has the right to obtain information as to any relationship of his hospital to other health care and educational institutions insofar as his care is concerned. The patient has the right to obtain information as to the existence of any professional relationships among individuals, by name, who are treating him.

9. The patient has the right to be advised if the hospital proposes to engage in or perform human experimentation affecting his care or treatment. The patient has the right to refuse to participate in such research projects.

10. The patient has the right to expect reasonable continuity of care. He has the right to know in advance what appointment times and physicians are available and where. The patient has the right to expect that the hospital will provide a mechanism whereby he is informed by his physician or a delegate of the physician of the patient's continuing health care requirements following discharge.

11. The patient has the right to examine and receive an explanation of his bill regardless of source of payment.

12. The patient has the right to know what hospital rules and regulations apply to his conduct as a patient.

No catalogue of rights can guarantee for the patient the kind of treatment he has a right to expect. A hospital has many functions to perform, including the prevention and treatment of disease, the education of both health professionals and patients, and the conduct of clinical research. All these activities must be conducted with an overriding concern for the patient and, above all, the recognition of his dignity as a human being. Success in achieving this recognition assures success in the defense of the rights of the patient.

FIGURE 1.1 The Patient's Bill of Rights adopted by the American Hospital Association (Reprinted with the permission of the American Hospital Association.)

education. This role is "the process of promoting, organizing, implementing, and evaluating health education programs, as well as planning with other health care institutions and community agencies to define the role and responsibility of each organization to meet the health education needs of the populations they serve" (American Hospital Association, p. 1). "The major emphasis of health education is health promotion, which includes health maintenance, disease and trauma management, and the improvement of the health care system and its utilization" (American Hospital Association, p. 2). Also, in 1975 the Blue Cross Association released its *White Paper on Health Education.* This publication not only endorsed patient education but also urged third party reimbursement for patient education costs (Somers, p. 9).

On June 23, 1976, President Ford signed into law the National Consumer Health Information and Health Promotion Act (P.L. 94–317). This law provides for a national program of "health information, health promotion, preventive health services, and education in the appropriate use of health care." The Secretary of Health, Education and Welfare was instructed to develop national goals in each of these areas and to support programs to meet the goals. The Office of Health Information and Health Promotion was established within the office of the Assistant Secretary for Health. The Task Force on Consumer Health Education, a combined effort of the American College of Preventive Medicine and the National Institutes of Health, shortly thereafter presented recommendations on policies for and implementation of consumer health education on a national scale. "Through health education programs, hospitals and other health care institutions can contribute to important health care goals, such as improved quality of patient care, better utilization of outpatient services, fewer admissions and readmissions to inpatient facilities, shorter lengths of stay, and reduced health care costs" (American Hospital Association, p. 2).

In recent years, various patient bills of rights have emerged. Such statements recognize the rights of patients to expect and to receive appropriate standards of care. These statements have further recognized the right of patients to receive health education. The American Hospital Association adopted its Patient's Bill of Rights in 1972. Eight of the twelve rights listed deal with informing clients (Fig. 1.1). The National Association of Children's Hospitals and Related Institutions (NACHRI) adopted The Pediatric Bill of Rights in 1974. Canon XI states: "Every person, regardless of age, shall have the right to ask pertinent questions concerning the diagnosis, the treatment, tests and surgery done, on a day-to-day basis in a hospital setting" (NACHRI). Similarly, the Los Angeles Children's Hospital adopted its own Pediatric Bill of Rights. Article III states: "I have the right to expect my Doctors and Nurses to teach me and my family all we need to know about my illness so we can help me to recover and stay

well" (Fig. 1.2).

The Joint Commission on Accreditation of Hospitals has also underscored the rights and responsibilities of patients. In its written accreditation standards, the right of patients to "information" is addressed. The Commission states: "The patient has the right to obtain from the practitioner responsible for coordinating his care, complete and current information concerning his diagnosis (to the degree known), treatment, and any known prognosis. This information should be communicated in terms the patient can reasonably be expected to understand" (Joint Commission on Accreditation of Hospitals, p. xi).

Guidelines of the Joint Commission specify that criteria for education should be established. The guidelines further require evidence that the patient has learned or has demonstrated knowledge. Requirements related to patient education are imposed on many hospital departments and thus indicate that a multidisciplinary approach would be optimally effective in meeting the hospital's patient education needs (American Hospital Association, p. 3).

Adequacy of patient education has also become the object of legislation. Some states, by law, require physicians to explain in clear language the possible consequences and complications of certain procedures, such as surgery and special tests. Informed consent is a growing trend based on the patient's need to know and to understand his care and treatment before giving his formal approval. Patient education responsibilities are part of the professional practice acts for several health care professions, including medicine, nursing, dietetics, and pharmacy. Failure to insure that the patient is adequately informed about his care places both professionals and hospitals in danger of liability (American Hospital Association, p. 11).

The patient's responsibility in health care should also be recognized. The Joint Commission emphasizes that "a patient is responsible for following the treatment plan recommended . . . . This may include following the instructions of nurses and allied health personnel as they carry out the coordinated plan of care and implement the responsible practitioner's orders, and as they enforce the applicable hospital rules and regulations" (Joint Commission on Accreditation of Hospitals, p. xiii).

These developments, coupled with increased consumer awareness, further the accountability of health care organizations and providers. Failure to meet these obligations fully furthers liability on the part of the institution and its staff, and with liability come the potential costs of litigation and negative public relations for failure to meet expected requirements or standards.

Today's health care standards require proof of the quality and quantity of care given to patients. Consequently, great emphasis is being placed on appropriate documentation of care. This includes the need to document not only "what was taught" but also to indicate "what was learned."

Currently there is growing emphasis on the "ecology of

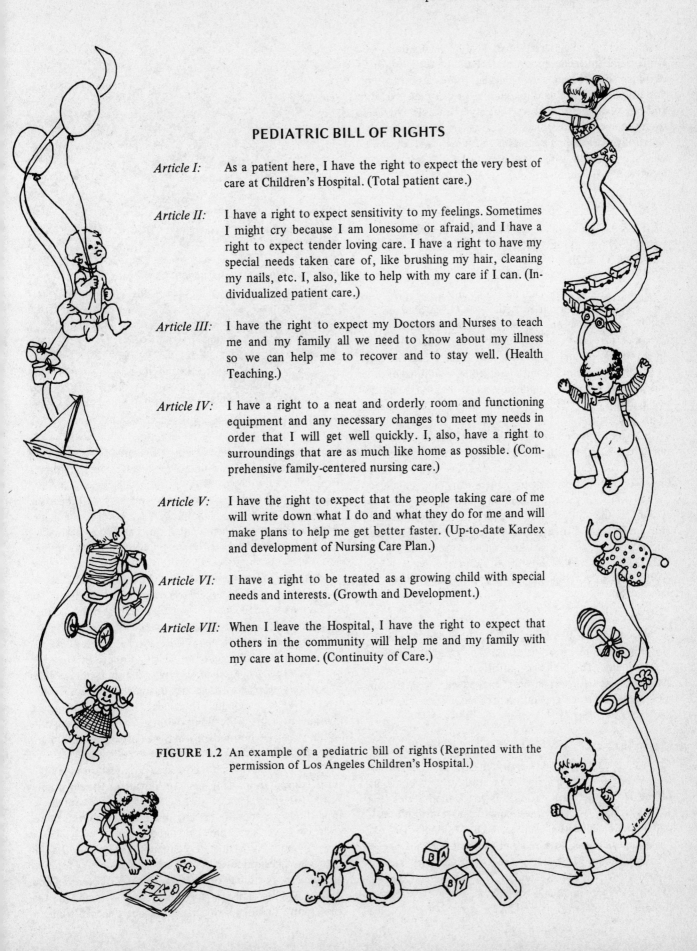

PEDIATRIC BILL OF RIGHTS

Article I: As a patient here, I have the right to expect the very best of care at Children's Hospital. (Total patient care.)

Article II: I have a right to expect sensitivity to my feelings. Sometimes I might cry because I am lonesome or afraid, and I have a right to expect tender loving care. I have a right to have my special needs taken care of, like brushing my hair, cleaning my nails, etc. I, also, like to help with my care if I can. (Individualized patient care.)

Article III: I have the right to expect my Doctors and Nurses to teach me and my family all we need to know about my illness so we can help me to recover and to stay well. (Health Teaching.)

Article IV: I have a right to a neat and orderly room and functioning equipment and any necessary changes to meet my needs in order that I will get well quickly. I, also, have a right to surroundings that are as much like home as possible. (Comprehensive family-centered nursing care.)

Article V: I have the right to expect that the people taking care of me will write down what I do and what they do for me and will make plans to help me get better faster. (Up-to-date Kardex and development of Nursing Care Plan.)

Article VI: I have a right to be treated as a growing child with special needs and interests. (Growth and Development.)

Article VII: When I leave the Hospital, I have the right to expect that others in the community will help me and my family with my care at home. (Continuity of Care.)

FIGURE 1.2 An example of a pediatric bill of rights (Reprinted with the permission of Los Angeles Children's Hospital.)

health" and the conservation of health related resources. While some influences may be a result of the popularity of fads, people seem to be placing more importance on "do-it-yourself" health care, such as proper diet, exercise, and physical fitness. However, society as a whole still needs to recognize and to value health as a national resource. Hopefully the growing awareness and sense of responsibility of today's health care consumers signal the beginning of progress toward this end.

GENERATING A PATIENT EDUCATION PROGRAM: THE CHILDREN'S HOSPITAL EXPERIENCE

Continued home care and health maintenance programs are especially important in pediatrics. Often children are totally dependent on others for care. Nonexistent or improper care at home can result in continuation, recurrence, or initiation of health problems, repeated visits to health care facilities, and increased expenditures of time and money. At worst, the disruption of necessary care can result in a shortened life expectancy or in a reduced quality of life.

Dealing with large numbers of pediatric patients and their families, the professional staff of Children's Hospital has become increasingly aware of and sensitive to the need for improving the continuity of patient care and enhancing the methods of patient and family instruction. The staff recognizes that hospitalization is traumatic for both child and family, and also that patients and families may often misunderstand or forget instructions provided by the staff. Our Homegoing Education and Literature Program (H.E.L.P.) was developed in response to these problems.

ABOUT CHILDREN'S HOSPITAL

As the "birthplace" of the H.E.L.P. concept, Children's Hospital was a major influence on the system's design and development. The following information is presented to acquaint you with our institution; you may wish to compare the similarities and differences between your setting and ours.

The History

From its beginning in 1894, Children's Hospital, Columbus, Ohio, has grown from a nine bed institution to become one of the largest pediatric facilities in the United States (Fig. 1.3). Through its many achievements and contributions in patient care, education, and research, Children's Hospital has established itself as a leader in pediatric health care.

Each year the 313 bed hospital provides primary, secondary, and tertiary care to about 170,000 children: approximately 15,000 inpatient admissions, 50,000 emergency room visits, and over 105,000 visits to the forty-six spe-

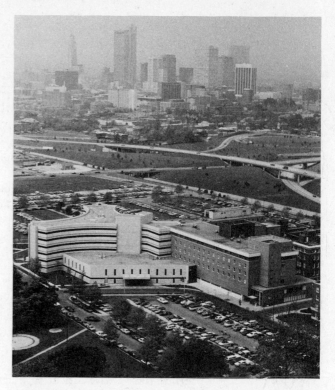

FIGURE 1.3 The Children's Hospital, Columbus, Ohio

cialty outpatient clinics and five satellite community clinics. Serving children under 19 years of age, Children's Hospital is fully departmentalized; the departments include medicine, pediatric surgery, otolaryngology, orthopedics, dentistry, psychiatry, radiology, laboratory medicine, thoracic surgery, neonatal medicine, and anesthesiology. Children's Hospital is the major child care facility among the twelve hospitals serving the Columbus metropolitan area—about one million people. The Hospital also serves as a regional referral center, receiving acutely ill or injured youngsters via helicopter or ambulance from other areas of Ohio and from the surrounding states.

Children's Hospital has been the pediatric teaching affiliate of the Ohio State University College of Medicine for over 30 years. As such, each year the hospital provides educational services for approximately 500 medical students, 100 postgraduate physicians, and many students of the allied health professions. With seven affiliated schools of nursing, the hospital provides pediatric clinical experiences for nearly 900 student nurses annually.

The Children's Hospital Research Foundation is a nonprofit corporation dedicated to research. Recent topics of investigation include birth defects, cancer, nutrition, drug therapy, genetics, learning disabilities, lead poisoning, epilepsy, Reye's syndrome, and child abuse.

As a university-affiliated community hospital, the institution takes pride in its tradition of providing care to all children, regardless of financial status. Over two million dollars of free care is given each year. Located in the center-city, Children's Hospital has made a special commitment to deal with problems resulting from poor housing, inadequate sanitation, improper diet, psychosocial stress, and other difficulties of the underprivileged.

Approximately 70% of the inpatients and 90% of clinic and emergency room patients are from central Ohio. The remainder are referred from throughout Ohio and from the surrounding states, with occasional patients from foreign countries. Most patients are English speaking with a mid-western background.

The Philosophy

A philosophy embodying the belief in and commitment to organized patient/family education is basic to any effort in program development and patient teaching. Without this belief and commitment, patient education programs will wither. Ideally, such a philosophy should be visible at every level of the organization—from top management to the staff nurse and allied health workers, and beyond.

The philosophy of Children's Hospital includes a commitment to patient education recognizing that "all children should have access to preventive health care and should be educated concerning health issues and health care systems" (Fig. 1.4). The hospital has a formalized goal to "promote the health and well-being of local, regional, and national populations through the provision of community-based

---

STATEMENT OF PHILOSOPHY

A hospital's philosophy is a statement of the fundamental beliefs which underly an institution's determination of mission, role, goals and actions and which continually influence the development and interpretation of policy.

We recognize that life is a cyclical process and that the health of a mother can affect the health of her unborn child. Each child who is wanted and born to a healthy mother will begin life with a better chance for health and productivity. Similarly, the quality of life for every individual as well as for future generations, can be enhanced through the early development of health-promoting and preventive behavior. We believe, therefore, that:

- All Children should be born well; and that the combined resources of our society should be organized to promote continual improvements in the health of each successive generation.

- All Children should have access to preventive health care and should be educated concerning health issues and health care systems.

- All Children should have good nutrition.

- All Children should live in a safe and healthful social environment.

- All Children should live in an environmental setting where adequate resources are available to provide the basic needs to ensure physical and intellectual health.

- All Adolescents and young adults should live in a societal setting that recognizes their special health and social needs.

- Adequate health care resources should be available to ensure that high-quality health care is accessible to all acutely sick Children.

- All chronically ill Children should have access to those social and medical resources which will enable them to function at their optimum level.

FIGURE 1.4 Statement of the philosophy and objectives of Children's Hospital, Columbus, Ohio. (Adapted from the American Academy of Pediatrics philosophy.)

PHILOSOPHY OF THE DIVISION OF NURSING

We, the members of the Nursing Department, believe in the dignity and worth of each individual and strive to maintain optimum health of our clients and to provide comprehensive nursing care to all children. Comprehensive nursing care involves maintaining a sensitivity to the individual patient's physical, psychosocial, and spiritual needs, while recognizing him as a unique family member. Our care is directed toward maximum restoration and promotion of the individual's health and encompasses utilization of available family and community resources and the coordinated contributions of allied health team members. We recognize that nursing care is influenced by the rapid social and technological advancements occurring within our world. We strive to be attuned to advancements and trends and to initiate change through self-evaluation, continued education, and research.

FIGURE 1.5 Statement of the philosophy of the Nursing Division, Children's Hospital, Columbus, Ohio

programs aimed at prevention, treatment and education."

The nursing administration of Children's Hospital identifies patient education as an integral part of health and healing and as a responsibility of all health care workers. The philosophy of the Division of Nursing indicates that care is to be directed toward maximum restoration and promotion of the patient's health (Fig. 1.5).

THE BEGINNING OF H.E.L.P.

Attempting to deal with the need for patient and family education, nursing staff members evaluated existing pamphlets and teaching materials. Disappointingly, we found that most of the needs of our patient population could not be served by available materials. The Children's Hospital Nursing Department, therefore, developed the Homegoing Education and Literature Program (H.E.L.P.), a system of developing and distributing teaching aids. The primary objectives in this endeavor were:

1. To provide understandable information for patients and families relative to prevention, therapeutics, diagnostic testing, and health care maintenance

2. To provide organized information to support the knowledge and approach of those performing patient education

3. To provide the patient and family with written reference for reinforcement of teaching after leaving the health care facility

We were fortunate to have within our ranks of knowledgeable and dedicated employees, several exceptionally talented and highly motivated people who created the H.E.L.P. concept for developing teaching materials. Using

their ingenuity and knowledge of nursing and patient needs, these people masterminded this innovative approach. At times the task became arduous, due largely to the lack of information in the literature. However, the eagerness of the coordinating personnel was matched with responsiveness from nursing and hospital staff members who provided the necessary input in designing the system, in developing the individual teaching aids, and in evaluating the program.

The Help in Helping Hands

Just how do Helping Hands help? The answer is, "in a variety of ways."

Helping Hands help *patients and families* by:

- Providing a *written resource* of information given by the physician and nurse, for use at home

- Providing *step-by-step instruction* for difficult procedures

- Providing *reminder* information about health guidance topics, such as immunizations

Helping Hands help *nurses and other health professionals* by:

- Providing a ready and *standardized reference* for the teaching of various topics

- Assisting in *explaining* difficult or confusing procedures to patients/families

- *Saving time* through prewritten, rather than handwritten, instructions

- Providing *chart documentation* which specifies content of instruction. (The prewritten information also reduces time spent in documentation of teaching session.)

Helping Hands help *physicians* by:

- *Providing* the patient/family with *written* instructions for *home reference*

- Supporting physician instruction and *aiding compliance* with instructions

- Informing the physician about the *detail of instructions* given to patients (which is particularly useful to referring physicians.)

- *Decreasing phone calls* to/from patients/families for information or clarification

- Helping to *insure home follow-up and compliance* after agency care intervention

- Helping patients to *keep follow-up appointments*

Helping Hands help *paraprofessionals* by:

- Providing a *ready reference* of information needed by patients/families concerning diagnostic tests or other procedures

- Assisting in *preparing* patient/family for accurate tests or procedures

Using the Helping Hands

Of course, the success in using the Helping Hands depends on several factors. First, each staff member must recognize his responsibility to initiate and to carry out needed individual patient teaching. Failure to recognize such responsibility means that individual patient teaching needs will likely be unidentified and unmet. Further, to be most effective in patient education, the staff must possess basic knowledge about teaching principles. The staff must also *know about the system* and understand its use. Unless all are acquainted with their availability and use, the materials will go unused, and patient teaching will be less effective. Finally, the *system must be usable,* with effective mechanisms for cataloging, ordering, and revising the materials.

It is important to understand that the purpose of the Helping Hands is to serve as an adjunct resource to the staff's patient education endeavors. In no way should the Helping Hands replace the individual staff-patient instructional contact. The written materials must *not* be substituted for the teacher-learner interaction in which individual needs are assessed and responses to teaching evaluated. Rather, they should be used to supplement and complement this patient–staff interaction.

THE ROLES IN GENERATING A PATIENT EDUCATION PROGRAM

For a patient education program to be successful, it must be recognized and supported by the leaders of the health care facility. Since nurses are probably the primary health teachers in most settings, it seems appropriate that the Nursing Administrator, nursing leadership personnel, and staff nurses assume a highly visible leadership role in promoting the efforts of this type of program.

The Role of the Nursing Administrator

The role of a nursing administrator in developing patient education programs is primarily one of support and guidance. She assists in identifying the scope of the project and the resources available, determines factors concerning the program's structure and process in relation to the entire department and hospital, sets priorities among other projects, selects staff, and monitors outcomes to insure that predetermined objectives are met.

Progressive, imaginative, and practical approaches are needed in problem solving and in goal attainment for patient education. The nursing administrator should recognize and promote creative, innovative activities directed toward improvement of patient care, including health education. Creativity, which often blooms as a result of praise and appreciation, may also be thwarted by discouragement. All of us generate more and better ideas if our efforts are appreciated.

Insuring the skill and knowledge of nursing staff to fulfill patient education expectations capably is a responsibility of the nursing administrator. Thus, continuing education must be supported and provided to the staff. Continuing education should be aimed at improving the nurse's ability to teach patients and to use teaching materials effectively.

Organizationally, the nursing administrator (in our setting titled Associate Administrator and Director of Nursing) is responsible for communicating needs, problems, direction, and achievements to the chief executive officer of the hospital or health care facility. Further, the nursing administrator recommends specific programs to meet objectives and requests allocations of resources sufficient to accomplish these programs. In our situation, these resources included office space, access to library resources, and budgetary allocations for personnel, supplies, and equipment.

The nursing administrator serves as an interpreter to physicians and allied health personnel of the nursing role in patient education. An enthusiastic orientation to the program will raise interest and participation in the program and can generate both support and innovation for patient education on a hospital-wide basis. Good "salesmanship" promotes acceptance and use of patient education programs.

The difference between merely recognizing a viable idea and producing visible results is a good manager. Sound leadership is essential for development of a patient education program. Though the responsibility for program development may be assigned in a variety of ways, the nursing administrator must insure appropriate leadership for the growth of the patient education program.

The Role of the Staff Nurse

Teaching is applicable to the four modes of nursing intervention—prevention of disease, promotion of health, maintenance of health, and modification of patient behavior. We believe that staff nurses must be actively involved in planning, providing, and evaluating teaching for individual patients. Thus, education of patients is identified as a function of each nurse's role and each nurse is held accountable for planning and providing patient education. Further, staff nurses are active in identifying needed patient teaching materials and in developing these materials with assistance from the H.E.L.P. coordinator.

There are few, if any, jobs in which ability alone is sufficient. Needed also are loyalty, sincerity, enthusiasm, and cooperation. Ample doses of these ingredients contribute to the overall effectiveness of each person and to the progress of patient education.

COST VERSUS BENEFIT

Since patient education is regarded as basic to all aspects of patient care at Children's Hospital, separate patient charges for the Helping Hands have not been established. Identifiable factors justifying the establishment and continuation of the program were (1) improved quality of care, (2) reduction of potential liability, (3) reduction of potential patient health complications, (4) improved staff satisfaction, and (5) enhanced patient satisfaction. Derek Bok, president of Harvard University, once stated, "If you think education is expensive, try ignorance." We believe the same idea applies to patient education. Theoretically, patient education can increase the quality of health care and present potential cost savings to the health care system and its public. Further research, however, is needed to verify these assumptions.

"The justification for health education and health promotion depends partly on assumed economics, but, even more, on the conviction that good health demands individual knowledge, individual responsibility, and individual participation in making informed choices about one's life. Such individual participation ranges from institutional policy making to actual health care and behavior changing activities" (Somers, p. xxv).

The effectiveness of most current health promotion programs and practices is unknown. Much research is needed to identify specific, long-term results. "However, we learn only by doing and measuring, not by doing nothing. The practice of health education can no more be put off until 'all the data are in' than can the practice of medicine" (Somers, p. xxvi).

PATIENT EDUCATION: THE ESSENCE OF CARING

Our experience in developing the Homegoing Education and Literature Program has not been without problems. However, most difficulties have been surmounted, and the results have been very positive and gratifying in terms of the responses of our nurses, physicians, patients and of health care professionals in other settings. Our experience is still in an intermediate phase. Further work remains in the areas of research on teaching problems and program evaluation. To date our attempts in these areas have lacked depth due to time and financial limitations, however evaluative research is now underway.

Nevertheless, our general findings conclude that the benefits of our H.E.L.P. system are significant to the health professional and to the patient. We believe the system warrants replication in other settings. Although our teaching aids were developed for use in a pediatric medical center, the concept itself may be directly applied to nearly any type of setting or client population. Furthermore, many of the specific teaching materials may be modified for use as applicable to the individual caseload or setting.

Due to the dearth of practical information guides in patient education, we feel obligated to share our experience in the hope of providing useful information to others facing the challenge of educating patients. We hope that our experience may motivate, encourage, and assist you in fulfilling *your* role in patient education. Hopefully, this book will aid initial planning and eliminate some of the pitfalls in developing your system. Our goal is to promote *your* ability to meet *your patient's* health education needs by providing a fresh approach and a realistic handbook.

The following chapters discuss the systems and methods used to develop our program, including instructions for organizing the system, developing the actual patient teaching materials, educating staff, and evaluating the program. Many of the actual Helping Hands used at Children's Hospital appear in Part II of this book.

A conceptual background of the teaching process is helpful in developing a patient education system. The following chapter deals with the theoretical components of patient education, vital to the effective delivery of patient education.

Patient education is an integral part of caring. Ours is the challenge of helping people to realize that the more they learn about health, the healthier they may be. We hope this book will help you meet this challenge.

SELECTED READINGS

American Hospital Association. *Statement on the Role and Responsibilities of Hospitals and Other Health Care Institutions in Personal and Community Health Education.* Chicago: American Hospital Association, 1974.

Green, Lawrence W. "The Potential of Health Education Includes Cost Effectiveness." *Hospitals* 50 (May 1, 1976): 57–61.

Health Maintenance Organization Act of 1973. 93d Congress.

Holder, Lee. "Education for Health in a Changing Society." *American Journal of Public Health* 60 (December 1970): 2307-2313.

Johnson, Jean E.; Kirchhoff, Karen T.; and Endress, M. Patricia. "Easing Children's Fright During Health Care Procedures." *American Journal of Maternal Child Nursing* 2 (July-August 1976): 206-210.

Joint Commission on Accreditation of Hospitals. *Accreditation Manual for Hospitals.* 1978 ed. Chicago: Joint Commission on Accreditation of Hospitals, 1978.

Lee, Elizabeth A. and Garvey, Jeanne L. "How Is Inpatient Education Being Managed?" *Hospitals* 51 (June 1, 1977): 75-82.

National Association of Children's Hospitals and Related Institutions. *The Pediatric Bill of Rights.* Wilmington, Del.: National Association of Children's Hospitals and Related Institutions, 1974.

National Consumer Health Information and Health Promotion Act of 1976. 94th Congress.

National Health Planning and Resources Development Act of 1974. 93d Congress.

Redman, Barbara K. "Patient Education As a Function of Nursing Practice." *Nursing Clinics of North America* 9 (December 1971): 573-580.

Redman, Barbara K. *The Process of Patient Teaching in Nursing.* St. Louis: C.V. Mosby Co., 1976.

Sharp, Alice E. "Four Steps to Better Patient Teaching." *RN* 37 (May 1974): 62-63.

Shaw, Jane S. "New Hospital Commitment: Teaching Patients How to Live with Illness and Injury." *Modern Hospital* 121 (October 1973): 99-102.

Simonds, Scot. *Current Issues in Patient Education.* New York: American Association of Medical Clinics, 1974.

Somers, Anne R., ed. *Promoting Health: Consumer Education and National Policy.* Germantown, Md.: Aspen Systems Corp., 1976.

Storlie, Frances. "A Philosophy of Patient Teaching." *Nursing Outlook* 19 (June 1971): 387-389.

Ulrich, Marian and Kelley, Kenneth. "Patient Care Includes Teaching." *Hospitals* 46 (April 16, 1972): 59-65.

chapter 2
The Challenge of Patient and Family Teaching

Laurel Ratcliff Talabere

"Just because you've said something doesn't mean it's been learned."

Carl Rogers

Health education is both a consumer expectation and a professional responsibility. Today, health consumers want and expect information about the human body and its functions, managing illness, and maintaining health—and they expect this information in straightforward, understandable terms. The potential of health education in promoting better health care and in improving cost effectiveness is only beginning to be realized (Green, p. 57). Unfortunately, most health education efforts fall short of this potential. Programs are often fragmented and vary considerably in scope, depth, and effectiveness (Redman, p. 212). They lag behind both the advances in disease management and the increases in consumer demand.

Where does this leave you, the person who gives health care and values health education? You recognize patient teaching as essential to the maintenance of health and to the management of illness. You know it provides that important link between what the health professional says and what the patient does (Fig. 2.1). And yet, in the day-to-day delivery of health care, patient teaching often gets shortchanged. Simply handing a patient some prescriptions is an all too frequent discharge routine. So are the hurried instructions given to the patient who has his hat in hand and one foot out the door. All of us have had a similar experience and vowed not to let it happen again—and yet it does. What can be done to be more effective? How can our teaching make more of a difference?

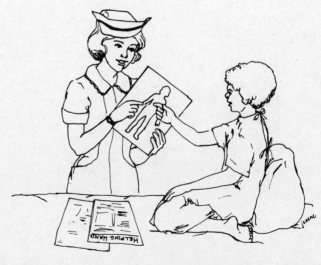

FIGURE 2.1 Patient education: The link between health professional and patient/family

These concerns are the focus of this chapter. In it, patient teaching concepts are discussed and some practical suggestions which you can use in your daily practice are presented.

WHO IS THE TEACHER?

If you *give* health care, you *teach* health care. It is not a matter of choice. All of us are role models for patients and families. The choice is whether we are effective or ineffective health teachers.

THE SCOPE OF HEALTH TEACHING

A consumer health education task force, established by the National Institutes of Health and the American College of Preventive Medicine, has identified six broad categories of health education: (1) patient education, (2) school health education, (3) occupational health education, (4) community programs, (5) national programs, and (6) media programs (Somers, p. 54). From these six categories it can be seen that health education spans the continuum of the health-illness experience. It ranges from anticipatory guidance to the management of complex therapeutic regimens. The focus may be on maintaining health or on managing acute or chronic health problems. The setting can be inpatient, outpatient, community, or home. Nevertheless, there are general principles that undergird all aspects of health teaching; these will be discussed in detail later in this chapter. Let's take a brief look at some of the specific areas of health teaching.

Anticipatory Guidance

Anticipatory guidance means providing direction for events that are *expected* to occur but have not yet happened. Much of the health teaching that involves parents and children is anticipatory and is related to developmental events. Thus, safety measures can be taught in anticipation of certain predictable behaviors related to the child's developmental age. Dental hygiene is taught in relation to our knowledge about the role of plaque in causing dental caries (*Cleaning the Teeth and Gums*).[1] Immunization information is presented in relation to predicted immunity levels (Fig. 2.2) (*Immunizations*).

Both the *timing* and *content* of anticipatory guidance must be related to the *developmental age* of the child. If anticipatory guidance is given too early, it loses relevance and therefore is ineffective in changing behavior. On the other hand, guidance given too late, as in the case of safety measures, may have tragic consequences. When working

[1]Note: All Helping Hands referred to in this and succeeding chapters are referenced in the following way: (*Helping Hand Title*). These Helping Hands are included in Part 2 of this book (see page 178 for contents of Part 2).

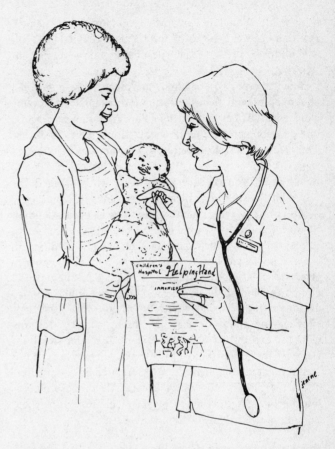

FIGURE 2.2 Anticipatory guidance: This mother is learning about immunizations.

with a patient who has developmental delays, it is necessary to use estimated developmental age rather than chronological age. Marcene Erickson's book, *Assessment and Management of Developmental Changes in Children,* is an excellent reference for determining levels of development in infants and children.

Preparation for Procedures

Preparatory instruction is another type of health teaching. The focus is on a situational event, such as a diagnostic test, a treatment, or a surgical procedure which the patient will be experiencing. Often this kind of event is intrusive—an unwelcome entry into the body. The stress level of the patient is frequently high and may interfere with his ability to understand and to remember what is being taught. Therefore, you must be direct and explicit. The initial teaching session should include only essential information. However, you need to allow opportunity for discussion during the first session and afterward so the person's specific needs can be met. Questions must be answered honestly if a trust relationship is to be maintained.

Preparation for having an I.V. started illustrates these points well (*Having an I.V.*). This is a procedure that is feared by many children and adults. The fact that it will hurt a bit should be acknowledged rather than denied. Pointing out the benefits of the I.V. is acceptable, but this should not be used to evade questions about the unpleasant aspects.

Patients, especially children, are much more concerned about the present than the future. For example, if a young child asks, "Will it hurt?", the following response provides limited support: "Yes, a little, but don't worry about it. Tomorrow you'll feel better." A more appropriate and supportive response would be: "Yes, a little, but I'll stay with you and you can squeeze my hand tightly" (Fig. 2.3).

In addition to giving straightforward answers, you should describe briefly but accurately the steps involved. Children may need more than verbal information about a procedure. A play situation which simulates the actual procedure can provide important sensory information. Such an experience gives the child an opportunity to manipulate the hospital equipment and supplies which will be used in his care. By demonstrating the procedure on a doll first and then allowing the child to "play this back," the child learns what to expect and also retains control of the situation. He has the opportunity to express *nonverbally* those feelings that are too difficult or too frightening to verbalize. Thus, the child is more likely to integrate the information into his thought processes through a "hands-on" experience than if only verbal information were given.

Home Management of Health Problems

Instructing the patient and the family in the ongoing management of health problems at home is a third kind of

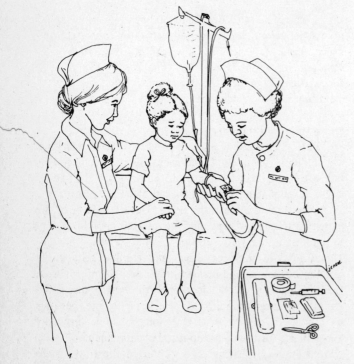

FIGURE 2.3 Preparation for procedures: This child is being supported during an intrusive event.

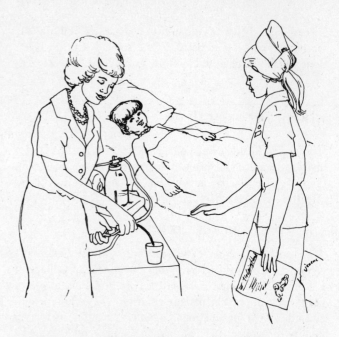

FIGURE 2.4 Home management: This mother is learning to suction her child's tracheostomy before taking him home.

health teaching. This teaching occurs after a particular health problem has been identified but before the patient and the family are given the responsibility to manage it on their own (Fig. 2.4). The health problem may require relatively simple management, such as the administration of eyedrops, or it may be more involved, such as care of a urinary diversion. The health problem may be short term, such as observing a child with a mild concussion, or it may be long term, such as giving postural drainage to a child with cystic fibrosis (*Eye Drops, Your Child's Urinary Diversion, Head Injury, Postural Drainage*). The content and complexity of the teaching varies with the patient and the condition. Perhaps the greatest challenge in teaching home management is to make it both realistic for the family and therapeutically effective.

Follow-up Care

A fourth kind of health teaching is follow-up teaching. During this type of teaching situation, you evaluate the patient's knowledge, skills, and attitudes *after* he has had sufficient opportunity to apply and to integrate these into his patterns of living (Fig. 2.5). Follow-up teaching may be done in one session, but more commonly it is an ongoing process that provides reinforcement and redirection as the patient's needs and behaviors change. Follow-up teaching deserves special consideration for these reasons: (1) Learning usually takes place gradually over time rather than all at once. (2) Often follow-up teaching is done by someone other than the initial teacher. For example, a clinic or office nurse or a community health nurse is likely to do the follow-up teaching for what was originally taught in the

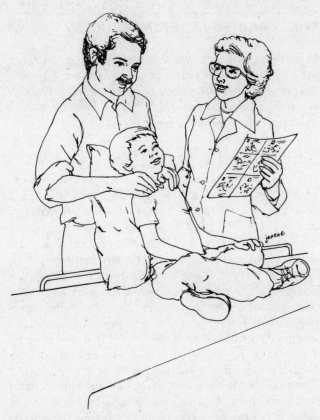

FIGURE 2.5 Follow-up care: The physical therapist watches as a father reviews his postural drainage technique.

hospital. (3) Forgetting, which occurs naturally over time, can be compounded by a lack of reinforcement in the home situation. (4) Follow-up teaching can be a potent motivating factor because it emphasizes the patient's accountability. For these reasons, follow-up teaching requires deliberate planning and excellent communication. It is the final and perhaps most important step in effective patient education.

PLANNED VERSUS SPONTANEOUS TEACHING

Most of us relate health teaching to a *planned* session between the patient and health professional. We anticipate and prepare for planned teaching. We know in advance what we want to present and discuss. There is a certain security in planned teaching because we are ready for it.

We are probably less aware of the powerful impact that we have through our day-to-day practice. Like it or not, we are role models for patients and families all of the time. If you consider your health care behaviors in this light, a new dimension is added to even routine skills.

Proper or improper technique in a procedure can reinforce or undermine a planned teaching session. For instance, as you demonstrate how to take a temperature, you emphasize the importance of staying with an infant while the rectal thermometer is in place (*Taking a Temperature*).

However, the family sees another nurse leave the infant for a few moments. The parent is quite likely to notice this discrepancy but may not question it. The parent may reason: "A nurse knows how to take a temperature. If each nurse does it differently, the differences must not be important." Therefore, the parent may assume that it really doesn't matter which way it is done.

This kind of situation can be magnified many times in a complex medical center where each patient is in daily contact with many health professionals and students, each of whom gives somewhat different information and opinions. Here, consistently high standards of practice assume a significant teaching function. We can view this mandate for high quality care as an added burden or as an important opportunity to help the patient to learn.

The occasions for *spontaneous* teaching in any setting are endless. Consider the number of situations in a given day in which you can teach health care. For example, you can teach breast examination while giving a woman patient her bath. You can explain the action of a medication as you give the medicine. You can discuss the importance of adequate fluid intake as you encourage an asthmatic to drink liquids. Capitalizing on these spontaneous opportunities takes a minimum of extra time, but the effect can be great, particularly if other staff members are making the same effort.

Whether we are engaging in *planned* or *spontaneous* teaching, being a health teacher is an impressive responsibility. It demands skill. It demands knowledge. It demands commitment. And it offers us the chance to make a positive difference in the health and well-being of our patients.

WHO IS THE LEARNER?

Perhaps this can best be determined by asking, "Who needs to learn?" "Who will be taking the responsibility for managing the patient's health care?"

The learner may be the patient himself, a parent, a babysitter, or a friend. Often there is more than one learner. It is important in the beginning to identify all the learners so they can be included in your teaching plans. Certain complex care situations, such as home care of a child with a tracheostomy, require at least two learners. This is necessary so the learners can share the responsibility for care, as well as provide mutual support.

THE PATIENT AS THE LEARNER

The patient, whenever possible, should be the primary learner; that is, the person who will assume most or all of the care. "Only by using that powerful untapped resource—the patient—only by giving him the knowledge and responsibility to care for himself, can we convert our present 'illness care' system to a 'health care' system . . . . " (Winslow, p. 213).

Self-management is an important concept to emphasize. You want to get across the idea that the patient can control and influence his health problem, that what he does or does not do *can* make a difference. Young children and elderly patients alike can take an active role in managing their health problems. For instance, asthmatic children as young as 5 years of age have learned to give themselves adrenalin and thus become "asthma experts" (Dyer, p. 17). Young children can learn to manage their diabetes with insulin injections and urine testing (*Rotating Injection Sites, Giving an Insulin Injection, Urine Testing*).

A patient benefits greatly from participating in his health care as much as possible within the limitations of his age and ability. Sometimes it is difficult to get this idea across to well-intentioned persons who may overprotect the patient or may interfere with the patient's attempts to assume more of his care. For example, it is not unusual to see a chronically ill child develop dependent behavior patterns. This dependency is often reinforced by the child's parents because they feel guilty. They compensate for this guilt by doing more for the child than is necessary, which actually discourages the child's normal thrust toward independence. This overprotective response can seriously jeopardize the child's need and right to become his own person and health care manager. Therefore, the development of self-management skills from the time a health problem is identified needs to be encouraged. For example, the toddler with cystic fibrosis can begin to hold his own aerosol mask and the school-age child can begin to administer self postural drainage. This is a significant step toward allowing the patient to become a partner in his own health care—which is both his right and his responsibility.

THE PATIENT'S NETWORK

As you try to determine who the potential learners are, consider your patient's network: his family and friends. Ask yourself and your patient: Who are the family and extended family members? Who of these could and would be available? What does a child's school teacher need to know? Could an adolescent's friend be involved?

There are several factors you need to consider in selecting a potential learner. These factors are (1) the willingness of the person to participate in your patient's health care, (2) the geographic location of that person in relation to your patient, (3) the person's resources including time, energy, and transportation, and (4) your patient's feelings toward having this person involved in his care. Whenever possible, these additional learners should remain secondary; that is, they should assist and support the patient in managing his health problem, but they should not do for the patient what he can do for himself.

THE TEACHING-LEARNING PROCESS

Teaching-learning is a two-way street that requires active participation by both you and your patient. You become a teacher only when the patient becomes a learner. Together you form a twosome or a *dyad*. You are interdependent in the teaching-learning relationship.

TEACHING AND LEARNING DEFINED

Teaching is a special kind of communication that produces learning. It involves various activities, both verbal and nonverbal, that change a person's knowledge, skills, or attitudes. Teaching takes into account the perceptions and feelings of the learner as well as his specific needs. It responds to feedback and evaluates the outcome.

Through health teaching you give the patient appropriate alternatives for handling a health-illness situation. To be most effective you must individualize these alternatives and must be realistic about what is possible. The best of teaching content will be useless unless it is perceived by the patient as a better alternative. It must be seen as having more advantages than disadvantages.

Learning is the development of new behavior patterns that result from acquiring new knowledge, skills, or attitudes. It involves new ways of doing things or new ways of relating to oneself, to others, or to the environment. To learn, one must *want* to learn because learning is active, not passive. To learn is to change. Health beliefs and behaviors are the targets of this change (Redman, p. 22).

HEALTH BELIEFS AND BEHAVIORS

The beliefs and behaviors of the patient that are related to health and to illness are the focus of the teaching-learning process. At times both a belief and a behavior are appropriate and adequate for the situation and, therefore, need to be supported and reinforced (Fig. 2.6). For example, an adolescent patient who had been hospitalized with diabetes returned to the clinic for his follow-up appointment. He was taking his insulin regularly and said he believed this had made him feel much better. In this case positive feedback to the patient means approval from you, the health teacher. Approval reinforces this desired belief and behavior.

Sometimes a particular behavior is appropriate and needs to be supported, but the belief needs to be changed. For example, the mother of a failure-to-thrive baby was seriously questioning her ability to feed her infant. She believed that her behavior—that is, her feeding technique— was causing her baby's condition. After assessing the mother's feeding technique, the nurse found that she was doing an excellent job. The child was later diagnosed as having cystic fibrosis with serious digestive problems. The mother's behaviors in feeding the baby were adequate and

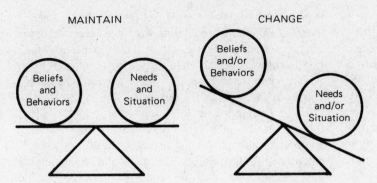

FIGURE 2.6 Health beliefs and behaviors: To maintain or change?

needed to be reinforced. However, her belief that the child's failure-to-thrive was her fault needed to be changed.

At other times neither the behaviors nor the beliefs are satisfactory. An example of this situation is the family of a child with a tracheostomy. Often when parents are first told that their child will have a tracheostomy when he goes home from the hospital, they believe that they cannot possibly manage his care. New knowledge and skills are needed to produce new behaviors which will enable the parents to provide safe and supportive care. Usually the initial doubts can be changed into confidence if adequate time is allowed for the family to express their fears and if the teaching-learning process fosters the development of new knowledge, skills, and attitudes.

RELATED CONCEPTS

The teaching-learning process involves interaction and exchange between teacher and learner: the health professional and patient. Let's explore two ideas that are central to this view of health teaching.

Systems Theory

Systems theory is a concept that provides valuable insight into the teaching-learning relationship. *Human beings are open systems.* A person takes in information and energy from his environment (input), reacts to it (throughput), and gives out information and energy (output). Whenever an open system receives input, there is potential for change "which makes possible nursing intervention to facilitate the promotion, maintenance, and restoration of health" (Sills and Hall, p. 24). *We all have the potential for change,* and this has tremendous significance for patient education.

Health teaching, from a systems perspective, can be described as providing input to the patient for the purpose of changing health-illness behaviors. This change (learning) actually occurs when the patient reacts to the input (teaching) so a different output (behavior) results. This new behavior represents a new way of responding to the environment and a new alternative for handling a health-illness situation (Fig. 2.7).

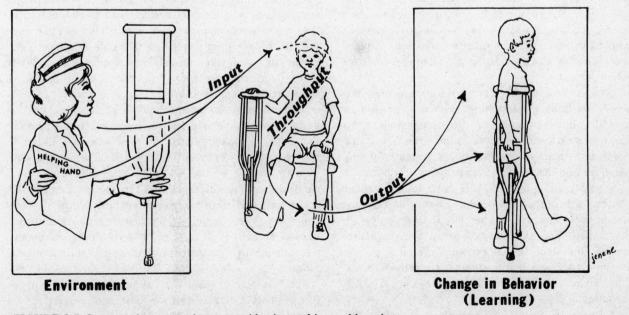

FIGURE 2.7 Systems theory: An important idea in teaching and learning

The Nursing Process

The nursing process is another concept that supports this view of health teaching as interaction and exchange. *Process* refers to a systematic set of actions that are directed to a goal. *Nursing process,* then, is the orderly method of interacting with a patient in which nurse and patient work together toward a mutual goal. When the nurse and patient work together, the perceptions, values, and expectations of each influence the behaviors of the other. This results in a constantly changing interaction in which "the nurse must be continually observing and measuring the changing behavior" of both the patient and herself (Daubenmire and King, p. 517).

The nursing process provides a guiding framework for health teaching. The steps in the nursing process are (1) assessment, or the collection of data to determine a patient's situation, (2) planning, or the analysis of data by the nurse and patient to identify the patient's needs and priorities, (3) intervention, or the direction of a patient toward solving or managing a health problem, and (4) evaluation, or the collection of data to determine whether the goal was reached (Turner, pp. 12–28). These same steps are used in the teaching-learning process.

SIMILAR COMMUNICATION SKILLS

We defined teaching as that special kind of communication skill which produces learning. Now let's compare it with interviewing, informing, and counseling. All are interpersonal skills that you use daily. These communication skills overlap, but they are not interchangeable. An important difference is in the purpose.

The purpose of *interviewing,* which often includes history taking, is to gather information. It is an important prerequisite of teaching because it provides essential baseline data. For example, before teaching a parent how to bathe an infant, you would want to find out about the parent's previous experiences with infant care. Interviewing, in the context of health teaching, can be one of several tools for collecting data.

The purpose of *informing* is to give information. It is frequently confused with teaching. In fact, it fits with an earlier and more traditional view of teaching in which the learner was passive and received information much the same way as a funnel receives water. The goal of informing is to give facts or ideas. A change in behavior, if it occurs at all, is secondary. For instance, you can inform a patient that he has high blood pressure, but he may or may not understand what this really means. In one study only 23% of the patients had a correct, or partly correct, understanding of the term, "blood pressure" (Petrello, p. 38). Obviously, if your patient does not understand the information, he cannot act on it to effect a change in his health care behavior.

The purpose of *counseling,* an important adjunct to teaching, is to lend support or advice. Particularly in stressful situations, counseling may be necessary before teaching can be effective. For example, a parent who is feeling guilty about his child's ingestion of an overdose of aspirin will probably need to share these feelings before you can teach about safety measures.

Health teaching draws on many interpersonal skills. It focuses on the beliefs and behaviors of the patient so appropriate alternatives for managing health care can be determined. Interviewing, informing, and counseling are not teaching, but they are similar communication skills that support teaching efforts.

YOUR RESPONSIBILITIES AS THE TEACHER

The teaching-learning process is active and ongoing. Both you (the teacher) and your patient (the learner) have responsibilities that are vital to a successful outcome. These responsibilities follow identifiable, sequential steps as shown in Figure 2.8.

MAKE IT RELEVANT

Relevant teaching means that what is taught has meaning for the patient in terms of his own life experiences, his environment, and his particular learning needs (Talabere, p. 20). This requires an assessment of the patient and others in his network so learning needs and readiness can be determined.

Assess the Learning Needs

During your assessment discussion with your patient, both of you have the opportunity to delineate the scope and depth of the teaching needed. This provides valuable data from which you can plan an individualized and relevant teaching-learning experience. The data that you collect during this discussion should be supplemented and validated by observations of your patient's behaviors during the actual teaching sessions.

Both you and your patient should begin by discussing and deciding what is appropriate and necessary to learn. What *you* think your patient needs to know and what *he* thinks he needs to know may vary widely. The learner may underestimate what is needed, as in the case of the parent of a child with a gastrostomy tube. The mother thought she could wait and learn to change the tube on the day the child was to go home. Or the learner may overestimate what is needed, as in the case of a recovered pneumonia patient's parent who wanted to learn auscultation of breath sounds.

You, the teacher, may also misjudge the amount of information that is needed to prepare your patient for an event that seems commonplace to you. Giving a patient a

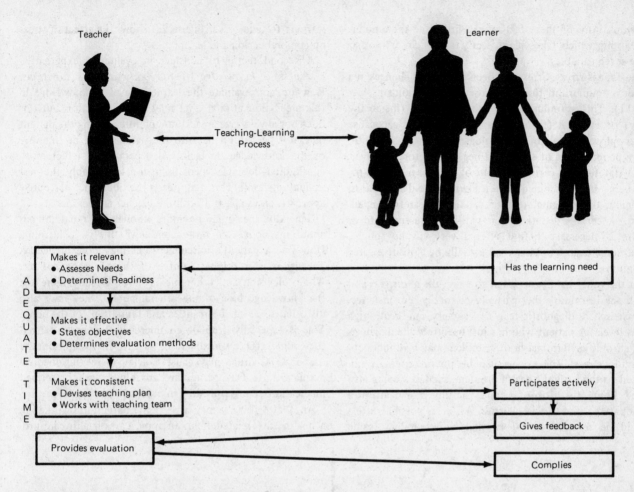

FIGURE 2.8 Steps in the teaching-learning process

"routine" injection is an example of this. In young children, for whom intrusive events can be so frightening, injections are by no means routine. Specific, step-by-step preparation, support, and an opportunity to "play it out" by giving a doll an injection are needed. (For more information about play as a method of teaching, see page 34.) It is also easy to be overzealous and teach more than is needed or desired. For example, a child who is to have a cystogram does not need or want a detailed explanation of the urinary system. Instead the child needs to know how this procedure will feel and what will be expected of him (*Having a Cystogram*). Those with less experience in health teaching are likely to "overteach" because they tend to equate the patient's learning needs with their own.

Also consider the personal needs of the patient and family when arranging the teaching session. Many well-planned teaching sessions have not taken place because teacher and learner could not get together; work schedules, transportation problems, and child care requirements can all interfere. Ask about work schedules. It may be necessary to arrange for a family member to take a few hours off from work. Many employers are very cooperative if notified in advance; a phone call from you may help. Check on

transportation. You may need to assist the patient or family in making special arrangements, or you may want to refer them to a social agency for assistance. In some communities the local Red Cross chapter can transport patients or family members. Inquire about child care. Often a neighbor or friend can assist if arrangements are made ahead of time. In all these areas, advance planning will be time well spent.

Determine Readiness
After you assess the learning needs, evaluate the readiness of your patient to participate in the teaching-learning process. There are two aspects to readiness: experiential readiness which is related to a person's previous and present experiences of living and emotional readiness which is related to a person's level of motivation (Redman, p. 22).

Experiential Readiness
When you evaluate experiential readiness there are a number of factors to consider: (1) stress, (2) knowledge of the body and its functions, (3) previous experiences in caring for others, (4) physical and mental capacities, (5) cultural influences, (6) language, and (7) the pattern of family rela-

tionships. Any of these factors can influence the amount of learning which takes place. Let's take a closer look at these seven variables.

The first is *stress*. Stress has been defined as changes in a person's equilibrium that are caused by a stimulus (Selye, p. 311). This stimulus can be either internal (inside the body) or external (from the environment). It can cause either physiological or psychological changes or both. Many people think of stress as a negative factor. However, Selye states that a certain amount of stress is necessary for well-being and has coined the term *eustress* to describe this. Learning, or changing, requires a stress greater than eustress. A certain dissatisfaction with the present state of affairs is necessary before alternatives will be sought. Thus, some degree of stress can actually be a positive force in learning.

On the other hand, too much stress results in *distress* and can block learning, either partially or totally. For instance, events such as diagnostic tests and surgery can create high stress levels. A patient who has just been told the diagnosis of a chronic or terminal health problem may be under considerable stress. There may also be potent stressors unrelated to the patient's health problem, such as moving into a new home, the birth of a child, the illness or death of a grandparent, or financial worries. As far as possible, stress should be reduced to a level that allows at least some learning to take place. Figure 2.9 shows the effect of stress on comprehension and learning.

A second factor to consider in evaluating experiential readiness is *knowledge of the body and its functions*. How do you evaluate the learner's level of knowledge in this area? Educational level may be an indicator, but this does not always give an accurate picture. Asking the patient may not be helpful because the patient may be unaware of the knowledge he lacks. Also people are reluctant to admit their deficits. Open discussion is probably the best evaluation tool. This requires a flexible and perceptive approach on the part of both the teacher and learner.

Generally speaking, the more knowledge a patient has about his body, the more conducive this is to learning. However, a patient's misconceptions may pose difficulty. Television is a primary source of these misconceptions. While television and other media have certainly increased the knowledge base of the general public, they have also distorted some of the realities and limitations of the body. This is especially true of commercials that present over-the-counter (OTC) medications as cure-alls. Inappropriate use of OTC drugs may cause a delay in seeking medical evaluation. If OTC drugs are combined with prescribed medications, dangerous drug interactions can result.

Another difficulty may arise if the patient has worked in a health care related field. In some cases health care pro-

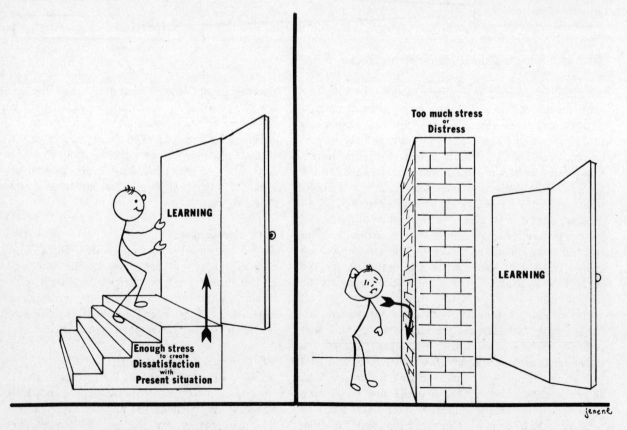

FIGURE 2.9 Stress: Its effect on learning

fessionals are reluctant to accept health teaching because they feel they should know. In other cases we are reluctant to give health teaching because we assume they know. In either case the patient's right to receive quality health teaching is compromised.

Previous experiences in caring for others is a third factor. You can usually determine these experiences through direct questioning. Find out about parents' experiences with well and ill children. Ask if a child has had experience with an ill grandparent or other family member. The learner's positive perceptions about earlier experiences build confidence and skills which can be meaningful in the present situation.

Give the learner credit and recognition for these previous achievements rather than starting the teaching at an arbitrary beginning. For instance, a mother who is learning to care for her infant with a myelomeningocele feels overwhelmed and insecure. This is her second child. The mother comes from a large family in which she is the oldest child. The nurse draws on these previous experiences and helps the mother to focus on applying the many infant care skills she has already learned. As this is done, the care requirements for this second baby, while still very real, become less threatening. If the nurse had begun teaching basic bathing and feeding techniques without identifying the mother's earlier child care experiences, the mother may have viewed the baby as different in all its needs.

Previous experiences can also be negative influences on learning. The learner may feel responsible for an illness which did not improve, which became worse, or which even resulted in death. This sensitive area should be explored carefully, especially if there seems to be unusual resistance to learning.

Another factor is the *physical and mental capabilities* of the learner. Of concern here are any impairments that may interfere with necessary behaviors. For instance, a parent with arthritis can hardly be expected to do postural drainage treatments. A patient with a visual handicap may need special assistance to insure that medication labels are read correctly. A learner who cannot read does not benefit from any written materials—and illiteracy is a larger problem than many of us realize. Pictorial representations, such as a heart on the bottle of digoxin to convey "heart medicine" or the chart that illustrates the postural drainage positions (*Postural Drainage*), are appropriate alternatives.

Cultural influences are an "integral part of providing total health care services to people" (Leininger, p. 5). A person's perceptions of health and illness shape his response to health and illness. We are all strongly influenced by our cultural identity. Therefore, understanding your patient's cultural viewpoint—his beliefs, values, and style of living—is a necessary prerequisite to effective health teaching. This is especially true when your cultural orientation differs from that of your patient.

In the United States where there are many ethnic groups, *ethnocentrism* is likely. Ethnocentrism is the tendency for each of us to believe that our own culture or way of doing things is superior. Ethnocentrism on the part of you or your patient can block the teaching-learning process. As health care providers we must develop a cultural sensitivity that enables us to recognize and respect another's health beliefs and practices.

Many ethnic groups or subcultures have their own traditional health care practices. These include the Appalachian people (Tripp-Reimer and Friedl, pp. 48–49), the American Indians (Primeaux, pp. 60–61), and the Mexican-Americans (White, pp. 32–33), among others. Even if illness causes a member of an ethnic group to seek medical attention from the dominant culture, the home care prescribed by the professional may be modified or supplemented by the patient. The appropriate strategy in such a situation is to recognize a home remedy as a given health care alternative and to evaluate its effectiveness nonjudgmentally. You should seek to alter only those practices that are potentially harmful. For example, rubbing a child's chest with goose grease to relieve congestion is perfectly safe although probably ineffective. There is no reason to change this particular behavior unless it replaces or hinders other health care measures. On the other hand, an asthmatic who smokes strong tobacco to the point of choking may indeed compromise his health. This behavior should be changed if possible (Wigginton, pp. 231, 234).

Middle-class Americans also practice health beliefs that may be detrimental. Many use vitamins as a solution to dietary inadequacy. This solution has created another problem, namely vitamin overdose, which is a common kind of poisoning in children under 5 years of age (Johnston, p. 80).

Many traditional health beliefs are very positive, and we would do well to accommodate them in our own practices. For instance, many ethnic groups place great emphasis on family ties and include the family as well as the sick person in health care.

The sixth factor in evaluating experiential readiness is *language.* In most areas of the United States, communication is a problem of paramount importance for the patient who speaks little or no English. The patient's stress level and sense of isolation will be considerably increased. First, find out if another family member speaks English. If not, perhaps someone in your agency or institution can serve as an interpreter. Many cities have an organized group of volunteers who serve as a language bank. Also, officials at your closest international airport may be able to direct you to appropriate translators.

Even if your patient does speak and understand English, he may not understand the "medicalese" that we health professionals often speak. Be conscious of the words you choose during your teaching sessions as well as in your daily care. Terms and abbreviations such as "I&O," "N.P.O.," and "ambulate" can be confusing and lead to misconceptions which may frighten and concern your patient.

The *patient* may also use terms which we need to clarify. For example, does "low blood" mean anemia or hypotension? Does "miseries" mean physical pain or depression? Effective communication requires attention to the barriers created by different languages as well as the more subtle barriers created by variations in perceptions and understandings in the English language.

The last factor is *the pattern of family relationships.* Families differ in development, composition, values, and perceptions of health and illness, all of which influence relationship patterns. In assessing family patterns it is important to focus on strengths as well as weaknesses. The following questions will help you identify strengths (Otto, pp. 92-93):

1. What strengths do you see in the family?

2. Can the family identify its own strengths and resources?

3. Does the family have hidden strengths and resources?

4. How can the family use its strengths and resources to the best advantage?

5. Can the family identify a change in strengths and resources after teaching has been completed?

You can assess weaknesses by using the same questions, except substitute "weaknesses" for "strengths and resources". The answers to all these questions have important implications for the family's present and future health practices. These answers also tell us something about the family's ability to adapt to or cope with changes.

The adaptive family is able to handle the tensions and anxieties of daily living and can maintain a state of reasonable equilibrium. "The best adapted family is one that uses mild, firm, consistent discipline, is rational, evidence-oriented, and objective. It looks to future goals, is self-confident, trustful, and enjoys new experiences" (Petrillo and Sanger, p. 47). If a stressful event does occur, the adaptive family perceives the event appropriately and mobilizes resources to offset a crisis.

From time to time, families meet events that throw them off balance. Additional support may be needed before equilibrium is regained. Some families, however, are in disequilibrium much of the time. These families are considered to be maladaptive. Because much of their energy and time is crisis oriented, there may be few resources available for demands that seem less critical, such as learning about health and illness. Characteristics of maladaptive families may include frequent mood swings, distorted perceptions of strengths and weaknesses, threats and

sometimes physical abuse, rigid family roles, and reluctance to accept appropriate help. Families with these patterns need special consideration if teaching is to be relevant to their needs. Therefore, in planning for teaching, it is essential to assess family relationships. They have a significant bearing on the family's ability to assimilate and to comply with the teaching-learning process.

Emotional Readiness

Motivation or emotional readiness is also influenced by a number of variables which include: (1) the setting, (2) the patient's priorities, (3) the organization of your presentation, (4) whether goals are realistic or idealistic, and (5) the type of reinforcement that you give (Redman, pp. 40-42). Let's look at these five factors and consider ways in which motivation in the teaching-learning relationship can be enhanced.

First, arrange *the setting* so that the environment is conducive to learning. An area that is separate from distractions is ideal, but often space is limited. You can modify your patient's immediate environment by turning off the television, drawing the curtains, and sitting down next to your patient.

Second, begin with your *patient's priorities.* Usually these concerns relate to prognosis and the implications for life style. For example, leukemia patients may be more concerned about the immediate consequences of chemotherapy, such as hair loss, than about longer term considerations. Health professionals, on the other hand, may think it is important to begin with information about the disease itself. Ask your patient what he would like to learn first.

Third, *organize your information* so it follows a logical pattern. Proceed from simple to complex, from present to future, from cause to effect, from problem to solution. Arrange the information to avoid boredom (too many single steps) or frustration (too few steps or steps that are too complicated).

Fourth, *be realistic about goals,* and help the family or patient to be realistic. Set subgoals so the material can be divided into "manageable doses." Doing too much too fast increases stress, decreases learning, and creates untold frustration.

You may wish to consider a contract between you and your patient. Decide on goals that are agreeable to both of you. Determine what steps are needed and how much time is required to reach each goal. Then set a specific target date for each goal and put this in writing. This technique is especially useful if the teaching is complex or extends over a period of time. For example, an obese adolescent girl may find a weight reduction program more successful if the goals are realistic and set in a specific time frame and if a reward of her choice will be given for fulfilling the contract (Wang and Watson, pp. 46-48).

If lack of time is a problem, it may be more realistic to arrange for outpatient teaching, either through a clinic or by a community health nurse, rather than trying to teach everything in detail before the patient leaves the hospital.

Fifth, *give positive reinforcement* frequently. Remember that your nonverbal behavior conveys as much as your verbal statements. Your feedback answers the patient's question, "How am I doing?" Your feedback also communicates that you *care* about how your patient is doing. Making your teaching relevant is your first responsibility as a teacher. It requires time, thought, and effort. Having taken these steps to assess readiness, you are now ready to assume your second responsibility as a teacher—making your teaching effective.

MAKE IT EFFECTIVE

With effective teaching, maximum learning is possible. To be effective, you need to direct the beliefs and behaviors of your patient toward appropriate alternatives for handling a health-illness situation. This requires the structuring of goals or teaching-learning objectives that can be measured. Written objectives enable you to determine whether the patient has met these goals or needs further teaching.

Teaching-Learning Objectives

Objectives should focus on the desired behaviors of the learner. Therefore, you should state these objectives in behavioral terms that precisely describe what is expected of the learner. Each objective should present a single, specific behavior.

Behaviors and behavioral objectives fall into one of three categories: (1) cognitive, which show knowledge or mental ability, (2) psychomotor, which show skills or physical ability, and (3) affective, which show attitudes or feelings. Behavioral objectives give you a framework for measuring your patient's knowledge, skills, and attitudes about health and illness.

In writing a behavioral objective, the first step is to decide which category of behavior you are measuring, cognitive, psychomotor, or affective. Second, determine as precisely as possible what your patient should know, do, or feel. The data that you obtained in assessing your patient's needs are incorporated here. For example, a primipara with no previous infant care experiences needs to learn how to feed her baby satisfactorily before leaving the hospital. To be precise, it is helpful to divide feeding behavior, which has many aspects, into specific behaviors. These specific behaviors might relate to positioning, rate of feeding, bubbling, and so forth.

The third step is to put the objective into words. To do this, select a verb that states what your patient should know or be able to do. Consider what kinds of behaviors you can actually measure and observe. It is important to choose a verb that is specific rather than general, one

Specific Verbs (Few Interpretations)	General Verbs (Many Interpretations)
To compare	To appreciate
To demonstrate	To believe
To describe	To feel
To differentiate	To know
To identify	To realize
To inject	To understand
To insert	
To list	
To recognize	
To state	

FIGURE 2.10 Writing behavioral objectives: A comparison of specific and general verbs

that has few rather than many interpretations. Compare the verbs listed in Figure 2.10. For example, let's look at the difference between the verbs "to understand" and "to state." You want to teach your patient, who is on a high potassium diet while taking diuretics, about appropriate food sources. If the objective reads, "to state foods high in potassium," you can determine if your patient achieves the objective by whether or not he can state the correct foods. If, on the other hand, the objective reads, "to understand about foods high in potassium," measurement becomes more difficult. "Understanding" is a general and subjective term that means different things to different people. You can see that the verb is a key word and should be selected carefully.

The fourth and last step is to add qualifying words to the objective so you can be even more specific. For instance instead of writing that your patient is "to state foods high in potassium," you could say that your patient is "to state five foods that he likes that are high in potassium." Now the objective is even more precise and more easily measured. It is also individualized.

Writing objectives is similar to building the frame of a house. It requires planning and takes time. Writing objectives can be tedious and repetitious. But it shapes the teaching-learning process and thus is a primary determinant of the outcome. Without establishing objectives, teaching tends to be haphazard and difficult to evaluate, and you are likely to be less effective.

Ways to Evaluate

Now that you have determined your patient's needs, and stated them in behavioral objectives, how can you actually evaluate whether or not learning has taken place? There are three methods in particular that lend themselves to the evaluation of patient education: (1) verbal measurement or *discussion,* (2) written measurement or paper-and-pencil *tests,* and (3) *observation* which includes demonstration. In choosing one or more of these methods, consider the advantages and disadvantages of each; these are summarized

Method	Advantages	Disadvantages
Discussion	• Flexible • Gives immediate feedback to learner	• Subjective • Variable
Tests	• Standardized • Objective	• May intimidate the learner • Delayed feedback to the learner • Requires advance preparation
Observation	• Evaluates skills and attitudes	• May make the learner ill at ease

FIGURE 2.11 Evaluation methods

in Figure 2.11. (Refer to Chapter 7 for a detailed discussion of evaluation methodology and techniques.)

A common error in education is to think about evaluation at the *end* of the teaching-learning process, rather than at the *beginning*. Although a specific evaluation method is applied after the teaching-learning process is completed, you need to plan carefully for evaluation before you begin teaching. By formulating behavioral objectives and selecting evaluation methods before you teach, you will be able to focus your teaching on specific goals and to measure whether or not these goals have been reached.

MAKE IT CONSISTENT

We have discussed ways to make teaching *relevant* and *effective*. Your third responsibility is to be *consistent*. Consistency means that what you teach today is in agreement with what you taught yesterday. It means that what you are teaching fits with what others are teaching. Inconsistencies are confusing. They may interfere with the learner's trust in those caring for him—"Who can I believe because everyone tells me something different?" They may interfere with your effectiveness—"Since everyone does it differently, it probably doesn't matter."

The Teaching Plan

"A consistent approach requires an overall teaching plan that is specific, concise, and accessible to all health professionals involved . . . " (Talabere, p. 21). The plan should be easy to follow, should facilitate documentation, and should reflect the progress that is being made. The teaching plan should be organized so it includes the following:

TEACHING PLAN

CHILDREN'S HOSPITAL
COLUMBUS, OHIO

Instructions for Use

1. Identify the procedure(s) or area(s) of knowledge to be taught. Enter this in the first column.

2. State the desired parent or child behaviors. These should tell what you expect the parent or child to be able to do after the teaching is completed.

3. Under Performance of Achieved Behaviors indicate *S* for satisfactory performance or *R* if repeat instruction is needed.

4. Under Date and Instructor place date and the initials of the instructor.

Procedure/ Knowledge to be Taught	Desired Behavior of Parent(s)/Child (Learning Objectives)	Performance of Achieved Behaviors	Date and Instructor

FIGURE 2.12 An open-ended teaching plan

1. A brief statement of the content to be taught

2. The behavioral objectives which specifically state the desired behaviors of the learner

3. An evaluation of the objectives—were they achieved or not?

4. The name of the teacher and the date the teaching-learning sessions took place

5. Methods of teaching may also be included

A teaching plan can be open-ended as in Figure 2.12. This format has the advantage of being flexible enough to be used for most health problems. A disadvantage is that increased staff time and effort is needed to complete the plan. The staff may need to develop skills in writing objectives and identifying content. Without these skills they may perceive this kind of a teaching plan as a barrier to teaching.

A standard teaching plan can be developed for a partic-ular health problem or procedure. An example is our initial teaching plan for cystic fibrosis shown in Figure 2.13. The advantages of the standard plan are its availability and the minimum preparation time required of staff. A disadvantage is the standardized format which may overlook or neglect individual learning needs.

We use both types of teaching plans at Children's Hospital. The first kind is used for less complex and/or less frequent health problems. The standardized type is used for health problems that are more involved and/or those that occur often.

The Teaching Team

The teaching team is comprised of all health care givers who are involved in your patient's care, as well as the patient and other learners. Each of these people needs to be informed about the content, objectives, and progress of the teaching plan. The most effective and practical way to keep the health care givers up to date is to place the

INITIAL TEACHING PLAN FOR CYSTIC FIBROSIS

CHILDREN'S HOSPITAL
COLUMBUS, OHIO

Instructions for Use

1. Under Performance of Achieved Behaviors indicate *S* for satisfactory performance or *R* if repeat instruction is needed.

2. Under Date and Instructor place date and your initials.

Procedure/Knowledge to be Taught	Desired Behaviors of Parent(s)/Child	Performance of Achieved Behaviors	Date and Instructor
1. Nature of CF*	1.1 Has read CF pamphlet(s)	1.1	1.1
	1.2 Describes briefly the disease process and primary organs affected	1.2	1.2
	1.3 States complications, especially respiratory infections	1.3	1.3
2. Increased need for nutrition and vitamins	2.1 States reason for this	2.1	2.1
	2.2 Describes ways to increase nutrition and vitamins: (a) high protein foods, (b) frequent feedings, (c) supplemental vitamins	2.2	2.2
3. Increased need for salt replacements	3.1 States reason for this	3.1	3.1
	3.2 Describes ways to do this: (a) pretzels (b) saltines	3.2	3.2
	3.3 Relates this to times of greater loss (i.e., fever, hot weather)	3.3	3.3

FIGURE 2.13 A standard teaching plan for patients with cystic fibrosis and their families. (Reprinted with the permission of the *Journal of the Association for the Care of Children in Hospitals.*)

Procedure/Knowledge to be Taught	Desired Behaviors of Parent(s)/Child	Performance of Achieved Behaviors	Date and Instructor
4. Psychosocial needs of child/family	4.1 Recognizes that child's needs for love, security, and protection should be balanced with needs for growing independence, peer group relationships, achievement	4.1	4.1
	4.2 Recognizes signs and problems of overprotectiveness; can discuss ways to offset this	4.2	4.2
	4.3 If siblings, parents can discuss what they plan to tell them and how they plan to involve them.	4.3	4.3
	4.4 Parents recognize own need to "get away"; can discuss babysitting arrangements	4.4	4.4
5. Genetics of CF*	5.1 States chances for *each successive* child having CF as 1 in 4	5.1	5.1
6. Infection control	6.1 States importance of up-to-date immunizations	6.1	6.1
	6.2 Recognizes need for vigorous aerosol treatment and postural drainage at home, even in the absence of respiratory distress	6.2	6.2
	6.3 Recognizes need for prompt medical advice when respiratory distress occurs.	6.3	6.3
7. Activity level	7.1 Recognizes that child can engage in normal activities within limits of tolerance	7.1	7.1
	7.2 Recognizes need for adequate sleep	7.2	7.2
	7.3 Identifies activities such as swimming that can improve respiratory functioning	7.3	7.3
8. Signs of respiratory distress and/or infection requiring medical consultation	8.1 States these signs as difficult breathing (dyspnea), turning blue (cyanosis), temperature ↑ 102° F	8.1	8.1
	8.2 Correctly describes assessment of these signs in infant or child	8.2	8.2
	8.3 States how to reach physician	8.3	8.3
9. Postural drainage**	9.1 Correctly demonstrates clapping and vibration for all eleven positions	9.1	9.1
	9.2 Does each position twice: claps 1 minute, vibrates for five exhalations, repeats clapping and vibrating	9.2	9.2
	9.3 Does all positions	9.3	9.3
	9.4 Recognizes need for postural drainage in the absence of acute distress	9.4	9.4

FIGURE 2.13 (Continued)

Procedure/Knowledge to be Taught	Desired Behaviors of Parent(s)/Child	Performance of Achieved Behaviors	Date and Instructor
10. Medication administration	10.1 States the primary action of each prescribed medication	10.1	10.1
	10.2 Gives correct dosage	10.2	10.2
	10.3 Applies a scheduling procedure to medication administration	10.3	10.3
11. Aerosol administration***	11.1 Places correct dosage of aerosol(s) into nebulizer	11.1	11.1
	11.2 Demonstrates correct administration of aerosol for time ordered	11.2	11.2
	11.3 States why aerosols precede postural drainage	11.3	11.3
	11.4 Reiterates procedure for mixing A-33 solution and for cleaning equipment daily with it	11.4	11.4
	11.5 Demonstrates correct assembly of equipment for home use	11.5	11.5
	11.6 Describes special precautions for installing ultrasonic nebulizer cable and maintaining patent orifices	11.6	11.6
	11.7 States how to reach pharmacist in case of equipment problems	11.7	11.7
12. Follow-up and community resources	12.1 Has in writing time and place of physician and/or clinical specialist appt., other clinic appts	12.1	12.1
	12.2 Has decided whether or not public health nurse is needed	12.2	12.2
	12.3 If school-age child, has read CF pamphlet for teachers; is aware that school nurse referral can be made	12.3	12.3
	12.4 Has information about CF Foundation and local parent group	12.4	12.4

*Initial information to be given by physician or clinical specialist
**To be taught by physical therapist
***To be taught by pharmacist

FIGURE 2.13 (Continued)

teaching plan in an accessible and visible place such as in your patient's chart or in the nursing care Kardex.

A duplicate of the teaching plan can be kept in your patient's room or, in the case of young children, given to the parents. Sometimes sharing the teaching plan with the patient or family can be an effective strategy to increase the patient's sense of involvement. It also communicates exactly what is expected. At other times, sharing the teaching plan can add to the stress and be perceived as overwhelming. To decide, you need to evaluate your patient's readiness carefully.

If the teaching plan covers several areas of care, or if it focuses on aspects that are unfamiliar to the teaching team, a health team planning conference will help to insure consistency. Such a conference provides an opportunity for the entire teaching team to review and to further develop the teaching plan together. Data about the patient and family as well as objectives and teaching content can be shared. It is also a good idea to decide which member of the team is responsible for which areas of teaching. This avoids both overlap and omissions. The team leader can be any member of the team, but it is helpful to select someone who has rapport with the patient and family and who has had previous patient teaching experience.

Sometimes it is helpful to bring the patient and/or family into the team planning conference, but first you need to give this careful thought. On one hand, this approach can increase patient involvement and compliance. The patient and family may also raise important points not previously considered. On the other hand, this approach may create unnecessary stress for the patient and/or family. They may feel outnumbered or overwhelmed by the health professionals or may fear embarrassment. If, after thoughtful consideration of the situation, you decide that the family or patient would benefit by involvement in the planning conference, directly ask the patient and/or family if they wish to participate in the conference—you may be surprised at the number of enthusiastic responses you receive.

ALLOW ADEQUATE TIME

In the hurried pace of everyday demands it is easy to postpone the teaching until "later." When this happens teaching becomes a last minute effort. How often have you wished for just a little more time?

Planning for adequate time is an important consideration in the teaching-learning process. For initial teaching, especially if it is complex, your patient may need several days to integrate new knowledge and skills adequately. You will need to decide which aspects of the teaching plan are essential to cover before your patient goes home and which aspects can be safely left for follow-up teaching at a later date.

If your patient is overwhelmed with a new diagnosis or with numerous tests, teaching may have to be delayed. This is another time variable to consider. Patients with perceptual or communication deficits may require extra time. Children have special time needs related to developmental stages and their shorter attention span.

LEARNER RESPONSIBILITIES

The teaching-learning process actually begins with the learner, for it is his need that is being addressed (Fig. 2.8). In this process the learner has responsibilities which are vital for him to assume if the teaching-learning is to be a two-way street. These responsibilities include active participation, providing feedback, and compliance.

ACTIVE PARTICIPATION

"Involvement is essential for learning and the more thoroughly the individual participates the more effective will be the learning which results" (Pohl, p. 18). Active learning is learning through doing. It provides the learner with a chance to "try on" new alternatives for dealing with his health problem.

The learner should be informed that you expect him to take an active role. Many people still view learning as a passive process; these individuals will need extra encouragement to get involved. Learning depends on wanting to learn. If the learner perceives the teaching-learning process as shared responsibility, he will involve himself more actively in the process.

PROVIDING FEEDBACK

Feedback provides information about "the way things are going." The role of the teacher in giving feedback is well known. This is part of the evaluation process. Equally important, but less emphasized, is the role of the learner in giving feedback. Learner feedback lends significant guidance to the teaching-learning process because it lets you, the teacher, know whether or not you are meeting your patient's needs.

Learner feedback is often indirect. In some cases it may be essentially nonverbal. There are several ways to obtain learner feedback. Consider the degree of attentiveness. Do comments and questions pertain to what you are saying or do they point in another direction? Pick up on patterns of discussion. Does the learner ask any questions? Does the discussion flow or does it jump from one subject to another? Watch facial expressions. Verbal and nonverbal cues provide valuable data about the impact of your teaching. Appropriate observation of these cues will enable you to make maximal use of the time and effort that you and your patient invest.

Encourage your patient to give you feedback. Explain to him that it helps you do a better job in teaching. Although this is changing, patients still tend to place health care givers on "authority" pedestals. They may be hesitant to tell us directly that we are not meeting their learning needs. They may even avoid asking important questions for fear of "sounding stupid." Only by promoting openness and seeking the learner's input can you be sure that you and your patient are moving toward the same goals.

COMPLIANCE

Patient compliance is the third responsibility of the learner. Compliance means that the patient is carrying out what has been learned. It includes appropriate application of knowledge, correct performance of skills, and acceptance of limitations. It occurs when your patient recognizes that what he has learned is an acceptable alternative to his health problem.

Compliance will be short-lived if the patient is not able to adapt his life style to accommodate his new knowledge, skills, and attitudes. In general, compliance decreases as the extent of behavior changes increases (Ball, p. 273). In other words, if we require too many changes of the patient at one time, the chances of his actually carrying out all the instructions are reduced. As health teachers we need to temper teaching-learning goals with realism and to avoid the pitfall of teaching too much too fast.

The responsibility for compliance ultimately belongs to the patient. It is the patient who has the final say in whether or not medications are taken or a diet is followed. If the health teacher tries to assume this responsibility, he may delude himself into thinking that he is the one who can achieve compliance. The patient must be made aware that he has the final choice in accepting or rejecting a health care alternative—that he is accountable for his own health care. Remember, the responsibility for teaching belongs to you, but the decision to comply belongs to the patient.

TEACHING-LEARNING METHODS

It was stated earlier in this chapter that beliefs and behaviors related to health and illness are the focus of health education. Changing or modifying these beliefs and behaviors is necessary when they are not satisfactory for a particular situation. Teaching-learning methods are the strategies and techniques that are used in the actual teaching-learning situation to achieve these changes in beliefs and behaviors. There are several frameworks that can be used; three of these are growth and development principles, conditioning techniques, and play.

PRINCIPLES OF GROWTH AND DEVELOPMENT

Providing individualized health education to children and their families requires careful consideration of cognitive and psychosocial development. The natural course of this development, as described by Piaget and Erikson, offers a framework that has particular applicability for health teaching. Sharing these concepts with parents can enhance their skills in promoting and reinforcing desired health care behaviors.

Piaget speaks of infants as sensori-motor beings. This means their cognitive development is shaped by sensory inputs and motor activity. From these multiple inputs the infant learns to associate regular images and sounds with people and objects. Thus the infant evolves from a neonate whose behavior is largely directed by reflex activity to one who coordinates touch and vision, differentiates himself from others, and formulates rudimentary concepts about the world around him. In addition to this amazing cognitive development, the infant has a psychosocial task of paramount importance: to establish a trusting relationship. This is facilitated when the infant's needs are met by consistent care-givers in a safe and comfortable environment.

A toddler is embarking on language development which opens many new doors to him. As he learns symbolic representation of the world around him, conceptual development proceeds rapidly. However, the ability to understand exceeds the ability to verbalize. Nonverbal alternatives for expressing feelings need to be provided, such as gross motor activity, which is an effective outlet for venting frustration. The toddler is very literal, therefore verbal explanations should be carefully selected. A toddler is struggling to achieve some measure of autonomy, so exploration of the environment and trial and error are important means of learning for him.

The preschooler is expanding his language skills and vocabulary and is learning to carry on meaningful conversations with others. His thinking is primarily in magical or "preconceptual" terms. Ritual and repetition assume great importance. For example a 5-year-old boy, who was to have chest tubes in place after surgery, was given a doll and a plastic catheter so he could see where a chest tube would be inserted. But inserting the catheter one time was not enough; he repeated this eight times before he verbalized that this was going to happen to him. He had a beginning understanding of the inside of the body, but needed the visual reinforcement of the body (the doll) and the equipment (the catheter). A simple drawing of the lungs inside a body outline would also have been a helpful learning tool for this preschooler. The Helping Hand, *Cardiac Catheterization*, shows how both a body diagram and a coloring game can be used to increase knowledge about the body.

School-age children are learning to conceptualize. This means they can engage in logical reasoning about concrete problems. Conceptualization can be facilitated by providing active interaction with the environment through the manipulation of objects and materials. A study of school-age children having their casts removed showed that giving sensory information about what the child could expect to feel and to hear was especially helpful in reducing stress (Johnson, Kirchhoff, Endress, p. 210). School-age children are striving for a sense of achievement. They are receptive to assuming increased responsibility for self care and should be encouraged to participate in planning their own health care. They enjoy socializing and are able to appreciate the viewpoints of others. Group learning, games, and peer interaction provide reality orientation and encourage expression of shared feelings.

Adolescents are learning to deal with abstract problems as well as concrete ones. They are able to deal with longer term implications and can consider the ramifications of various outcomes. However, they tend to think that anything can be "reasoned out"; therefore, their approaches to problems may be more idealistic than practical. Providing realistic options in terms of limitations will assist the adolescent in making appropriate choices. The primary psychosocial task of adolescence is to develop a sense of identity. As health care professionals it is important that we teach about normal physical, mental, emotional, and cultural variability so the adolescent can appreciate his own uniqueness. Also, it is essential for us to clarify with the adolescent his role and responsibility in managing his own health care.

The thrust of normal growth and development is toward increasing independence. In teaching children and their families we need to select approaches and content in order to promote a level of self-management in health care that is both age-appropriate and individualized to the child's and family's needs.

TECHNIQUES OF CONDITIONING

A second framework is operant conditioning. According to this view, learning occurs as a result of positive reinforcement, whereas negative reinforcement teaches the learner to avoid undesired responses. One approach to enuresis provides an example of conditioning. A pad is placed in the child's bed. When the child urinates, a loud alarm is triggered. Immediately the parents get the child out of bed and take him to the bathroom. The alarm helps the child to associate waking up with urinating. Eventually, the child learns to wake up *before* urinating; a dry bed and no alarm are the positive reinforcements. If the child wakes up *after* urinating, a wet bed and loud alarm are the negative reinforcements. In the absence of underlying pathology or severe emotional disorders, this technique of conditioning has been cited as one of the most effective methods of treating enuresis in many children (McKendry and Stewart, p. 1025).

Conditioning principles are used in behavior modification. Any of the following techniques may be selected: chaining, modeling, shaping, or fading.

Chaining is the technique of putting together more and more complex ideas into a chain of learning. For example, a person with diabetes may first learn about the separate ideas of dietary control of carbohydrates, urine testing to check for sugar in the urine, and insulin injections to improve carbohydrate utilization. Then the patient is taught to put these ideas together and to see the relationships among diet, insulin, and urinary glucose. In chaining, the emphasis is on increasing the complexity of knowledge.

Modeling, shaping, and fading emphasize increasing the complexity of skill. *Modeling* means showing the learner what to do through demonstration. *Shaping* begins with small, simple behaviors and gradually adds more complex behaviors. The following example illustrates both of these techniques. A mother is receiving her initial instruction in tracheostomy suctioning. First, the nurse demonstrates suctioning water from a cup. Then she shows the mother how to suction from a cup while rolling the catheter between her fingers. Next the nurse demonstrates the actual suctioning of the child's tracheostomy. After the nurse demonstrates or *models* each of these steps, the mother performs each step of an increasingly complex behavior (shaping).

Fading, a third technique, involves gradual withdrawal of teacher participation. Continuing with the preceding example, fading occurs as the nurse moves from both suctioning and holding the child, to holding the child while the mother suctions, then to turning both tasks over to the mother.

PLAY

Play, a third framework, is a child's means of communication. Play stimulates and organizes cognitive learning (Arnaud, p. 15); therefore it is a valuable adjunct to pediatric teaching. Through play a child moves toward mastery of a real, and sometimes painful, world.

One of the best and most practical references about the preparation of children for diagnostic and surgical procedures through play is *Emotional Care of Hospitalized Children* by Madeline Petrillo and Sirgay Sanger. This book, organized according to a developmental framework, contains both age-specific and procedure-specific guidelines that serve as models for teaching.

TEACHING-LEARNING TOOLS

The teaching-learning process can be greatly enhanced by the selection of appropriate tools. Learning is a multisensory experience. Inputs through a variety of means reinforce each other and can be cumulative in effect. For example, discussing the effects of a particular therapeutic regimen on an internal organ is rather abstract. Showing a picture of a bronchiole before and after a bronchodilator is given makes a graphic point about the action of this medication. Visual aids are one tool that can be a definite asset. They need not be elaborate or expensive. But they must enhance rather than distract from your teaching. There is a wide range of materials which vary considerably in scope, depth, and quality. Whether they are a help or a hindrance depends on what you choose and how you use it.

The Helping Hands have been carefully developed to make teaching as relevant, effective, and consistent as possible. These teaching aids provide reinforcement in two ways: through written explanations that are direct, simplified, and specific (refer to Chapter 4), and through illustrations that accurately depict important points (refer to Chapter 5). The Helping Hands were designed with the following criteria in mind (Pearson pp. 30–31):

1. Is the tool appropriate for the age and ability of your patient? Consider developmental level as well as chronological age.

2. Consider both general intelligence and educational level.

3. Is the information specific to your patient's learning needs?

4. Will the tool promote active participation by the learner? Will it increase discussion or questions? Will it stimulate the practice of skills?

5. Does the tool present information in an interesting way that appeals to the senses? If it's a visual aid, is it clear or cluttered? Realistic or idealistic? Accurate or misleading?

6. If it is a tool that you are purchasing, is it flexible enough to serve the needs of different patients?

7. Does the tool save you time and money?

There are other excellent tools available as well. By applying these guidelines you can select the best learning tools for your patients' needs and build a reservoir of high quality, patient-specific materials.

MEETING THE CHALLENGE

Health teaching is an integral part of health care. If we are to meet this challenge, it is the responsibility of each of us, individually and collectively, to provide relevant, effective, and consistent health education for the patient and his family. This requires us to have a planned approach that includes the following: assessment of patient needs and readiness, formulation of appropriate and specific objectives, selection of an evaluation method, development of the teaching plan, use of teaching-learning methods and tools, and evaluation of the outcome. Your patient, as a partner in his own health education, has the responsibility to participate actively, to give you feedback, and to carry out his newly learned behaviors. Together you have made that important link between what you teach as a health professional and what your patient does in managing his health care.

The Helping Hands are a significant contribution to patient and family teaching. The next chapter illustrates how you can create and implement a similar patient education program in your setting.

SELECTED READINGS

Arnaud, Sara. "Polish for Play's Tarnished Reputation." In *Play: The Child Strives Toward Self-Realization.* Washington, D.C.: National Association for the Education of Young Children, 1971.

Ball, W. L. "Improving Patient Compliance with Therapeutic Regimens." *Canadian Medical Association Journal* 3 (August 3, 1974): 268-273.

Daubenmire, M. Jean and King, Imogene M. "Nursing Process Models: A Systems Approach." *Nursing Outlook* 21 (August 1973): 512-517.

Dyer, Bonnie. "Asthmatic Kids—Independence: One Giant Step." *Pediatric Nursing* 3 (March–April 1977): 16-23.

Erickson, Marcene L. *Assessment and Management of Developmental Changes in Children.* St. Louis: C.V. Mosby Co., 1976.

Erikson, Erik. *Childhood and Society.* 2nd ed. New York: W.W. Norton & Co., Inc., 1963.

Green, Lawrence W. "The Potential of Health Education Includes Cost Effectiveness." *Hospitals* 50 (May 1976): 57-61.

Havighurst, Robert. *Developmental Tasks and Education.* New York: David McKay Co., Inc., 1952.

Hughes, Cynthia Bach. "An Eclectic Approach to Parent Group Education and Care." *Nursing Clinics of North America* 12 (September 1977): 469-479.

Johnson, Jean E.; Kirchhoff, Karen T.; and Endress, M. Patricia. "Easing Children's Fright During Health Care Procedures." *American Journal of Maternal Child Nursing* 2 (July–August 1976): 206-210.

Johnston, Maxine. "Folk Beliefs and Ethnocultural Behavior in Pediatrics." *Nursing Clinics of North America* 12 (March 1977): 77-84.

Leininger, Madelein. "Cultural Diversities of Health and Nursing Care." *Nursing Clinics of North America* 12 (March 1977): 5-18.

Lewis, Oscar. "The Culture of Poverty." *Scientific American* 215 (October 1966): 19-25.

McKendry, J. B. J. and Stewart, D. A. "Enuresis." *Pediatric Clinics of North America* 21 (November 1974): 1019-1028.

Murray, Ruth and Zentner, Judith. *Nursing Concepts for Health Promotion.* Englewood Cliffs, N.J.: Prentice-Hall, 1975.

Otto, Herbert A. "A Framework for Assessing Family Strength." In *Family-Centered Community Nursing: A Sociocultural Framework.* Edited by Adina M. Reinhardt and Mildred D. Quinn. St. Louis: C.V. Mosby Co., 1973.

Pearson, Betty. "Learning Tool Selection." *Supervisor Nurse* 6 (March 1975): 30-31.

Pender, Nola J. "A Conceptual Model for Preventive Health Behavior." *Nursing Outlook* 23 (June 1975): 385-390.

Petrello, Judith. "Your Patients Hear You, But Do They Understand?" *RN* 39 (February 1976): 37-39.

Petrillo, Madeline and Sanger, Sirgay. *Emotional Care of Hospitalized Children: An Environmental Approach.* Philadelphia: J.B. Lippincott Co., 1972.

Pohl, Margaret L. *The Teaching Function of the Nursing Practitioner.* 2d ed. Dubuque, Iowa: Wm. C. Brown Co., 1968.

Porter, Anne Lynn, ed. "Symposium on Diabetes: Patient Education and Care." *Nursing Clinics of North America* 12 (September 1977): 361–445.

Primeaux, Martha H. "American Indian Health Care Practices: A Cross-Cultural Perspective." *Nursing Clinics of North America* 12 (March 1977): 55–65.

Redman, Barbara Klug. *The Process of Patient Teaching in Nursing.* 2d ed. St. Louis: C.V. Mosby Co., 1972.

Rogers, Carl L. *Freedom to Learn.* Columbus, Ohio: Charles E. Merrill Publishing Co., 1969.

Selye, Hans. *The Stress of Life.* New York: McGraw-Hill Book Co., 1956.

Sills, Grayce M. and Hall, Joanne E. "A General Systems Perspective for Nursing." In *Distributive Nursing Practice: A Systems Approach to Community Health.* Edited by Joanne Hall and Barbara Weaver. Philadelphia: J.B. Lippincott Co., 1977.

Smith, Carol R. "Patient Education in Ambulatory Care." *Nursing Clinics of North America* 12 (December 1977): 595–608.

Smith, Dorothy L. *Medication Guide for Patient Counseling.* Philadelphia: Lea & Febiger, 1977.

Somers, Anne R. "Consumer Health Education—To Know or to Die." *Hospitals* 50 (May 1, 1976): 52–56.

Swezey, Robert L. and Swezey, Annette M. "Educational Theory as a Basis for Patient Education." *Journal of Chronic Diseases* 29 (July 1976): 417–422.

Talabere, Laurel R. "The Development and Implementation of a Cystic Fibrosis Teaching Plan." *Journal of the Association for the Care of Children in Hospitals* 5 (Fall 1976): 18–24.

Tripp-Reimer, Toni and Friedl, Mary Cardwell. "Appalachians: A Neglected Minority." *Nursing Clinics of North America* 12 (March 1977): 41–45.

Turner, Mary N. "Nursing Process: An Operational Framework for Nursing Practice." In *Nursing of Families in Crisis.* Edited by Joanne Hall and Barbara Weaver. Philadelphia: J.B. Lippincott Co., 1974.

Wadsworth, Barry. *Piaget's Theory of Cognitive Development.* New York: David McKay Co., Inc., 1971.

Wang, Rosemary Y. and Watson, Joellen. "Contracting for Weight Reduction—Making the Sacrifices Worthwhile." *American Journal of Maternal and Child Nursing* 3 (January–February 1978): 46–49.

White, Earnestine Huffman. "Giving Health Care to Minority Patients." *Nursing Clinics of North America* 12 (March 1977): 27–40.

Wigginton, Eliot, ed. *The Foxfire Book.* Garden City, N.Y.: Anchor Press/Doubleday, 1972.

Winslow, Elizabeth Hahn. "The Role of the Nurse in Patient Education—Focus: The Cardiac Patient." *Nursing Clinics of North America* 11 (June 1976): 213–221.

chapter 3
Developing a Viable System

Rose-Marie Duda McCormick

"You do not need the acquirement of fresh knowledge half as much as to put into practice that which you already possess."

Frances De Salignac

Our Homegoing Education and Literature Program developed as a result of a need for organization of patient/family teaching aids. Our health professionals were concerned because the teaching aids they needed were either too expensive or unavailable. The storeroom manager was concerned about the dusty pamphlet inventory which "didn't move" because no one knew it was there. The patients and parents were probably the most concerned because after they left the hospital, they had difficulty remembering the instructions they had received.

We had been trying to get around to the project of organizing the order, storage, distribution, and filing systems of preprinted materials, but it seemed that with every feeble attempt, a roadblock was met head on. If it wasn't money, it was storage space; if not the ordering system, then the distribution system. Who was going to do it? How should it be done? Where should we look for guidance? It took some time, but finally we developed a system: The Homegoing Education and Literature Program (H.E.L.P.).

Why should a patient education system be a priority project? The answer is simple. As the cost of health care rises, patient education becomes more and more important. It has become less expensive to keep a patient *out* of the hospital than to pay for his care while he is *in*. Recognizing this fact, insurance companies are beginning to pay for patient education. But, for an institution to receive reimbursement for the teaching given, evidence must be shown that patient teaching aids are available and used. For a product to be used, it must be available and readily accessible. *A system is part of the solution.*

Building a system is much like constructing a building. Erecting a building requires a blueprint, supplies, tools, and person-power. The blueprint maps out how to attain the end result—a sturdy building; and the construction supervisor determines exactly what steps are taken and in what order. This is analogous to building a system: this chapter gives you the blueprint and tools, it is up to you to provide the supplies and the person-power. Are you ready to begin? Let's go.

WHO?

"Who?" is a good question. Who should be responsible for setting up a patient teaching aid system? You will need to answer this question before beginning your program.

The "whos" you choose should be determined by the purpose and scope of your program. If all you need is a system for organizing currently available materials, a person skilled in filing and distribution systems can probably do the job. But if you need to "create" new materials, the primary "whos" will probably be a program director, a program coordinator, an illustrator, and many reviewers.

THE PROGRAM DIRECTOR

In most settings, the responsibilities of the program director can be incorporated into one of the administrative positions already in existence. But, in our situation, a program director position was necessary since the Helping Hand concept was being created "from scratch." As our program progressed and changed, so also did the responsibilities of the director so the part-time position was maintained.

THE PROGRAM COORDINATOR

When we first envisioned this program we realized the only way it could be accomplished was with one person coordinating the efforts; without this, the project of developing teaching aids would certainly fail. In selecting the program coordinator, we believed that the most important qualities to look for were creativity, knowledge of various diseases and conditions, experience with patient and staff teaching, skills in written expression, and the ability to get along with all types of people. Fortunately, we had such a person —a nurse.

Although your program coordinator does not necessarily need to be a nurse, we found that it is advantageous for several reasons. Nurses are usually the hub of patient activities, they are natural coordinators. If you disagree, just observe a patient unit: the physicians ask nurses about the patients, the dietitians, respiratory therapists, and physical therapists confer with the nurse, the families and the patients consult her. Of course this isn't a one-way street—the nurses are conferring, coordinating, and directing at the same time. Nurses also have a working knowledge of the entire health care system, as well as of the total scope of patient care. So, because a nurse has learned some of the skills of coordination, and because her contact with various levels of hospital staff and patients/families is pre-established, the decision is quite easy: a nurse coordinator.

THE ILLUSTRATOR

Another very important person is the illustrator. Since illustrations are a valuable addition to the communication of thoughts and directions, this person's talent and efforts are vital to the success and usefulness of the teaching aids.

When we first began our program, we did not have the services of an illustrator. So we scanned magazines, news-papers, and advertisements for pictures of people, places, and things; and we used a lighted x-ray box to aid in tracing. With these devices and our belief that illustration is vital, we created some good pictures, but nothing compared with the illustrations we have now.

We were fortunate that the mother of one of our special patients was willing to volunteer her time to help us in our efforts. Although she did not have years of experience as an illustrator and had not "studied with the Masters," she *did* have artistic talent, creativity, excellent interpersonal relationships, enthusiasm, and the ability to capture all this in "caring" illustrations of real life experiences. She worked as a volunteer for a year before being hired on a part-time basis.

Hopefully, you will be lucky enough to find such a person, but if not, don't despair. There are plenty of ready-to-use aids on the market today, as discussed in Chapter 5. These aids, plus a little creativity and ingenuity, will go a long way in developing adequate illustrations.

THE SIGNIFICANT OTHERS

The significant others involved in the program are too numerous to mention by title, but the primary groups are: nurses, physicians, patients and families, pharmacists, dentists, physical therapists, respiratory therapists, dietitians, social workers, occupational therapists, activity therapists, clergymen, paramedical, and ancillary personnel. Just about anyone who has knowledge of and/or experience with patient teaching and medical information can contribute to the development of teaching aids by supplying information, by assisting in writing the teaching aids, and in reviewing drafts throughout the process. Also, of utmost importance are the services of an efficient and dedicated secretary/typist. Without help with typing, distribution, and organization, the program becomes more difficult and time-consuming to maintain.

JOB RESPONSIBILITIES

The responsibilities developed for our director, coordinator, and illustrator are presented here for informational purposes (exerpted from our actual job descriptions). You may wish to use these as models in developing your own. The scope of our program required a part-time director, a full-time coordinator, and a part-time illustrator. Depending on the needs of your program, the number of people and/or the time spent may need to be modified. But, whomever you select, the persons should be able to fulfill the specified requirements.

The Director

1. Directs the activities of Homegoing Education and Literature Program and coordinates these with the

Nursing Department, medical staff, and other departments to provide quality homegoing instructional materials for the patients and families

a. Organizes systems for the proper implementation, utilization, and periodic re-evaluation of the Homegoing Education and Literature Program teaching aids

b. Evaluates the program to identify achievements, to provide data for forecasting and planning, and to recommend and/or to implement necessary changes to enhance the program

c. Maintains statistics for H.E.L.P., including Helping Hands developed and other pertinent information

d. Develops annual objectives and prepares a written annual report on projects, programs, and activities

e. Participates in fiscal planning and control, recommending budgetary plans related to the Homegoing Education and Literature Program

2. Directs and supervises the Homegoing Education and Literature Program, coordinator, and illustrator

3. Participates in the planning and implementation of patient education programs and promotes continuing education related to patient education.

a. Participates in the writing of internal and "external" publications of patient education-related materials

b. Participates in planning for research related to patient/family education materials

4. Reports regularly, verbally and in writing, to the director of nursing regarding H.E.L.P.

5. Carries out personal and professional responsibilities as required by the health care facility

The Coordinator

1. Coordinates the development of the program teaching aids (Helping Hands) used for supplementing and/or reinforcing instructions given to patients and families

a. Evaluates and coordinates the selection of teaching aids to be developed with members of nursing staff and other departments

b. Researches and reviews literature on aspects of patient care and instructional methods; consults with appropriate hospital personnel in the writing of Helping Hands

c. Coordinates the Helping Hand draft critiques of medical and nursing representatives and revises teaching aids as necessary

d. Coordinates the illustration of written instructional materials with the program illustrator

e. Coordinates distribution of finalized Helping Hands

f. Coordinates the periodic re-evaluation of the teaching aids

2. Maintains accurate records of all activities in the development of Helping Hands and prepares a monthly report

3. Provides or coordinates staff development sessions for personnel on the use of teaching aids and methods of teaching

a. Participates in orientation and inservice programs on the importance of teaching, teaching methods, and use of the Helping Hands

b. Acts as liaison between Nursing and other hospital departments regarding the use of Helping Hands

4. Reports to the program director on progress, accomplishments, and problem areas

5. Carries out personal and professional responsibilities as required by the health care facility

The Illustrator

1. Plans, coordinates, and evaluates illustration, design, and format of the Helping Hands

a. Designs appropriate illustrations for the Helping Hands with emphasis on portraying realism with warmth (nonclinical), reinforcing important points of written instruction, providing clarity of written instructions through illustration, and projecting (through illustration) a caring attitude of those providing health care to patients and families

b. Designs and prepares layout and "paste-up" of all Helping Hands

c. Revises illustrations on Helping Hands as necessary to meet the changing needs of patients/families and health care practitioners

d. Acts as advisor and consultant to the program director and coordinator and to appropriate others in the area of graphic production

2. Collaborates and consults with hospital personnel, patients, families, and outside sources in the illustration, design, and printing of Helping Hands

a. Consults with appropriate health care practitioners and patients/families to determine types and technical aspects of illustrations needed for specific Helping Hands

b. Consults with nursing personnel to obtain assistance and permission to use appropriate models for illustration

c. Acts as liaison between H.E.L.P. and the Children's Hospital Print Shop and outside printing services in matters relating to the printing and production of Helping Hands

3. Meets regularly with the program director and coordinator to discuss the progress of projects and to plan future Helping Hands

4. Carries out personal and professional responsibilities as required by the health care facility

---

DETERMINING THE SCOPE OF THE PROGRAM

Probably the best way to start a project such as this is to ask the question "Do we really need a system for developing and distributing patient education materials or is our current system adequate?" To answer this question, you will have to do a little investigating of your own.

GATHERING INFORMATION: THE INFORMAL SURVEY

First, find out if there is a system for supplying patient education materials. If there is, determine if any supply and storage problems exist. Then, observe in each area to see if teaching aids are easily accessible to staff. While on your tour, make a list of the teaching aid topics that are available in the units/clinics.

While you are gathering information about the system and the currently available materials, find out about the needs of the staff. Talk with the nurses, especially those who care for and teach patients and families daily. Ask them about which patient education materials they have, which they use, what they need, and if they have an interest in developing patient education materials. Start developing a list of topics that might be addressed in the teaching aids.

Talk with patients/families and ask them what type of information they would find helpful. If they have had previous hospitalizations, ask about what written information would have helped them at home.

Talk with the staff physicians. Find out if they are having problems with patients following their instructions. Do the patients/families understand when to call them? Do the procedure demonstrations need to be followed by written instructions to which patients/families can refer at home? Would written instructions save them time? Also ask if they would be willing to review and to critique the teaching aids developed. Make a list of their suggestions and add these to your list.

Talk to the staff dentists. Do their patients need instructions about dental hygiene? Are special instructions necessary for patients taking medications such as penicillin or anticonvulsant medications? Are instructions needed for patients who have had tooth extractions? Do parents know when their child should have the first dental examination? Ask also if they will review the teaching aids.

And there are other people to be consulted. Talk with the respiratory, physical, and occupational therapists. Ask the pharmacist, dietitian, social worker, and chaplain. Talk with the paramedical personnel, technicians, aides, and ward clerks. Ask them what problems patients/families encounter. Were patients prepared for return visits to have diagnostic tests? Was another appointment necessary because the mother did not understand that her child was *not* to eat or drink after midnight? Are some of the patients uncooperative because no one told them what to expect? List the problems; you may find that written instructions would be helpful.

Talk with public health nurses, school nurses, industrial health nurses, and other health professionals. Are there areas of concern where parent education is needed? Are the former patients having trouble in school because problems were not anticipated or identified when they left the hospital? Are new things taking place at this hospital or in the community which need reinforcement through written instructions.

Hopefully by the time you finish gathering information you will have created interest in patient/family education, or at least you will have aroused curiosity. Now it's time to compile your list of topics so you can formally survey the needs. (You might want to supplement your list by reviewing the procedure books of the nursing department and other hospital departments, adding to your list any procedures the patients/families would be doing at home.)

In developing the list of topics, try to determine the specific nature and the title of the teaching aid. Use titles which most patients would understand (for example, "Taking Temperature, Pulse, and Respirations" rather than "Vital Signs"). List all of the proposed topics in alphabetical order for use in your Teaching Aid Survey. You may find our Master Index (page 44-46) helpful in compiling your list.

SURVEYING THE NEEDS: THE FORMAL SURVEY

There are several ways to approach the organized gathering of data. One way is on a one-to-one basis, as we used in the informal survey; this is probably the most effective method, but it is very time consuming. Another way is questionnaire style—by distributing a teaching aid survey. Judging from our experiences, the questionnaire is probably the least effective approach. There is usually a lack of or "lag" in response in completing a questionnaire—it seems to be the last thing on people's long "to do" list. Perhaps this is due to the impersonal nature of this form of data collection.

A third way, and the approach we found most successful, is through small group meetings (ten or fewer participants). In small groups, the presenter is usually more comfortable in discussing the material, and the participants are more comfortable communicating questions and comments. Also, in small group sessions, you can determine the interest in the program and the amount of support the teaching aid program will receive.

The participants in our small groups were usually nurses from the same unit; we scheduled a unit conference to discuss H.E.L.P. and to survey the needs. We also presented the information in the Nursing Management Committee meeting conducted by the director of nursing; it is important for the staff to know that the nursing leadership supports the program.

To record the opinions and suggestions of the participants accurately, have them complete a teaching aid survey during the meeting (Fig. 3.1). This assures return of the information, since surveys can be collected at the end of the meeting.

THE TEACHING AID SURVEY

The teaching aid survey is useful in gathering information and in determining the scope of your program. You need not spend a lot of time constructing this data collection tool; just be sure that the recorded information is useful, and that the results can be objectively tabulated.

To develop the actual survey, determine the information you wish to obtain and design a format. You may find that our survey suits your needs (Fig. 3.1). Before actually conducting the survey in a meeting, test it on one of your colleagues. How much time does it take to comfortably complete the survey? Be sure to allow this much time during the meeting.

How to Use the Survey

When you give the teaching aid survey to the group participants, explain exactly how to use the survey. We used the following guidelines:

Unit. Have the person completing the survey give his/her unit, area, or department of assignment.

HELPING HAND SURVEY

Unit: _____

Date: _____

Signature (optional): _____

Patient/Family Teaching Aids	How Important to You?						Anything Available or in Use Now?		Comments
	High	Above Avg.	Avg.	Below Avg.	Low	No Interest	Yes	No	
Allergy to Dust									
Allergy to Mold									
Urine Testing									
Tracheostomy Care									
Immunizations									
Medications									
etc.									
Others:									

FIGURE 3.1 The Teaching Aid Survey

Patient/Family Teaching Aids	Participant 1					Participant 2					Participant 3					Participant 4				
	H	A/A	A	B/A	L	H	A/A	A	B/A	L	H	A/A	A	B/A	L	H	A/A	A	B/A	L
Baby Bath					X			X			X									X
E.C.G.			X			X								X			X			
Mold Allergy	X									X				X				X		

Results	Participant 1	Participant 2	Participant 3	Participant 4	Totals
Baby Bath	1	3	5	1	10
E.C.G.	3	5	2	4	14
Mold Allergy	5	1	2	3	11

FIGURE 3.2 Compiling the Survey Results. From the results of the four participants, E.C.G. is first priority; Mold Allergy, second; and Baby Bath, third.

Date. Note the date the survey is completed.

Signature (optional). Encourage signatures of participants.

Patient/family teaching aids. This is the list of proposed topics compiled from the informal survey. Encourage participants to suggest other topics, and note these in the blank spaces on the survey.

How important to you. The person should indicate how important it is to her whether a teaching aid on this topic is made available. The response assumes that if an aid were made available the person would *use* it. (Note: This information will help you give priorities to the teaching aid topics following the survey tabulation.)

Anything available now? Is the participant aware of or does she use any teaching aids on these topics at this time.

Comments. Encourage the survey participant to comment freely. For example, cite the name of a teaching aid currently in use or indicate interest in assisting in development of a teaching aid.

How to Compile the Survey Results

Before tallying the results of the teaching aid survey, determine what information you wish to obtain. If you want a general overview, compile all the information together; if you want to know what is needed for a certain group, tally it by unit. One way to compile the results is as follows:

1. Assign numbers to the six categories (High = 5, Above average = 4, Average = 3, Below average = 2, Low = 1, No interest = 0).

2. Use these numbers as you review and tally each survey. For ease in compiling results, have one person read the results and another record the data.

3. Add the numbers for each topic and assign a "total score" to that topic (Fig. 3.2).

4. Rank the topics according to priority; highest number is top priority. (You may be surprised with the results —a topic you thought would rank low may appear at the top of the list.)

5. Interpret the results and make this information available to the survey participants.

Although this method gives a clear picture of the priorities at the time of the survey, you will probably find that the teaching aids will not be developed in this exact order. Some may be "rush" projects; others may lose their priority status. Nothing is static. So, use this list as a general guide rather than as an inflexible priority system.

After compiling the data from the teaching aid survey, you will need to develop a filing and numbering system for the proposed teaching aids. This sounds simple enough, until you start thinking about it and asking others for their suggestions and input. Then, you realize no two people think exactly alike when it comes to filing.

DEVELOPING A FILING SYSTEM

Developing a logical, easy-to-use filing system is one of the most difficult and time-consuming tasks we faced in beginning our program. There should be one correct, logical method of filing, right? One might think so. But, it seems that each person has his own "mental file system" so the development of an acceptable, usable, efficient system becomes a monumental task.

Several months of research, trial and error, and just plain "heavy thinking", were required before we finally developed a suitable method. A variety of publications were reviewed to find examples of indexing. The medical librarian and the medical records librarian were consulted for advice. Books about how to organize topics were sought, but not found. Nowhere could we locate a guide for developing our index, so, we fashioned our own. Hopefully, the same system will work for you.

THE INDEXING SYSTEM

Several methods were suggested for indexing and filing, and after considering these, we eliminated all but three. Our plan was to put these alternatives to a vote, and use the system that the majority of our staff selected. The three alternatives were:

Alphabetical order. File *all* written instructions, regardless of topic, alphabetically (no subdivisions).

Body systems. File all instructions alphabetically under the most appropriate body system (e.g., circulatory, digestive, respiratory, and so forth).

Five major categories. File instructions alphabetically under one of the following categories: diseases, conditions & surgery; procedures; diagnostic tests; child care/ health information, and medications.

There were several anticipated problems with each of these methods, but the first two seemed to pose the most difficulties. The major problem with the alphabetical method was confusion. For example, would "How to Take Temperature, Pulse, and Respirations" be under "T" for TPR, or "V" for vital signs? Would "Care of Teeth and Gums" be under "D" for dental care or "T" for teeth? We found, in talking with many health professionals, that although their ideas differed in the matter of filing, most did *not* use the strict alphabetical system for their own strict alphabetical system for their own filing purposes.

The body systems method posed a different problem. Many procedures, diagnostic tests, and medications are used for several systems-related illnesses or conditions. Also many illnesses affect or are affected by several body systems. For example, would "Care of the Child with Cystic Fibrosis" be listed under the digestive or respiratory system? Or would "Having an X-ray" be under the skeletal or respiratory system, or both? No matter what method was selected, we preferred that each topic appear only under one category. Therefore, the body systems method would be very difficult to implement.

Placing topics into the five major categories, seemed to be the most promising approach. With this method, all the proposed topics could easily be listed under one category only. But, this system did not solve all problems. There were several proposed teaching aids that combined information belonging in several categories. But, if there is a question about which category the topic should be assigned to, a survey could be taken of the nurses and physicians who will most likely use that particular topic, and the majority rules.

CHOOSING THE SYSTEM

We were fairly certain about which alternative would be preferred. However, we wished to meet the needs of our staff who would be using the system in providing patient education. Therefore, all three alternatives were presented to a group of 40 nursing management members. After discussing the pros and cons of each alternative, a vote was taken. The third alternative, the five categories, received overwhelming approval; so this was the index/filing system we adopted.

Perhaps the results would be different for your setting, or perhaps you will devise a better system than any of those presented. That's fine. The most important point is to carefully devise and choose a system which meets the needs of your staff and client population, and then stick with it. Any subsequent change is very disruptive to all who use the system; so, it's best to "get it right the first time."

OUR MASTER INDEX/FILING SYSTEM

Our master index is divided into five major categories, and each of our Helping Hands is listed under one of these (Fig. 3.3). You may decide to use different titles for your subdivisions or designate additional categories; but for the sake of simplicity, we decided to limit the number of categories to five.

The following explanation of each category may be useful:

Section 1: Diseases, Conditions, and Surgeries. This category is fairly self-explanatory. It includes information on diseases and surgeries and also on conditions such as scabies, head lice, and hydrocarbon ingestion. In general, anything that alters the health of the individual is included in this category.

The key word in this category is "curative." For example, does "Treatment of Head Lice" belong under diseases, conditions, and surgeries or under procedures? Since the treatment is for a condition (curative) it belongs under this section.

Section 2: Procedures. All treatments, procedures and "hands on" type care, such as cast care, ear irrigations, and changing a dressing are included in this section.

Section 3: Diagnostic Tests. This category includes all diagnostic tests, such as x-ray and barium enema; and all home preparations for tests, for instance, using atropine drops in preparation for an eye exam. There is usually little confusion about what belongs in this category.

HELPING HAND MASTER INDEX

Section 1   Diseases, Conditions, and Surgeries

- HH-I-1   Allergies, Cottonseed
- HH-I-2   Allergies, Dust
- HH-I-3   Allergies, Flaxseed
- HH-I-4   Allergies, Karaya or India Gum
- HH-I-5   Allergies, Mold
- HH-I-74   Allergy to Stinging Insects
- HH-I-6   Amblyopia
- HH-I-7   Anemia, Iron Deficiency
- HH-I-9   Anemia, Sickle Cell
- HH-I-10   Arthritis
- HH-I-8   Aspirin Ingestion
- HH-I-11   Asthma
- HH-I-83   Asthmatic Breathing Exercises
- HH-I-12   Beta Strep Infection
- HH-I-80   Burns, Daily Skin Care
- HH-I-81   Burns (Preparation for Surgery)
- HH-I-13   Cardiac, Preparation for Surgery
- HH-I-14   Cardiac, Care After Surgery
- HH-I-15   Cerebral Palsy (Daily Care, Ambulation, Nutrition, Equipment)
- HH-I-31   Chicken Pox
- HH-I-16   Circumcision
- HH-I-17   Cleft Lip Repair
- HH-I-18   Cleft Palate Repair
- HH-I-30   Colds
- HH-I-82   Craniostenosis
- HH-I-19   Croup
- HH-I-20   Cystic Fibrosis
- HH-I-21   Dental Surgery
- HH-I-22   Dental, Local Anesthesia
- HH-I-23   Diabetes
- HH-I-25   Injection Sites, Rotating
- HH-I-26   Insulin, Giving
- HH-I-24   Insulin Reactions
- HH-I-27   Urine Testing
- HH-I-28   Diaper Rash
- HH-I-29   Diarrhea
- HH-I-32   Ears, Plastic Tubes
- HH-I-33   Ear Surgery, Care After
- HH-I-34   Enuresis
- HH-I-35   Epilepsy
- HH-I-36   Eye, Artificial
- HH-I-37   Eye Surgery, Having
- HH-I-38   Eye Surgery—Outpatient
- HH-I-39   G6 PD Deficiency
- HH-I-40   Gastroenteritis
- HH-I-41   Head Injury (Inpatient)
- HH-I-42   Head Injuries (Emergency Room)

- HH-I-75   Hemophilia
- HH-I-43   Hepatitis
- HH-I-44
- HH-I-67
- HH-I-69   Hernia Repair, Inguinal
- HH-I-68   Hernia Repair, Umbilical
- HH-I-45   Hydrocarbon Ingestion
- HH-I-84
- HH-I-76   Hypertension
- HH-I-85   Hypospadius
- HH-I-46   Impetigo
- HH-I-47   Lead Poisoning
- HH-I-48   Leukemia
- HH-I-49   Lice, Head—Treatment and Prevention
- HH-I-50   Lung Diseases
- HH-I-88   Myelomeningocele
- HH-I-51   Myringotomy
- HH-I-52   Nephrectomy
- HH-I-54   Otitis Media
- HH-I-55   Outpatient Surgery
- HH-I-77   Paraplegia
- HH-I-56   Pinworms, Treatment
- HH-I-78   Pyelonephritis
- HH-I-86   Pyloric Stenosis
- HH-I-58   Reimplant of Ureters
- HH-I-53   Reye's Syndrome
- HH-I-57   Rheumatic Fever
- HH-I-59   Scabies
- HH-I-60   Scoliosis
- HH-I-61   Seizures
- HH-I-62   Spina Bifida
- HH-I-73   Surgery, Preparing for (Home)
- HH-I-87   Surgery, Preparing for (Inpatient)
- HH-I-63   Surgery, Short Stay
- HH-I-64   T & A, Having a
- HH-I-72   T & A, After a
- HH-I-79   Urinary Tract Infection
- HH-I-65   Vaginitis
- HH-I-66   Venereal Disease
- HH-I-70   V-J Shunt
- HH-I-71   Vomiting
- HH-I-89
- HH-I-90

Section 2   Procedures

- HH-II-16   Arm Restraints
- HH-II-38   Artificial Respiration
- HH-II-7   Bandage, Changing a Gauze
- HH-II-1   Blood Pressure
- HH-II-47   Breast Milk, Collection of
- HH-II-2   Cast Care

FIGURE 3.3 Helping Hand Master Index (• indicates that Helping Hand is available as of 2/1/79).

HH–II–35	Catheterization, Explanation of
• HH–II–39	Catheterization, Intermittent—Female
• HH–II–49	Catheterization, Intermittent—Male
• HH–II–15	Catheterization Record, Intermittent
HH–II–42	Catheter, Indwelling, Care of
HH–II–43	Catheter Irrigation
HH–II–5	Crede of Bladder
• HH–II–6	Crutch Walking
• HH–II–8	Dressings, Wet to Dry
• HH–II–9	Ear Irrigations (Washings)
HH–II–10	Enema
HH–II–11	Exercise, Range of Motion
• HH–II–37	Fever, How to Reduce a
• HH–II–41	Gastrostomy Tube Feedings
• HH–II–12	Gastrostomy Tube, Changing a
HH–II–13	Gavage Feedings
• HH–II–44	Intermittent Positive Pressure
• HH–II–17	I.V., Having an (Intravenous)
• HH–II–40	Isolation, Protective for Children on Radiation Therapy or Chemotherapy
HH–II–19	
• HH–II–33	Ostomy Care, Child
• HH–II–4	Ostomy Care, Infant
• HH–II–20	Postural Drainage (Child)
• HH–II–21	Postural Drainage (Infant)
• HH–II–34	Radiation Therapy
HH–II–36	Rectal Stimulation
HH–II–22	Rectal Washout, Under 2 Years
HH–II–23	Rectal Washout, Over 2 Years
HH–II–32	Splinting, Application of
• HH–II–24	Suctioning Nose—Bulb Syringe
• HH–II–25	Suctioning, Nose and Mouth
• HH–II–26	Sutured Wound, Care of
• HH–II–18	Temperature, Axillary
• HH–II–27	Temperature, Taking a
HH–II–28	Temperature, Pulse and Respirations, Taking
• HH–II–29	Tracheostomy Care (Daily Care, Equipment, Suctioning, Childhood Illnesses, Emergency Care)
HH–II–48	Traction (For Fractured Femur)
• HH–II–30	Urinary Diversion, Child
• HH–II–31	Urinary Diversion, Infant
HH–II–46	
HH–II–50	

Section 3   Diagnostic Tests

HH–III–1	Amniocentesis
HH–III–10	
HH–III–15	Arteriogram
• HH–III–13	Atropine Drops for Eye Exam
• HH–III–2	Barium Enema
HH–III–18	Barium Swallow

• HH–III–16	Bone Marrow Test, Having a
• HH–III–3	Cardiac Catheterization
• HH–III–33	Clear Liquid Diet (For Test Preparation)
• HH–III–19	CT Scan
• HH–III–4	Cystogram
HH–III–20	
• HH–III–14	"E-Game" (Eye Exam)
• HH–III–5	E.E.G.
HH–III–21	
• HH–III–6	E.C.G.
HH–III–22	
• HH–III–12	Gallbladder Test
• HH–III–7	Glucose Tolerance Test
• HH–III–11	I.V.P.
HH–III–23	
• HH–III–31	Milk & Chocolate Free Test Diet
HH–III–24	Myelogram
• HH–III–8	Nuclear Medicine Laboratory
• HH–III–32	Pinworm Test
HH–III–25	Pneumoencephalogram
• HH–III–26	Stool Specimen, Collection of
• HH–III–9	Upper GI Series
HH–III–30	Urine Culture, Taking a
HH–III–20	Urine Specimen—24-hour
HH–III–27	Urine Specimen—Clean Catch
HH–III–28	Ventriculogram
• HH–III–17	X-ray
HH–III–29	
HH–III–34	
HH–III–35	

Section 4   Child Care/Health Information

HH–IV–1	Basic Diet
• HH–IV–2	Bathing Your Baby
• HH–IV–3	Birth Control Pills—Sunday Start
• HH–IV–23	Birth Control Pills—5-Day Start
• HH–IV–24	Birth Control—Diaphragm
• HH–IV–25	Birth Control—Foam
• HH–IV–26	Birth Control—IUD
• HH–IV–40	Body Outline: Infant/Toddler—Female
• HH–IV–41	Body Outline: Infant/Toddler—Male
• HH–IV–42	Body Outline: Preadolescent—Female
• HH–IV–43	Body Outline: Preadolescent—Male
• HH–IV–44	Body Outline: Adolescent—Female
• HH–IV–45	Body Outline: Adolescent—Male
HH–IV–19	Bowel Control, Older Child (Suppository Method)
HH–IV–28	Diet, Toddler
HH–IV–5	Feeding Baby (Bottle)
HH–IV–6	Feeding Baby (Breast)
• HH–IV–7	Formula, Preparing Baby's
HH–IV–33	Growth and Development—Infant
HH–IV–34	Growth and Development—Preschool

FIGURE 3.3 (Continued)

HH-IV-35	Growth and Development—School Age	HH-V-9	Cotazyme
HH-IV-36	Growth and Development—Preadolescent	HH-V-10	Decongestants
• HH-IV-20	Immunizations (General Information)	HH-V-11	Diamox
• HH-IV-21	Immunizations, Rubella	HH-V-12	Digoxin
• HH-IV-22	Immunizations, Rubeola	HH-V-13	Dilantin
HH-IV-8	Infant Care	HH-V-15	Diuretics
HH-IV-9	Infant Stimulation	HH-V-16	Ducolax
• HH-IV-10	Pediatric Nurse Associate	• HH-V-18	Ear Drops
HH-IV-11	Play Activities (Normal Play)	HH-V-19	Erythromycin
HH-IV-31	Play Activities (Confined to Bed)	• HH-V-14	Eye Drops
HH-IV-32	Play Activities (Confined to Home)	• HH-V-20	Eye Ointment
HH-IV-30	Poisoning (Plants, Household Materials)	HH-V-21	Furadantin
HH-IV-27	Premature Infant, Care of	HH-V-22	Gantrisin
HH-IV-12	Safety, Farm	HH-V-23	Inhalants
HH-IV-13	Safety, Infant and Toddler	• HH-V-17	Injections, How to Give
HH-IV-14	Safety, Older Child	• HH-V-24	Ipecac, Syrup of
HH-IV-29	Self Feeding Skills	HH-V-26	Keflex
HH-IV-15	Sex Education	HH-V-28	Lomotil (C-5)
• HH-IV-4	Teeth and Gums, Cleaning Your	HH-V-29	Medications, How to Give
HH-IV-16	Toilet Training	• HH-V-27	Medications, When to Give
HH-IV-17	Toys, How to Choose	HH-V-30	Metamucil
• HH-IV-37	University Hospital, Going to	HH-V-31	Metronidazole (Flagyl)
HH-IV-38		HH-V-33	Mycostatin (Oral Suspension)
HH-IV-39		• HH-V-34	Nose Drops
		HH-V-35	Phenobarbital
Section 5 Medications		• HH-V-32	Prednisone
		• HH-V-25	Sodium Valproate
HH-V-1	Aarane	HH-V-36	Steroids (Oral)
• HH-V-46	Adrenalin, How to Give	• HH-V-37	Sulfonamides
HH-V-2	Aerosols, How to Give	HH-V-38	Suppositories, Rectal
HH-V-3	Aldomet	HH-V-39	Suppositories, Vaginal
HH-V-5	Antibiotics	HH-V-42	Syringes, Oral—Using
HH-V-6	Anticonvulsants	• HH-V-43	Syringes, Glass—Using
HH-V-44	Antihistamine	HH-V-40	Tetracycline
HH-V-7	Apresoline	HH-V-41	Theophylline
• HH-V-4	Aspirin Dosage Schedule	HH-V-47	
HH-V-45	Carbamazepine (Tegretol)	HH-V-48	
HH-V-8	Codeine-Containing Medicines		

FIGURE 3.3 (Continued)

Section 4: Child Care/Health Information. This section includes information on diet, growth and development, safety, and prevention. In general, it is our miscellaneous section, but "preventive health care" is the key phrase. For example, should immunization and birth control information be included in this category or in the section on medications? Since both topics are "preventive" in nature rather than "curative" they are listed under Section 4: Child Care/Health Information.

Section 5: Medications. All information on how to give medications, such as nose drops and medication schedule, as well as on specific medications are included in this section.

This type of indexing system also lends itself easily to expansion. For example, if the therapeutic dietitians or respiratory therapists wish to add information to the system and want to keep it apart from the other categories, Section 6: Therapeutic Diets and Section 7: Respiratory Care, could be added later.

Numbering the Teaching Aids

The system used for numbering the teaching aids should correspond with the current paper flow system in your setting. At Children's Hospital a double letter and number system is used for forms and other printed materials. For example, in the forms NU-90 or ER-10, the letters represent the originating department (NU is Nursing; ER is

Emergency Room), and the numbers represent the number given to that particular form.

Since our Helping Hand system is somewhat more complex, a third number was added—the Roman numeral indicating the specific category. (For example in HH-II-3, the "HH" stands for Helping Hand, "II" indicates Section 2, and "3" signifies the number assigned to that particular Helping Hand.) This type of form number not only helps in ordering but also assists in filing since the section number is designated.

In devising your numbering system, determine first if a system exists currently for other forms; if so, tailor your system accordingly. If there is no current system, you are free to use ours or to create your own.

In our master index/filing system for the Helping Hands (Fig. 3.3), note that several spaces are open in the numbering system. We left these blank to insure that additional Helping Hands would appear in proper alphabetical numbering order. However, we have since found this to be somewhat confusing and actually unnecessary. If we had to do it over, we would first list all topics alphabetically in the appropriate category and then assign chronological numbers. If another topic was added later, the number following the last "HH" number would be assigned. This topic would be placed in alphabetical order on the next printing of the master index. (For example, HH-II-41 Gastrostomy Tube Feedings; HH-II-12 Gastrostomy Tube, Changing a). Again, the most important point is: *do not change systems or form numbers after they have been established unless it is absolutely necessary.*

Updating the Master Index

The Master Index should be updated periodically; every 3 months is usually sufficient. With each update, add the titles of the newly developed teaching aids as well as the requests received. If necessary, rearrange the list so titles are in alphabetical order. Place a large dot (•) or asterisk (*) by each teaching aid currently available. Distribute the updated index to all persons on your distribution lists and to others as appropriate.

(*Note:* We have included all requested topics on our master index. Those with a dot are available; the others are still in developmental stages. The reason for distributing this type of list is to represent the total scope of the program. You may wish to distribute a list of only those teaching aids currently available. This is certainly acceptable, but the first few lists may be quite skimpy and unimpressive.)

THE SYSTEM "TOOLS"

The system for developing teaching aids can easily become confusing and chaotic without a few organizational tools.

Beside the master index, the additional tools you will need are the topic flow chart and folder, the project status chart, the monthly report, the model file, the unit/clinic files, and the reference manuals. You should design and make the most of these tools before beginning your teaching aid development efforts; the two exceptions are the unit/clinic files and the reference manuals which should be prepared after several teaching aids are available.

TOPIC FLOW CHART AND FOLDER

The topic flow chart and topic folders are very important tools in the organization of this system. The flow chart can assist in keeping track of the development of the teaching aid, and the folder is useful for organizing research articles, critiques, and other information about the particular teaching aid.

The Topic Flow Chart

Before you prepare a topic flow chart, determine the steps in developing the teaching aid from beginning to completion. Assign a number to each step and design a topic flow chart. You may use our topic flow chart (Fig. 3.4) as a model. (Our actual "steps" are discussed in detail in Chapter 4.)

To complete the topic flow chart, record at the top of this chart the name of the teaching aid, the date the research is started, and a reasonable date for completion of the teaching aid. As you progress, note the date that each step is started on the date line below the step, and list the names of the persons involved in the "consultant" section.

These notes are a tremendous help in memory-jogging if a topic gets put aside for a while. Also, when several teaching aids are being developed at the same time, it is easy to forget the exact level of progress of each topic, and the chart serves as a reminder. However, for the topic flow chart to be effective, the information must be kept current.

The Topic Folder

The topic folder contains all information on research, names of consultants, drafts and critiques of teaching aids, and other important notes on the creation of the teaching aid. The folder serves as an information and resource file for that particular topic.

As soon as you have developed the list of proposed topics (after the teaching aid survey), begin to assemble a topic folder for each proposed teaching aid. To prepare a topic folder, print the name of the proposed teaching aid on the tab of a Manila folder. Then, staple one topic flow chart to the inside left flap (Fig. 3.5). Even before you actually start writing a teaching aid, you can collect information, note comments received, or record potential resources by using the folder and topic flow chart.

HELPING HAND TOPIC FLOW CHART

TOPIC:_____ TARGET COMPLETION DATE:_____

DATE STARTED:_____ ACTUAL COMPLETION DATE:_____

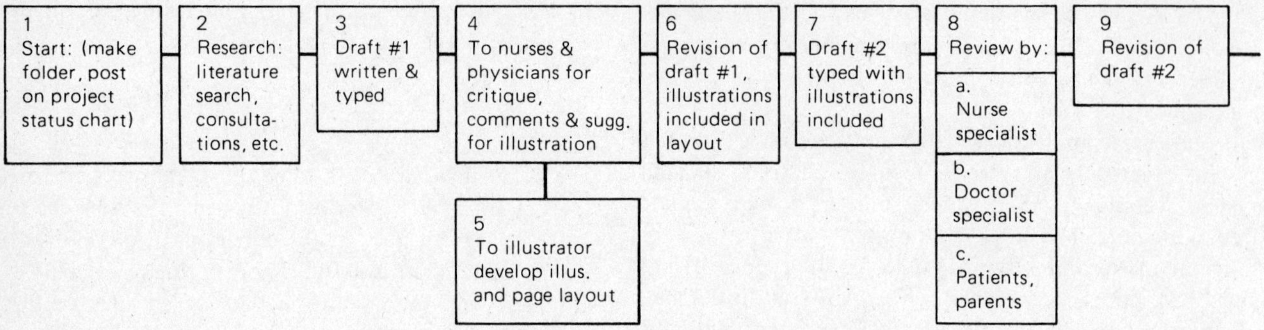

| 1 Start: (make folder, post on project status chart) | 2 Research: literature search, consultations, etc. | 3 Draft #1 written & typed | 4 To nurses & physicians for critique, comments & sugg. for illustration | 6 Revision of draft #1, illustrations included in layout | 7 Draft #2 typed with illustrations included | 8 Review by: a. Nurse specialist b. Doctor specialist c. Patients, parents | 9 Revision of draft #2 |

5 To illustrator develop illus. and page layout

DATES:_____

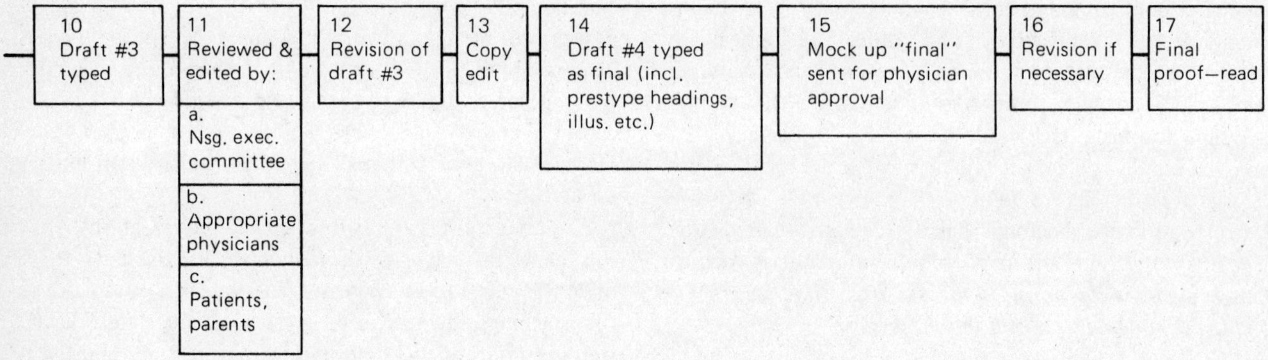

| 10 Draft #3 typed | 11 Reviewed & edited by: a. Nsg. exec. committee b. Appropriate physicians c. Patients, parents | 12 Revision of draft #3 | 13 Copy edit | 14 Draft #4 typed as final (incl. prestype headings, illus. etc.) | 15 Mock up "final" sent for physician approval | 16 Revision if necessary | 17 Final proof—read |

DATES:_____

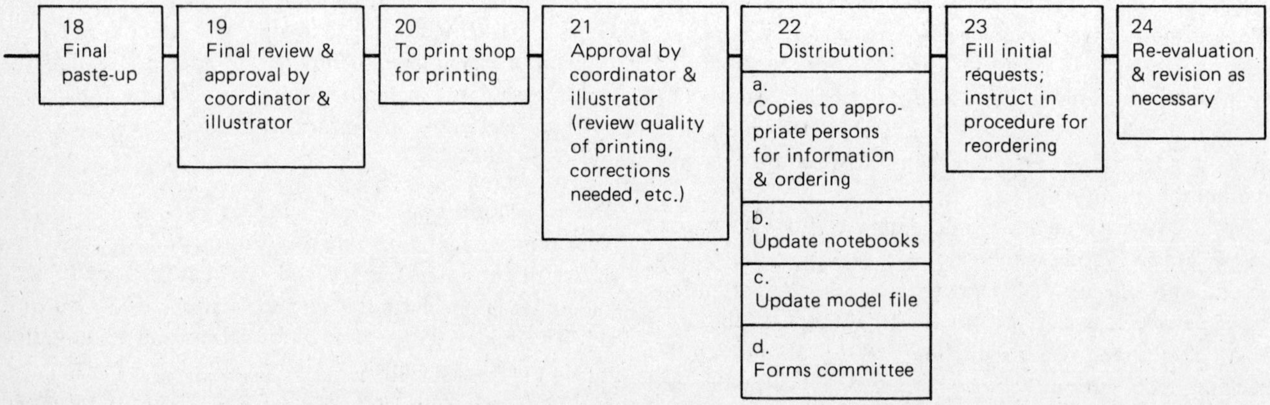

| 18 Final paste-up | 19 Final review & approval by coordinator & illustrator | 20 To print shop for printing | 21 Approval by coordinator & illustrator (review quality of printing, corrections needed, etc.) | 22 Distribution: a. Copies to appropriate persons for information & ordering b. Update notebooks c. Update model file d. Forms committee | 23 Fill initial requests; instruct in procedure for reordering | 24 Re-evaluation & revision as necessary |

DATES:_____

CONSULTANTS:_____

COMMENTS:_____

FIGURE 3.4 The Topic Flow Chart

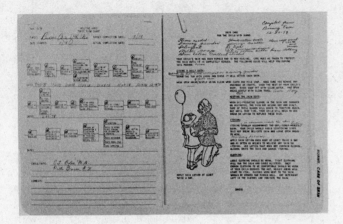

FIGURE 3.5 The Topic Folder

PROJECT STATUS CHART

The project status chart is useful in keeping track of progress (or lack of progress) on projects. The chart is also helpful as a communication tool, especially if there are several people involved with the project or if there are part-time people involved.

To make the project status chart, you will need: 18″ × 36″ white posterboard, a piece of clear acetate the same size or larger, and a "grease" pencil. First, determine exactly what you want to include on the chart; you may use ours as an example (Fig. 3.6). Then draw the lines, label the sections, and cover the chart with the acetate.

We developed the following guidelines for using the various sections of the chart:

Helping Hand description. List the titles (or topics) of the teaching aids being developed.

Work for (department). List the name of the person or department requesting the teaching aid. (This list serves as a quick reference in planning and communicating about the teaching aid. It also indicates if too much time is being devoted to one department or unit to the exclusion of others.)

Target completion date. Determine a reasonable date for completion. (We have found that we work more effectively and efficiently with designated deadlines. We seldom meet our deadlines exactly, but without them, we would have difficulty evaluating our progress.)

Project status: instructions. Note the progress level of each teaching aid. For example, "first draft being typed," or just "Step 3"; "third draft—to Nursing Executive Committee," or "Step 11." (Refer to the topic flow chart, page 48). Other comments or notes may also be included in this section.

Project status: illustrations. Note the stage of illustration development; for instance, "developing illustrations" or "being drawn by J. Smith." Other comments or notes may also be included in this section.

HELPING HAND PROJECT STATUS CHART

Helping Hand Description	Work for (Dept.)	Target Completion Date	Project Status		Completion Date
			Instructions	Illustrations	

FIGURE 3.6 The Project Status Chart

Completion date. Note the date the project is actually completed and teaching aid is distributed.

The information in the "project status" section will be changed frequently as progress occurs. The information in the other sections should remain on the chart until the project is completed. It is a good idea to post a copy of the topic flow chart next to the project status chart. This way the step numbers can be used in the "project status—instructions" section, rather than writing everything each time.

When the teaching aid is completed, transfer the information to a "monthly report" form. Then, erase that line on the chart and post the next project in its place.

THE MONTHLY REPORT

Just as committees keep minutes of meetings, a record of activities should be kept for this program. The monthly report form is a useful tool for both the person coordinating the development of the teaching aids, as well as for all other persons involved (especially those in administrative positions). It serves as a communication tool, a record of performance, a progress check, and a general plan. It can be helpful in budget and program planning and in justification of time and monies spent. Also, by keeping close account of your progress throughout the year, the request from the director to "compile an annual report" will cause no particular concern. You may wish

HELPING HAND MONTHLY REPORT

TO: _____   FOR MONTH OF: _____

FROM: _____   DATE OF REPORT: _____

Completed Projects

Helping Hand Title	Order Number	Requesting Dept./Person	Completion Date

Projects in Progress

Topic or Title	Requesting Dept./Person	Target Completion Date	Comments

COMMENTARY:

FIGURE 3.7 The Monthly Report

to adapt the model monthly report form shown in Figure 3.7.

To compile the monthly report, complete the information at the top of the form and then follow these guidelines:

Completed projects. This information is collected as the completed projects are removed from the project status chart. List the name of the teaching aid, the form number or reorder number assigned, the department or person who originally requested the aid, and the actual date of completion.

Projects in progress. This information may be taken directly from the project status chart. List the names or topics of the projects, the person or department requesting the teaching aid, the target date for completion of the projects, and any pertinent comments. (The "comments" section becomes especially useful when the target date has long since passed and the project is still "in progress." Many times the delay will be unavoidable, but an explanation is helpful.)

Commentary. This section is used for additional information or comments on the progress during the month(s). (For example, perhaps a particular person or group of persons was especially helpful in developing an instructional aid, or perhaps July and August vacations interfered with meeting deadlines. Such comments can be helpful to justifying needs and/or explaining progress.)

THE MODEL FILE

After the scope of your program is determined you should set up a model file. A model file contains mock-up teaching aid folders for each proposed topic. We have found that the most orderly and organized method of filing our teaching aids is with the use of hanging files and metal file drawers; our model file reflects this finding (Fig. 3.8).

A model file can serve several purposes. Before developing the Helping Hands, we set up a model file to visually demonstrate the scope of the program to the hospital staff and administrators. This approach aided in the "selling" of the program, since it is much easier for people to relate to an idea they can see and touch, rather than to an idea only on paper.

As each new Helping Hand is completed, we replace the "mock-up" folder with an actual folder containing several copies of the new Helping Hand. We use the model file during periodic rounds on the areas where unit/clinic files are located. Before making rounds, two or three teaching aid folders for each Helping Hand are prepared and placed in the model file. As we review the unit file, we suggest additional Helping Hands which are available and may be helpful. If the staff selects an additional topic, we remove one of the extra hanging files from the model file and place it in the unit file (Fig. 3.9). This method saves much time and also provides for immediate use of the new Helping Hand.

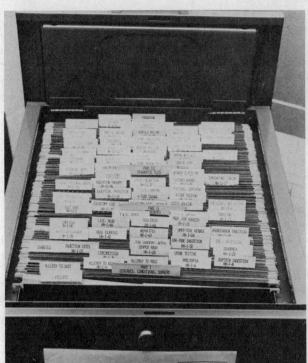

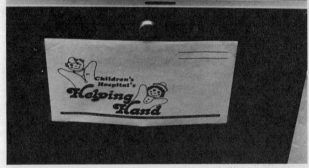

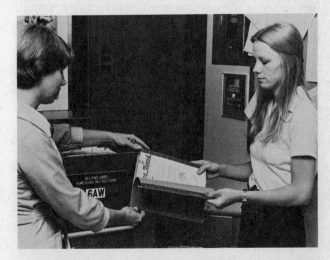

FIGURE 3.9 Making Rounds and Updating Unit/Clinic Files

We also use the model file in instructing health professionals and students in the use of the system. The health professionals can easily grasp the concept and use of the Helping Hands when the filing system is presented in this manner.

Setting up the File

These are the supplies we used in setting up our model file: a two-drawer metal file on casters, two hanging file braces, hanging file folders, two sizes of plastic file folder tabs and cards (4-inch for section dividers and 2-inch for teaching aid files), and plastic page protectors. First, we made the section dividers by cutting several hanging file folders in half. The section titles were typed in capital letters on colored paper (e.g., SECTION 2: PROCE-DURES), placed into the 4-inch plastic tabs, and then placed in the middle of the cut file folders (Fig. 3.10).

To make the teaching aid folder, the title and reorder number of each teaching aid is typed in capital letters on a *white* tab card. (The title should correspond with the index so it can be filed alphabetically.) This title card is inserted into a 2-inch plastic tab and is placed in the front flap of the folder (Fig. 3.10). To insure that one copy always remains in the folder, we place one copy of the completed teaching aid on the back inside flap of the file folder and cover it with a plastic page protector (Fig. 3.10). This reserve copy serves several purposes (especially if the supply is depleted); as a reference for staff members to review, a copy to duplicate if the need is urgent, and a reference for reordering additional teaching aids. Then the teaching aid folder is filed in alphabetical order after the appropriate section divider.

THE UNIT/CLINIC FILES

Unit/clinic files resemble the model file in that the section divisions are consistent from unit to unit. The only differ-ence is selection of Helping Hands in the files. Unit/clinic files probably will not contain *all* teaching aids developed; rather, the units will selectively choose those teaching aids suitable for the needs of their patient population.

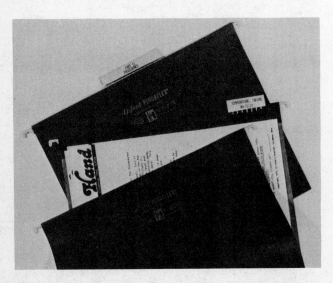

FIGURE 3.10 The Section Dividers and a completed teaching aid folder with Helping Hands

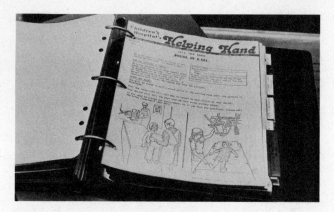

FIGURE 3.11 The Reference Manual

Locate a suitable file space in each unit/clinic. The file space may be an accessible desk drawer or file cabinet, or it may be necessary to purchase a cardboard hanging file box (Fig. 3.9) or a metal file drawer on casters. After a space is located, set up a file in the same way the model file was assembled.

THE REFERENCE MANUALS

Primarily, the reference manuals are used to aid staff members in selecting teaching aids for their units. Since all unit files do not carry the full complement of teaching aids, these reference manuals provide a "mini-file" for staff members to review periodically. Also, it is an important reference in developing new teaching aids. The reference manual should resemble the model file, except that it will be in notebook form (Fig. 3.11). We keep an updated copy of our master index in the front section of the manual and update the manual by adding the teaching aids as they are completed.

OTHER "PAPER TOOLS"

In our system, our "paper tools" also include stationery, memos, and lists. Use of these tools saves think-time, communication time, and adds to the overall organization of the program. Although not evident in this publication, each memo is a different color. The use of color-coding accomplishes several things: it is easily seen and recognized, and the recipient of the memo soon associates the color of the memo and the message contained.

The distribution lists are time-savers also. As the name implies, distribution lists indicate to whom each memo should be sent. If additional persons should receive a particular memo or teaching aid, these names can be specified at the time of distribution. It is important to keep the lists current; if your institution or setting is like many, there will be an addition and/or deletion of a name every month or two.

THE HELPING HAND STATIONERY

Almost as important as the content of your teaching aid is its overall appearance. Does it look inviting to read or does it look like every other page?

We wanted our Helping Hands to be distinctive, appealing, and easily recognized in our institution as well as elsewhere. We also wanted to increase awareness of their availability by providing the visual recognition. Therefore, in addition to illustrative considerations, discussed later in this book, we devoted considerable thought and effort to the design of the letterhead and envelope (Fig. 3.12).

The letterhead is printed in a medium blue ink on white paper. The envelopes, printed in blue ink on white envelopes, are used to organize the materials provided to the families during the hospital stay or clinic visit: (the Helping Hands, prescriptions given, return appointment slips and so forth).

TO DEVELOP A TEACHING AID

During the development of a teaching aid, most consultants and reviewers are approached on a one-to-one basis by the program coordinator. We have found this method to be most successful in the beginning stages of writing a Helping Hand since most people share more information verbally than they would in writing. But as the teaching aid goes through the final steps, it is easier to communicate through memos. We use three memos in the development stage: the editors' memo, the review/approval memo, and the re-evaluation memo.

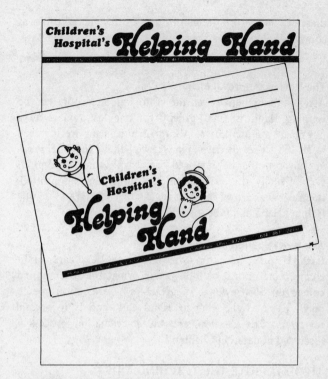

FIGURE 3.12 The Helping Hand Stationery

The Editors' Memo

After the teaching aid reaches the final stages and the editors are consulted, it is impractical to continue with the one-to-one contact. Therefore, we attach the editors' memo (Fig. 3.13) to the Helping Hand draft and distribute

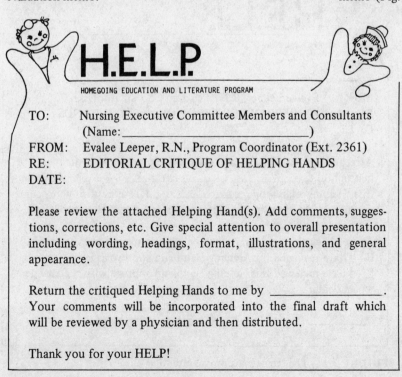

FIGURE 3.13 The Editor's Memo

these to the editors (a distribution list for the editors was compiled). Note that the memo includes a deadline date; we ask that the critiqued drafts be returned by this date.

The Review/Approval Memo

After the comments from the editors are incorporated, the Helping Hand is final—except for one last review by a physician representative. Although physicians are involved in all the stages of development, we believe the *final product* also should be reviewed from a physician's point of view. Usually the specialist in the topic area is consulted; the review/approval memo (Fig. 3.14) is attached to the Helping Hand and is sent to this physician.

The Re-evaluation Memo

Each Helping Hand is reviewed every 1–2 years, or as changes in the information occur. When the teaching aid comes up for review, we attach a re-evaluation memo (Fig. 3.15) to the Helping Hand and send it to several reviewers. The development and re-evaluation process is discussed in detail in Chapter 4.

TO DISTRIBUTE THE TEACHING AIDS

After the teaching aid has been approved and printed in final form, it must be distributed to the potential users for their information and review. There are several tools which make this easier and more systematic: the distribution/request memo, the forms committee memo, the reference manual update memo, and the distribution checklist.

The Distribution/Request Memo

There should be some type of communication each time a new teaching aid is finalized. Each institution has its own communication system, but for our purposes, we compiled a distribution list and use the distribution/request memo (Fig. 3.16). This memo serves two purposes: "advertising"— to inform staff members of new Helping Hands and "order blank"—to serve as a request for the new teaching aid. This double duty memo decreases time spent in "phone orders" and also provides a written record of the Helping Hand topics available in each unit/clinic. (Later the topics requested are transferred onto the unit/clinic request record (Fig. 3.21) and the distribution/request memo is discarded.)

The Forms Committee Memo

A copy of the completed teaching aid is also sent to our Forms Committee, which is responsible for the numbering and the paper flow systems at Children's Hospital. All printed forms used in the hospital are registered by this committee prior to implementation. Since our Helping

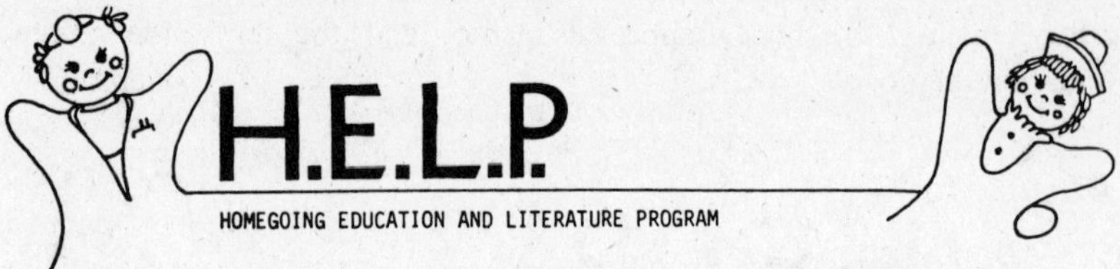

H.E.L.P.

HOMEGOING EDUCATION AND LITERATURE PROGRAM

TO:
FROM: Evalee Leeper, R.N., Program Coordinator (Ext. 2361)
RE: REVIEW AND CRITIQUE OF HELPING HANDS
DATE:

Attached is the final draft of the Helping Hand patient/parent instruction:_____ . We plan to print this Helping Hand by_____ . Please return your comments or corrections by this date to Evalee Leeper, Nursing Office.

Please check the appropriate box below. Thank you for your HELP!
☐ I have reviewed this Helping Hand and approve as is.
☐ I have reviewed this Helping Hand and approve with the changes indicated.

_____ (Signature of Physician)

FIGURE 3.14 The Review/Approval Memo

H.E.L.P.

HOMEGOING EDUCATION AND LITERATURE PROGRAM

TO:
FROM: Evalee Leeper, R.N., Program Coordinator (Ext. 2361)
RE: REEVALUATION AND REVISION OF HELPING
HANDS
DATE:

All Helping Hands are periodically revised and updated. We ask your assistance in reevaluating the attached Helping Hand.

Please answer the following questions and return to the critiqued Helping Hand to Evalee Leeper, Nursing Office by _____.

1. Does any of the information need to be updated? Yes _____
No _____
If yes, please comment and suggest change(s): _____

_____

_____

2. Does the Helping Hand include all necessary aspects of the topic? Yes _____ No _____
If no, please comment: _____

_____

_____

3. Is any part of the information confusing to patients/families?
Yes _____ No _____
If yes, which part? _____

_____

_____

4. Do the illustrations accurately represent the information?
Yes _____ No _____
If no, please suggest changes: _____

_____

_____

5. Are additional illustrations needed? Yes _____ No _____
If yes, please describe desired illustrations: _____

_____

_____

6. Please make additional comments or changes on the attached Helping Hand.

Thank you for your HELP!

FIGURE 3.15 The Re-evaluation Memo

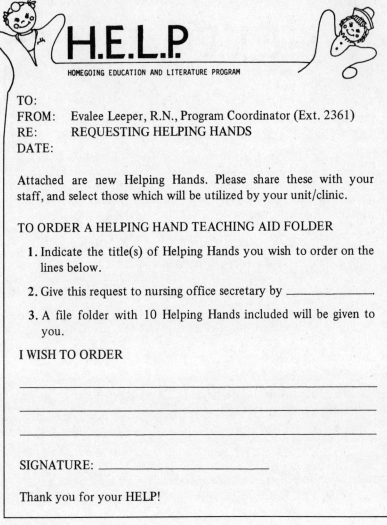

FIGURE 3.16 The Distribution/Request Memo

Hands have a standardized format and the details of coordinating the printing are the same for each, we requested and received "blanket approval" for the program. Therefore, to register a new Helping Hand, we attach a forms committee memo (Fig. 3.17) to the teaching aid and send this to the Forms Committee.

Updating the Reference Manuals

For the reference manuals to remain useful, they too must be kept current. Therefore, when the completed teaching aid is being distributed to the unit and clinic staff members, we send reference manual updates for all manuals. The new teaching aid is covered with a plastic page protector and labeled according to the index. The reference manual update memo (Fig. 3.18) is completed and attached to the Helping Hand. This is sent to all persons with a reference manual. (We also keep a distribution list of persons having reference manuals.)

The Distribution Checklist

The distribution checklist (Fig. 3.19) is simply a mental aid in the paper work process. It is easy to forget a step when so many things are happening simultaneously, so we developed this checklist. To use the checklist, we write the name and form number of the new teaching aid, and note the date that they were distributed to the units/clinics, Forms Committee, and reference manuals. We also note when the teaching aid folder is added to the model file, and when the master index is updated. These checklists can be kept in a notebook for ready use and reference.

TO FILL REQUESTS FOR TEACHING AIDS

After the new teaching aid has been distributed, we allow time for the staff to share the information. Soon the requests (distribution/request memo) are returned and the process of filling requests begins. To fill requests, we use

H.E.L.P.

HOMEGOING EDUCATION AND LITERATURE PROGRAM

TO: Forms Committee
FROM: Evalee Leeper, R.N., Program Coordinator (Ext. 2361)
RE: NEW OR REVISED HELPING HAND(S)
DATE:

The following Helping Hand(s) has/have been recently completed and distributed to the units. The original form is filed in the print shop.

Title	Form Number	New Form	Rev. Form
		☐	☐
		☐	☐
		☐	☐
		☐	☐

Thank you for your HELP!

FIGURE 3.17 The Forms Committee Memo

H.E.L.P.

HOMEGOING EDUCATION AND LITERATURE PROGRAM

TO:
FROM: Evalee Leeper, R.N., Program Coordinator (Ext. 2361)
RE: REFERENCE MANUAL UPDATE
DATE:

Please add this Helping Hand to your reference manual. File it in Section _____ after _____ .

Helping Hands can be ordered directly from the print shop by using the Helping Hand order form.

Thank you for your HELP!

FIGURE 3.18 The Reference Manual Update Memo

the teaching aid folder, the file/reorder memo, and the unit/clinic request record.

The Teaching Aid Folders

When requests for new Helping Hands are returned, begin to prepare the teaching aid folders. Assemble the unit/clinic teaching aid folders in the same manner as the model file folders (Fig. 3.8); refer to page 52 for directions.

The File/Reorder Memo

Rather than just "slipping" the folder into place in the unit/clinic file, give it to the person responsible for the operation of the area. Attach a memo indicating how to file the new teaching aid folder and how to reorder these and other teaching aids. We use the file/reorder memo (Fig. 3.20) for this purpose.

HELPING HAND
DISTRIBUTION CHECKLIST

DIRECTIONS: Note dates that steps are completed.

Helping Hand Title	Form Number	To Units/ Clinics	To Forms Committee	Update Manuals	Update Model File	Update Index

FIGURE 3.19 The Distribution Checklist

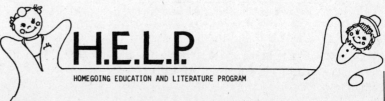

H.E.L.P.
HOMEGOING EDUCATION AND LITERATURE PROGRAM

TO:
FROM: Evalee Leeper, R.N., Program Coordinator (Ext. 2361)
RE: FILE FOLDERS AND REORDER SYSTEM
DATE:

Attached is the Helping Hand file you requested for use in your unit/clinic. Please inform your staff that this topic is now available.

TO FILE: File this folder in alphabetical order in Section _____ .

TO REORDER: Order additional Helping Hands directly from the print shop by using the Helping Hand order form.

Thank you for your HELP!

FIGURE 3.20 The File/Reorder Memo

HELPING HAND
UNIT/CLINIC REQUESTS

Helping Hand Title & Form No.	Unit/Clinic															
	6AE	6AW	5AE	5AW	4AE	4AW	4TN	4TS	3AE	3AW	3TN	3TS	2TN	2TS	ICU	OPD	ER

FIGURE 3.21 The Unit/Clinic Request Record

The Unit/Clinic Request Record

The unit/clinic request record (Fig. 3.21) serves as a quick reference in determining available teaching aids in the various areas of the hospital or facility. For instance, if you wanted to know how many units/clinics were using the teaching aid on cast care, you could refer to this record and have the information at a glance. A review of the record also indicates which units have an appropriate selection of teaching aids. (Perhaps they have not ordered many because only a few were suitable to their area. This may indicate a need to develop teaching aids in other topic areas.)

Since all our initial requests are filled from one source, the information on this record is easy to maintain. If your initial requests are filled in another manner or by several sources, the information will be more difficult (but still possible) to obtain.

PULLING IT ALL TOGETHER

Now you are buried in paper, and thoroughly overwhelmed with the "organized system" we promised to show you—right? All the papers and forms are stacked everywhere waiting to be used, and you are unsure about what comes first. Well believe it or not, even though the system is detailed and seemingly complex, it *is* organized and it *does* work.

Where should you begin? At the beginning of course. That is step 1 on the topic flow chart. Although all the steps you will take are mapped out on the topic flow chart (Fig. 3.4, page 48), perhaps a teaching aid checklist would be a helpful tool.

We do not use this particular checklist, because we have repeated this process so many times that we have it memorized; the topic flow chart serves as our primary guide. You may want to use the checklist during the development of your first few teaching aids, but after that, you probably will not need it either.

THE CHECKLIST

Step 1: Start

☐ Select a topic.

☐ Post the topic on the project status chart (P.S.C.) (Fig. 3.6, page 49); note topic, requesting department or person, and target completion date. Write "step 2" under "project status—instructions."

☐ Make a topic folder (Fig. 3.5, page 49).

☐ Note the topic, date started, and target completion date on the topic flow chart (T.F.C.) (Fig. 3.4, page 48).

Step 2: Research

☐ Begin research; review the literature, talk with consultants.

☐ Note references and consultants on T.F.C.

☐ Note date research is completed on T.F.C.

Step 3: Draft #1

☐ Refer to the appropriate framework guide (Chapter 4) and develop an outline for the proposed teaching aid. (You may want to do this prior to the research).

☐ Write draft #1.

☐ Have draft #1 typed.

Step 4: Review

☐ Distribute copies of draft #1 to several staff members who will be using this teaching aid. Have them comment on content and suggest illustrations.

☐ Note "step 4" on P.S.C.

☐ Note consultants on T.F.C.

Step 5: Illustration

☐ Give copy of draft #1 to illustrator for development of illustration and page layout.

☐ Note "step 5" on P.S.C. under "project status—illustrations."

Step 6: Revision

☐ Compile the comments of reviewers.

☐ Discuss revisions of the text and suggestions for illustrations with the illustrator.

Step 7: Draft #2

☐ Determine what illustrations should be included.

☐ Determine layout for draft #2 (to include illustrations)

☐ Have draft #2 typed according to layout.

☐ Tape *copies* of illustrations onto typed second draft.

☐ Note date on T.F.C.

Step 8: Review

☐ Distribute copies of draft #2 to several "resident experts" for critique of content and illustration.

☐ Note "step 8" on P.S.C.

☐ Note date and names of "resident experts" on T.F.C.

Step 9: Revision

☐ Compile the comments of "resident experts."

☐ Discuss illustration revisions with illustrator.

☐ Carefully review material; check for clarity, flow, consistency in layout, etc.

Step 10: Draft #3

☐ Design new layout if necessary.

☐ Have draft #3 typed.

☐ Tape copies of illustrations onto typed third draft.

☐ Note date on T.F.C.

Step 11: Review/Editing

☐ Distribute copies of draft #3 to editors. Use editor's memo (Fig. 3.13, page 53).

☐ Note "step 11" on P.S.C.

☐ Note date distributed on T.F.C.

Step 12: Revision

☐ Compile comments of editors.

☐ Discuss the revisions with illustrator if indicated.

Step 13: Copy Edit

☐ Copy edit material; read and review for sentence structure and flow, grammar, clarity, and so forth.

Step 14: Draft #4 (Final)

☐ Design new layout if necessary

☐ Have draft #4 typed.

☐ Use final headings and subtitles (i.e., prestype letters)

☐ Lightly tape copies of illustrations in appropriate places.

Step 15: Final Approval

☐ Copy the paste-up final onto letterhead stationery.

☐ Send paste-up to appropriate physician for review/approval. Use review/approval memo (Fig. 3.14, page 54).

☐ Note "step 15" on P.S.C.

☐ Note date sent on T.F.C.

Step 16: Revision

☐ Revise if necessary. (*Note:* if revision is indicated, make corrections and return it to physician for approval.)

Step 17: Proofread

☐ Carefully proofread material and correct errors.

Step 18: Final "Paste-up"

☐ Attach the final illustrations to the typed copy.

☐ Delete or erase fingerprints or other unwanted markings.

☐ Put form number on teaching aid.

Step 19: Review

☐ Coordinator and illustrator should look over teaching aid once again prior to printing.

Step 20: Printing

☐   Send teaching aid for printing.

☐   Note "step 20" on P.S.C.

☐   Note date sent on T.F.C.

Step 21: Approve Printing

☐   Review copied teaching aid for quality of printing. If it is unacceptable, determine the cause, make corrections, and have it reprinted.

Step 22: Distribution

☐   Have copies of teaching aid printed for distribution.

☐   Send copies of new teaching aid to all persons on distribution list and to others who have been involved in developing aid. Use distribution/request memo (Fig. 3.16, page 56).

☐   Send copy to Forms Committee. Use forms committee memo (Fig. 3.17, page 57).

☐   Update reference manuals. Use reference manual update memo (Fig. 3.18, page 57).

☐   Update model file

☐   Update master index

☐   Use distribution checklist (Fig. 3.19, page 58) to note dates of distribution

☐   Note date of distribution on T.F.C.

☐   Transfer information from P.S.C. to monthly report form (Fig. 3.7, page 50). Note actual completion date.

Step 23: Fill Requests

☐   Order enough copies to fill requests.

☐   Make teaching aid folders (see instructions, page 52).

☐   Attach file/reorder memo (Fig. 3.20, page 58) and give file folder to requesting person or department.

☐   Note that request was filled on unit/clinic request record (Fig. 3.21, page 59).

Step 24: Re-evaluation and Revision

☐   Periodically send teaching aids to "resident experts" for review. Use re-evaluation memo (Fig. 3.15, page 55).

☐   Compile comments and revise teaching aid.

☐   Note revision date on form.

☐   File new form in print shop.

   (*Note:* This checklist represents a very brief overview of the teaching aid development process, which is discussed in depth in Chapters 4 and 5.)

MAINTAINING THE SYSTEM

As you develop your system, thought must also be given to the maintenance; similar to a building, the most expensive system without maintenance will eventually fall apart. Consider the printing, reorder, and storage components of the system; if this part is too complicated or if it is faulty or collapses, your whole program is affected. Also consider the maintenance costs; if your costs exceed the value of the program to the institution, it may not be continued.

Maintaining a system also involves informing others of the program and encouraging the use of the product. It is much easier for administrators to continue a program that is used or is even "in demand" than one that is unused or unknown. These areas of system maintenance are discussed in this section.

PRINTING, REORDERING, AND STORAGE SYSTEM

To maintain your system, the teaching aids must be readily accessible. As you know, when staff ask for teaching aids, they usually need them yesterday. So, developing a well-oiled printing, reordering, and storage system will go a long way in meeting the needs of patients and staff.

The most important point is to tie into whatever system exists in your setting; find out how other forms are reordered and model your system after that. It may not solve all the problems, but at least the staff will not be taxed by learning a new system.

Before our Helping Hand Program, the system for printing, storage, and reorder of patient education materials was chaotic—actually nonexistent. Some of the printed materials which had been developed were printed in our print shop and others were printed by "outside" companies. The reorder system was not much better. Some materials were reordered through our print shop and some from outside companies, but there was no person or even department held responsible for this time-consuming task. The storage system was also in sad shape. Some teaching aids were in the storeroom, some in the nursing office, and some on the units at the bottoms of file drawers. We were asked to help, so we accepted the challenge and offered a simple solution—H.E.L.P.

Since the services of our in-house print shop are of generally high quality, relatively low in cost, and are conveniently located, this was our logical choice of printers (although we did consider outside printers before making the decision). Our print shop is the hub of the reorder system. When teaching aids are needed in the unit/clinics, a request is sent to the print shop. The request includes the name of the requesting person or department, the cost center (budget) number of the department, and the form number of the teaching aid. When a request is received, the print shop personnel select the appropriate Helping

Hand master (which is filed in the print shop) and make the number of copies requested. These copies are returned to the unit/clinic in the same manner as all other form requests.

A few Helping Hands must be printed outside the institution because of the inability of our print shop presses to handle double page (11″ × 17″) paper. The print shop also acts as the coordinator for this request and makes appropriate arrangements for printing.

For the most part, since almost all teaching aids are printed on request, there is no storage necessary. However, for those Helping Hands printed outside the institution or used in large quantities, some storage space is necessary. But again, since the print shop is the center of this system, they coordinate the storage and draw from this supply when requests are received.

BUDGETARY CONSIDERATIONS

Budgetary considerations are always necessary to discuss, for how many times have you been turned down because "it isn't in the budget." The development of our patient education materials was "not in the budget"; but, due to the concern and progressive thinking of our director of nursing and our hospital administrators, monies were found to support the program.

A goal of our program was to provide patient teaching aids in a cost-effective manner. Rapid changes in hospital spending are occurring due to changes in cost reimbursement factors, economic inflation, and the influence of consumers and government regulations. Our current costs of supplies and person-power may not reflect the actual costs at the time you read this book. However, we believe it is important to share certain specific considerations concerning costs.

To discuss costs, we need to establish a common frame of reference. As was mentioned earlier, patient education materials available from outside sources can be very costly. Pamphlets range from "free" to over $5.00 each; the average cost is about 25¢–35¢ per booklet. Therefore, if your facility cares for 25,000 patients a year and each patient receives one pamphlet, the cost will be $6250–$8750 per year; and the annual cost could be expected to rise as paper, printing, and mailing costs increase. To some this may seem to be reasonable cost for purchasing teaching aids. To others who may have little or no allocated funds, this may seem like a tremendous amount.

At present, each Helping Hand page costs approximately 1¢. Of course this 1¢ is the paper and printing cost alone and does not include the salaries of personnel involved in development of the Helping Hands. If salaries were considered, the cost of developing a Helping Hand would be considerably higher; but this development cost is a one-time expenditure.

For you, the initial costs of establishing a program such as this probably will be significantly less than our cost. We are giving you the tools, the "how to's," and the actual teaching aids (which have taken us 3 years to develop). So, you will be well on your way to developing an organized program without spending any more than the price of this book.

Person-power

As was mentioned earlier, the person-power required involves a director, coordinator, illustrator, and significant others. But there are several factors that can increase or decrease the salary cost: amount of time assigned to the program (part-time or full-time), actual salary, and fringe benefits.

The program director position may or may not be needed for your program. As discussed previously, these responsibilities can be incorporated into a presently existing administrative or staff position.

We have recommended that the person coordinating this effort be assigned only to this program. This is the ideal situation for the most rapid progression of the program, but of course it can be modified. For instance a part-time person could be hired for this position, or the task could be assigned to a full-time employee in addition to other responsibilities. The main problem with the latter approach is time management and setting of priorities. The development of teaching aids takes time. If there are other more pressing priorities, the program could get buried at the bottom of the list. Or even if the program is maintained, the teaching aids would be a long time coming.

Our recommendation, based on our experiences, is that a program coordinator position be established and maintained until the teaching aids are developed. At the point of completion, the person-power could be scaled down, but *not* eliminated. You should always have a coordinator for the program for the purpose of maintenance, staff development, and re-evaluation, or the whole system will fall apart.

To illustrate your teaching aids, there are a variety of methods you can use (many of these are discussed in Chapter 5). If you prefer original "tailor-made" illustrations, such as those that appear on our Helping Hands, you will need to find someone with artistic talents. If you search carefully, you may be lucky enough to find a talented person who is willing to volunteer time. Our illustrator volunteered her services for a year before being hired on a part-time basis. Before this, we either drew our own illustrations or used the services of our hospital medical illustrator who was already much in demand.

In a cost comparison, a volunteer illustrator is obviously the least expensive. The only expenditure is the cost of art supplies. If you cannot find a volunteer, the next best alternative is hiring a part-time illustrator. The most expensive method, we have found, is employing the services of a medical illustrator; this person usually charges an hourly rate which rapidly adds to the cost, considering the large number of illustrations needed.

Supplies and Equipment

The cost of supplies, equipment, and printing methods can also influence the total cost of your program. But with a bit of ingenuity, opportunism, and planning, you can reduce the cost considerably.

Most supplies need not be purchased especially for this project; most of the equipment can be gathered from unused or discarded items of others. Even the art supply list can be modified depending on funds available. For instance, when we started the program, we found a large table, several unused lamps, and a discarded x-ray viewbox; there was nothing wrong with these items except that they were not "new."

One supply expenditure will be your model file, although, depending on the size of your facility, you may not need this. Paper and other office supplies will be another cost, but usually this is "absorbed" into the operating budget of the facility. A paper copying method is also needed as you develop the teaching aid; this is probably the largest single cost.

The paper costs and printing method used for the final teaching aids are also significant expenses. An internal printing operation is probably least expensive. But, if you do not have access to your own printing source, you may have to use another means of reproducing the teaching aids, such as the services of an outside printing company; there are many companies available which charge reasonable rates (especially the smaller "quick print" companies). Learn how other forms in your facility are printed and supplied and try to tie in to the existing forms supply system if possible. This will help to insure maintenance of your teaching aid system. Types of printing processes and cost factors are discussed in depth in Chapter 5.

Actual cost calculations for developing a program such as this may be several thousand dollars, depending on variables such as the scope of your program, the size of your facility, and the methods you use. However, this will be several thousand well spent—and thousands less than you would spend on comparable materials from outside sources. If insufficient funding is a problem, try to justify the program by researching patient care problems resulting from lack of sufficient education; for example, repeat admissions or extended stays. Or look to the community, grants, private funds, physicians, or insurance companies for assistance. Don't let the cost factor dampen your spirits or stop your progress—the health and well-being of your patients are at stake.

PRESENTING (SELLING) THE PROGRAM

"Selling" the program may be one of the most difficult tasks you encounter, but, it is a task that must be done if your program is to be successful.

At Children's Hospital, the Homegoing Education and Literature Program needed to be approved and accepted by several committees, groups, and levels of personnel. We presented the program to the Medical Executive Committee (composed of departmental and section physician representatives), the Medical Staff Meeting (composed of the entire medical staff including both staff and local physicians), the Nursing Executive Committee (composed of nurses with administrative, teaching, and clinical expertise), Medical Records Committee, Forms Committee and the hospital administration, not to mention all the nursing staff members and various other groups of health professionals.

Determine the groups in your facility who should be informed about your program. Do your "homework" before presenting the ideas to committees or staff members. Intangible ideas can easily be disregarded, whereas, ideas on paper, presented in a logical, well thought-out manner, are better understood and accepted. So, be sure to present a well-designed package and be prepared to answer questions. Refer to the following guidelines as you organize your presentation.

Consider the audience. Who will be your audience? Before preparing your presentation, know the answers to the following questions: (a) What is the educational and vocational preparation of the group? (b) What level do they hold in the institutional hierarchy? (c) What are their day-to-day responsibilities and/or concerns for patient education? (d) What are the main interests or objectives of the group as a whole? (e) How does the program affect them? Use this information to gear the presentation to the interest and concerns of that particular group.

Present a clear, concise overview of the program. Organize your presentation with the audience in mind. Present only the information they need to know. Do not bore them with details about paper flow and tools used unless it is relevant to the group or unless someone asks. Include as many visual examples or samples of the product as appropriate.

Anticipate questions, concerns, problems and objectives and address these in the presentation. Recognize that each group member will have questions and concerns regarding the development of the program. For example, many will be concerned about the economic implications of development and maintenance of the program; others may subconsciously feel threatened by a program for educating patients; while others fearing change may try to deflate or to destroy the program rather than support it and make the necessary adjustments.

These questions or problems need to be addressed in the presentation, rather than hoping that no one will ask. For example, don't wait until someone asks, "What will this cost?" or "How do you propose we find time to orient the staff to the system?" Statements like this call other group members "to arms"; they join forces with the opposition which puts you on the defensive.

Include answers to these questions in the presentation. Visually compare the cost of buying pamphlets with the cost of developing your own teaching aids. However, do not deny that the program will cost something; after all, you can't get something for nothing. Also address time factors: "Of course there will be time involved in orienting staff to the program, but in the end, time will be saved. Less time will be needed for writing information by hand and for answering questions and reteaching patients, and less time will be spent on the phone, answering and re-explaining after the patient has left the facility."

By recognizing the concerns of others before the presentation, you will feel more confident knowing that you probably will be able to respond adequately to any question asked. Therefore, in preparing a presentation for a group, include not only the positive aspects of the program but also the possible questions, objections, or problems that might be raised.

Limit the length of the presentation to the time allotted. Before preparing the presentation, find out how much time has been allotted. Set aside part of that time for answering questions from the group. Develop the presentation with the time frame in mind.

Gain support. Before the meeting, try out your presentation in discussion with one or two people who will attend the meeting. Ask for tips on how to approach their group, and try to gain their support of the program before the presentation. If you are able to do this, you will probably feel more comfortable during the presentation, knowing you have some supporters in the audience who can positively influence their coworkers toward accepting the program.

Now that you have successfully presented and "sold" the idea, you are well on your way to developing a viable system. However, merely "selling" people on an idea does not insure success; it takes determination, perseverence, and just plain hard work. Hopefully, the information in this chapter and the rest of the book will make that hard work a bit easier.

Now you have the information needed for establishing and maintaining a system for developing and supplying patient education materials. But, a system is not enough. You still need to know the specifics for writing and illustrating the teaching aids. And you may also need to develop your staff in the area of patient education, or at least teach them how to use these teaching aids. Evaluating the program is also important: evaluation is necessary for improvement of teaching aids and the program as well. These topics—developing, teaching, and evaluating—are discussed in depth in the following chapters.

SELECTED READINGS

Hall, Joanne and Weaver, Barbara. *Distributive Nursing Practice: A Systems Approach to Community Health.* Philadelphia: J.B. Lippincott Co., 1977.

Kucha, Delores. "The Health Education of Patients: Development of a System, Part I." *Supervisor Nurse* 5 (May 1974): 8-21.

Kucha, Delores. "The Health Education of Patients: Development of a System, Part II." *Supervisor Nurse* 5 (June 1974): 8-15.

chapter 4

Writing a Helping Hand: The Art and Technique

Evalee Keck Leeper

"It is necessary to enter the child's world if we wish to understand others, or ourselves."

Arthur T. Jersild

Patient education is gathering momentum. Historically, many health professionals have been "caring for" patients rather than helping patients to care for themselves. We, at Children's Hospital, fervently believed that this mode had to be reversed, that we needed to enable patients to achieve and maintain their optimum health status independently. From this belief and commitment, the Home-going Education and Literature Program was born.

The project began with a review and evaluation of currently available materials. However, the more pamphlets we ordered and reviewed, the more money we spent. And, as more money was spent, the more concerned we became about the products being purchased. These pamphlets just did not meet our needs. Much of the available literature lacked readability and illustration, contained overabundant advertising, and cost money. Our specific concerns were:

Reading level. Reading level of most pamphlets (tenth to twelfth grade level) was higher than many patients or parents could understand. In contrast most Helping Hands have been designed at a sixth to eighth grade reading level.

Information presented. Some of the information in the available pamphlets was outdated or inappropriate; other information differed from that given at Children's Hospital. However, the information in each Helping Hand has been endorsed by appropriate staff of Children's Hospital and is reviewed and updated as necessary.

Illustration. In general, illustration was lacking. Many pamphlets presented instructions without illustration, while others contained inappropriate or tasteless "humorous" illustration. In comparison, Helping Hands have been illustrated to emphasize main points or messages. A human, caring message is portrayed; cartoon figures are rarely used.

Advertising. Many pamphlets (especially those available from private companies) included excessive advertising which detracted from the information presented. Helping Hands contain no advertisement or endorsement of products, except where brand names may help in explanation; for example, fever-reducing medication such as Tylenol, Tempra.

Number of topics discussed. Certain pamphlets dealt with a variety of topics making the material inappropriate, overwhelming, and/or difficult to read. Each Helping Hand discusses only one subject.

Availability of information. Pamphlet information was unavailable on many of the topics needed by our patients, families, and staff. New Helping Hands are specifically developed in response to requests and needs of staff members, patients, and families.

Order, storage, distribution, and filing system. A well-organized system for ordering, storage, distribution, and filing was at best difficult, and, at worst, impossible. Pamphlets were ordered from many suppliers: the length of time between order and delivery varied greatly, and there was a wide difference in the size of pamphlets. With the Helping Hands, an organized system is possible since all Helping Hands are printed internally on request. This simplifies ordering, storage, and distribution. Since all teaching aids are uniform in size, filing is infinitely easier.

Budgetary considerations. Along with the cost of living, costs of printed materials continue to escalate each year. Those pamphlets provided "free of charge" may also cost something in the future. Dividing the cost of materials ordered from various resources among the hospital units or clinics was difficult. In comparison, the cost of Helping Hands is much lower and more predictable; units/clinics pay only for Helping Hands that they order.

So, to meet the pressing need for suitable patient education materials we began the task of writing our own patient teaching aids. The acronym of our Homegoing Education and Literature Program (H.E.L.P.) inspired the name of our teaching aids—the "Helping Hands."

At Children's Hospital, we try to project an attitude of compassionate care to the public. Compassionate caring extends beyond the immediate needs of the child. Caring also extends to the parents or other caretakers. Caring is shown in *how* we perform our duties, as well as in *what* we do. The focus of the Helping Hands is to educate and to guide the parents (and significant others) in specific and total care of their child—to help people (patients) to gain independence in their care, thus freeing them from total dependence on health professionals.

The uniqueness of the Helping Hands is due largely to the experience and caring attitude of the writers. Collectively, our expertise comes from years of working with patients and families. The Helping Hands are not coldly clinical; a wholesome caring thread is woven into information that might have been written in a sterile, nonempathetic manner. This tone makes the instructions appealing to the readers, and lets the patients/families know that we understand their concerns and are trying to help them.

In this chapter, we will closely examine several Helping Hands. By reviewing the components of a Helping Hand, we hope to give you a useful model in developing your own teaching aids.

DEVELOPING A TEACHING AID

When the Homegoing Education and Literature Program was first established, we created a committee to develop and to review the teaching aids. Typical of many committee efforts, it flopped. In the committee situation, responsibility was too easily transferred—the "buck" too easily passed—and specific topic expertise was not always represented. So, we tried a different approach. We included the entire hospital staff in the committee (unofficially) and called them our "resident experts." These were our nurses, physicians, paraprofessionals, patients, and families.

We then selected several "resident experts" to write information about particular topics within their area of expertise. After several months of waiting, we decided that this approach was not effective either. Apparently, most of our experts, although very knowledgeable, were somewhat hesitant to put their thoughts and ideas on paper. So we went back to the drawing board and came up with a new approach—one that worked for us.

The role of the program coordinator evolved from that of a committee chairperson to the primary "doer." The coordinator is responsible for writing the first draft of the Helping Hand on the chosen topic. Thereafter, drafts of the teaching aid are given to several "resident experts" familiar with the topic; it is their responsibility to critique the information, to add additional needed information, to make corrections, and to eliminate unnecessary items. This approach has proven to be very successful; our staff is much more willing to critique written material than to write the information "from scratch."

There are a multitude of experts in every setting just waiting to be asked to help; you need only to be aware of the expertise around you and to draw on it. Enlist the help of nurses who teach patients daily, physicians who want their patients taught, patients and families themselves, and other professionals and paraprofessionals in the institution. Developing a teaching aid requires the input of more than one person; the coordinator's job should be just that—to coordinate the efforts of others.

GETTING STARTED

Before the development of a teaching aid can begin, a topic must be chosen. You can select a topic yourself using the information gathered in your teaching aid survey (p. 41), or you can respond to an urgent request. After the topic is chosen, complete the identifying information on the topic flow chart (Fig. 4.1). Then, on the project status

HELPING HAND TOPIC FLOW CHART

TOPIC: __HAVING AN X-RAY__   TARGET COMPLETION DATE: __5/31/79__

DATE STARTED: __3/5/79__   ACTUAL COMPLETION DATE: __5/24/79__

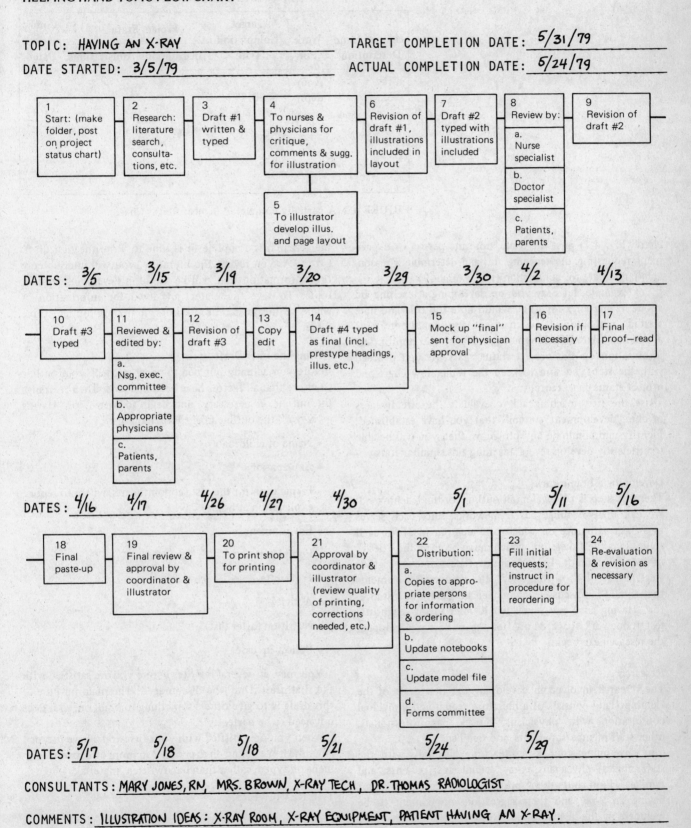

FIGURE 4.1 A completed Topic Flow Chart

PROJECT STATUS CHART

Helping Hand Description	Work For	Target Completion Date	Project Status		Completion Date
			Instructions	Illustrations	
X-ray	X-ray dept.	5/30/79			

FIGURE 4.2 A partially completed Project Status Chart

chart (Fig. 4.2) post the topic, note the person or department requesting the teaching aid, and determine a reasonable target date for completion (Fig. 3.6, p. 49).

For example, let's say you are developing a teaching aid about having an x-ray. You would note the title and date started on the topic flow chart and also would determine a deadline date. Then, you would post the appropriate information on the project status chart. As you proceed with the steps, be sure to keep the topic flow chart and project status chart current.

Use the first teaching aid to evaluate the effectiveness of the "development system" that you have established. Identify and eliminate any problems; then you will be able to efficiently develop several teaching aids simultaneously.

Developing a Framework
The next step is to develop an outline for the teaching aid. We call these outlines our frameworks, since each serves as a basic structure on which to shape our ideas for each topic. It is the "skeleton" which much be given the "flesh" of specific content. Use the appropriate framework guide (see pages 74–85), and select the framework elements that should be discussed in your teaching aid. For instance, for "Having an X-ray," you would refer to the diagnostic test framework (page 81). After the outline is developed, the research can begin.

Research
The research involved in developing the first draft of the Helping Hand consists of a literature search and individual consultation with physicians, nurses, paraprofessionals, other staff members, patients, and families.

In developing your x-ray teaching aid, talk with the staff nurses, physicians, x-ray technicians, patients, and families. Find out their problems and concerns about having an x-ray and their suggestions on content to be included in the teaching aid. Review the literature; read journal and magazine articles about x-rays. Keep all this information in the topic folder (refer to page 47). When the research is complete, it is time to write the first draft. (*Note:* As you review the literature, you will undoubtedly find information that will be useful in developing another topic. To save time later, jot down the information or where to locate it. Put the note in the appropriate topic folder.)

Writing the First Draft
Before you actually put pen to paper, recheck your outline to insure that all factors have been included. Then rearrange the outline, if necessary, and begin to write. For "Having an X-ray," the outline might look like this:

- Name of child/date
- Explanation
- Preparation for the test (appointments, where to report, explanation at home)
- Environment
- Equipment
- Procedure
- Activity
- Nutrition (after test)
- Follow-up care

You may do several rewrites before you are satisfied with the first draft. Don't be discouraged! The main purpose of this draft is to give others something to build on, so it does not need to be perfect.

When you are satisfied with your first draft, have it typed (Fig. 4.3). We found that people can more effectively comment on typed, rather than handwritten, material.

THE REVIEWERS

Following the completion of the first draft, give copies to several reviewers who are familiar with the topic. For "Having an X-ray," choose several persons who will be most

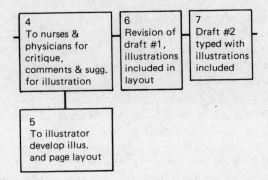

likely to use the final teaching aid: a nurse, physician, x-ray personnel, patient/family, and test scheduling clerks. In general, selection of more than five people to review the first draft becomes too time-consuming. Solicit their input and critique of the information. Ask reviewers to suggest illustrations.

Although you may *send* the material to the reviewers, we have had better success when the material is given and explained in person. A copy of the first draft should also be given to the illustrator to develop ideas for illustration. Allow a reasonable length of time for the reviewers to evaluate the teaching aid. Provide a deadline date—1–2 weeks is usually sufficient.

When you receive the comments from the reviewers, begin to compile the second draft. Discuss the revisions and illustration suggestions with the illustrator and determine which illustrations should be included. (For "Having

an X-ray" the illustrator could depict the patient in the room with the x-ray machines.) Then, include these illustrations in the layout of the second draft. Have the second draft typed and the illustrations pasted up according to the layout. (Refer to Step by Step Layout and Paste-Up, pages 134–135.) The second draft of the teaching aid now resembles the final product.

THE RESIDENT EXPERTS

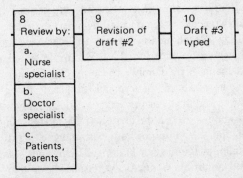

The second draft should be reviewed by your "resident experts" who are knowledgeable in the topic area. For "Having an X-ray" the "resident experts" might be the physician responsible for the X-ray department, a staff nurse on the orthopedic unit, an x-ray technician, and a patient/family who has experienced the procedure.

This review is primarily a content critique, so these reviewers should look closely at the content of the teaching

```
                                                      DRAFT #1

HAVING AN X-RAY PICTURE

Name of Child:_____    Date:_____

EXPLANATION:

An x-ray takes a picture of the inside of your child's body. It does not hurt.

PREPARATION FOR THE TEST:

· No special preparation is needed at home.
· Bring your child to the X-ray Department on (date)_____ at
  (time)_____ a.m. p.m.
· Give your x-ray request (pink slip) to the clerk at the desk.

EQUIPMENT:

A large camera that hangs from the ceiling will take the picture.

PROCEDURE:

· Your child will be asked to lie down on a table or stand hold very still.
· The parents are asked to leave the room.
· A technician will aim the camera and take the picture.
· You will be asked to wait a short time in the waiting room until the picture is
  developed. Then the technician will tell you either to return to your clinic or
  your doctor.

ACTIVITY:

No particular restrictions related to having an x-ray.

FOLLOW UP CARE:

Your doctor will tell you what your child's picture showed.

If you have any questions, please call _____.
```

FIGURE 4.3 First draft of *Having an X-ray*

aid, both the written word and illustration. The questions you might ask are: Is the content correct? Is it clearly written? Has anything been left out? Do the illustrations represent the information clearly and correctly? Are additional illustrations needed?

Input from patients and families who have had extensive experience with the topic can be very valuable at this point. The teaching aid may contain home care instructions that are feasible in a hospital setting, but impractical at home. Patients/families can make helpful suggestions about information needed based on their own past experiences.

In writing a teaching aid, there is a tendency to mention items that are of concern to the health professional and to overlook many of the family's concerns. One mother whose child was hospitalized for insertion of plastic tubes in his ears pointed out that her private pediatrician had given her much reading material on anatomy, physiology, and diseases of the ear; but nowhere was there a mention of shampooing, swimming, or bathing. The mother was more concerned about these practical considerations than anatomy. The opposite situation occurred with a mother who had been caring for her child's tracheostomy for over a year. She indicated that, for months following her child's surgery, she did not understand how and where the tube was located inside the throat. So in preparing our teaching aid, we added an anatomical drawing.

After you compile the comments of the "resident experts," read over the material carefully. Reading aloud to someone who has not read it before helps to identify statements needing clarification. Check the subheadings for clarity and make sure the information appears under the appropriate subheading.

Review this material with the illustrator and have a new layout designed if indicated. Have the third draft typed according to the layout and attach copies of the final illustrations to the typed material. This third draft should represent the best efforts of you, your consultants, and the illustrator.

THE EDITORS

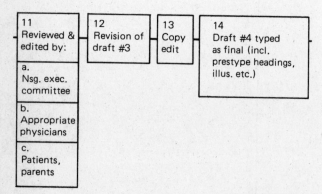

In the final stages of development, the teaching aid is reviewed by several editors who provide editorial critique

rather than content critique. They review the teaching aid for clarity, readability, grammar, punctuation, effectiveness of illustration, layout, and design.

We chose our Nursing Executive Committee as the primary "editing body" (composed of the director of nursing, associate director, clinical nursing directors, clinical specialists, and nurse clinicians). This group of administrative and clinical nurses is especially helpful in editorial critique because members have varied expertise; most members have not seen the new Helping Hand before and can review objectively; also many are generalists rather than specialists and can comment from the perspective of a patient, parent, or staff nurse. Their comments are extremely helpful since, when working so closely to a subject, we sometimes fail to see the obvious.

How to Submit the Draft to the Editors
Initially, we submitted the teaching aid to our editors in manuscript form (double spaced typing with illustrations separated from the text). We noticed a great lag in return of the critiqued papers, and many were never returned. We determined that part of this lag was due to the unappealing appearance of the teaching aids; administrative staff are usually so bogged down with reading material in manuscript form that the Helping Hands got buried with other paper.

So we decided to spruce up the teaching aid drafts and make them distinctly visible and interesting reading. Therefore, the third draft is typed in a manner similar to the final Helping Hand: typed material is single spaced and illustrations are included in the layout of the teaching aid rather than attached separately. This method has been extremely successful; we now receive most, if not all, of the critiqued teaching aids with suggestions for change and/or complimentary remarks (Fig. 4.4).

At this stage of development, one-to-one contact with the editors is impractical and often impossible because of conflicting work schedules. Therefore, it is wise to have a system for written communication with the editors. With the aid of a memo attached to each Helping Hand in need of editing, individual editors may review the teaching aid at their convenience (Fig. 3.13, page 53).

At this stage of development, patient or parent review is again sought. However, we select families for whom the subject of the teaching aid is a new experience. This gives us a parent's objective point of view. If the instructions are not clear to "new" parents, some changes may be indicated.

Writing the Final Draft
After the comments are received from the editors, revise the teaching aid appropriately. It is the responsibility of the program coordinator to determine which comments and criticisms made by the reviewers and editors should be included and which should be overlooked. "You can't

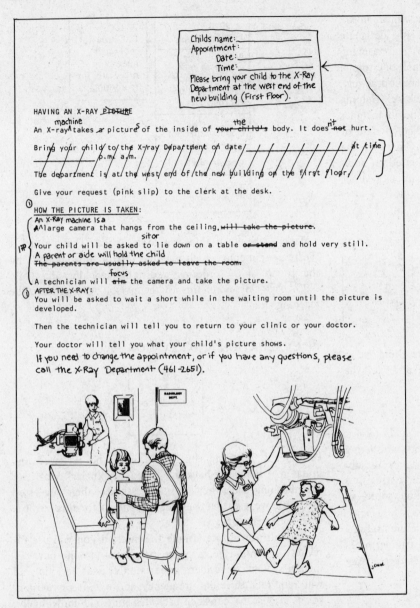

FIGURE 4.4 Third draft of *Having an X-ray* with editor's comments

please all the people all of the time" is an apt saying which applies to compiling the suggestions of others. For example, if there are ten suggested ways of revising the same sentence, the coordinator must judge which is the best statement of thought. Certainly all ten revisions cannot appear on the final teaching aid.

After the comments of the editors have been incorporated, the teaching aid is ready for copyediting, a method of preparing the material for final typing. The teaching aid is read again for sentence structure and flow, grammar, clarity, and consistency. We have found that the most effective way to do this is to read the material aloud to one or two other persons, or to read into a tape recorder and play it back. Typographical errors, which may be overlooked in silent reading, also become apparent when read aloud.

After a final check by the illustrator, the teaching aid is retyped into the final layout, the fourth draft. At this point, transfer type for headings and subtitles may be applied. Lightly attach copies of the final ink illustrations with cellophane tape on the back of the illustration. Now make a copy of this "mock-up" on your letterhead and send it to your "final" reviewers.

THE FINAL REVIEW AND APPROVAL

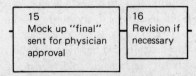

In establishing the Helping Hand Program, we recognized the need to work collaboratively with physicians in developing the Helping Hands. And, as a final review mechanism, we request that our medical director or his designate (usually chief of a department) review the final teaching aid before printing and distribution. Because one-to-one communication with this physician is often impractical, a memo is attached to the copy of the "mock-up" Helping Hand and sent (Fig. 3.14, page 54). The memo includes the name of the teaching aid and the projected date of publication. If this physician suggests no changes, the teaching aid is complete and may be distributed. If additional suggestions are made, the teaching aid is revised, rechecked by the physician, and then distributed.

THE FINAL STEPS

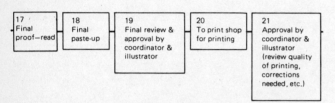

A few final steps are needed before the teaching aid is complete: proofreading, printing, and evaluation of the print job.

Proofreading

Very carefully review the final typed material. Look for typing errors, spelling errors, consistency in numbering steps, listing points or materials, and consistency in subtitles and underlining. There are usually few corrections at this point; but you will occasionally find some, so it's worth the effort.

After corrections have been made, the final illustrations may be permanently pasted up. Make sure that fingerprints or other unwanted markings are deleted. Your teaching aid is now ready to go to press (Fig. 4.5).

Printing

As far as you are concerned, your teaching aid is "perfect" when you send it for printing, but the quality of printing will affect its overall appearance. Carefully review the teaching aid after it is printed. If it is *not* acceptable to you, determine the cause, make corrections, and have it reprinted.

DISTRIBUTION

Now your teaching aid is ready for distribution to persons on your distribution lists, to others who have been involved in developing the teaching aid, and to those who have a reference manual. (Refer to pages 54–59 for sample memos.)

Soon after the teaching aid has been distributed, you will receive requests for teaching aid folders. Estimate the number of teaching aids you will need to fill the orders and have them printed.

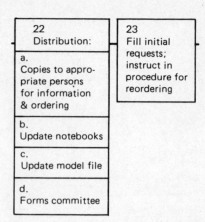

Make a labeled teaching aid folder (page 52) and attach a file/reorder memo which includes instructions about filing the folder and reordering additional teaching aids (Fig. 3.20, page 58). Send this to the person who ordered the teaching aid.

RE-EVALUATION AND REVISION

Periodically, each teaching aid should be reviewed and updated. Usually we have the "resident experts" look over the teaching aids they use and ask for their suggested revisions; we use the re-evaluation memo for this purpose (Fig. 3.15, page 55).

You will need to determine the method you will use for review—a committee, a procedure similar to the developmental system, or resident experts only. Each teaching aid will require a different frequency and extent of revision, so it is best to consider each teaching aid individually. However, for the most part, they can be divided into two groups—those needing minor revisions and those needing major revisions.

For "Having an X-ray" you might go to the chief radiologist, the x-ray technician, a staff nurse, and a scheduling clerk. If there are only minor revisions, no further review steps may be required. If major revisions are necessary, it is advisable to repeat steps 9 through 16 on the topic flow chart. In either case, a revision date should be noted on the revised teaching aid and the final proofreading should be completed (steps 17 through 22). Distribution of a revised form can be modified depending on the extent of the revision. Certainly the reference manuals, model file, teaching aid folders, and Forms Committee should receive the updated material; but unless the revisions are extensive, copies probably do not need to be sent to all persons on the distribution list.

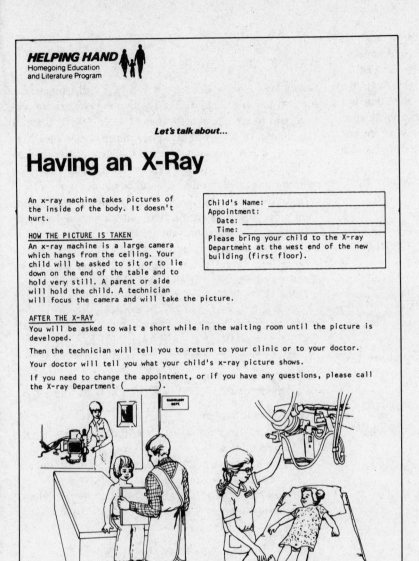

HELPING HAND
Homegoing Education
and Literature Program

Let's talk about...

Having an X-Ray

An x-ray machine takes pictures of the inside of the body. It doesn't hurt.

HOW THE PICTURE IS TAKEN

An x-ray machine is a large camera which hangs from the ceiling. Your child will be asked to sit or to lie down on the end of the table and to hold very still. A parent or aide will hold the child. A technician will focus the camera and will take the picture.

AFTER THE X-RAY

You will be asked to wait a short while in the waiting room until the picture is developed.

Then the technician will tell you to return to your clinic or to your doctor.

Your doctor will tell you what your child's x-ray picture shows.

If you need to change the appointment, or if you have any questions, please call the X-ray Department (_____).

Child's Name: _____
Appointment:
  Date: _____
  Time: _____
Please bring your child to the X-ray Department at the west end of the new building (first floor).

FIGURE 4.5 Final Helping Hand: *Having an X-ray*

As you can see, writing a teaching aid may not be quite as simple as it appears. While there may be times when you can produce a teaching aid without all the drafts and reviews outlined here, most will require this procedure to insure complete accuracy and a high standard of quality.

THE FRAMEWORKS

Our Helping Hand topics are divided into five specific categories: diseases, conditions, and surgeries; procedures; diagnostic tests; child care/health information; and medications. To promote consistency in the structure and writing of teaching aids within these groups and from one Helping Hand to the next, we devised outlines or frameworks.

The frameworks for each of the five major categories

include all the factors (topic subheadings) that should be considered in writing a teaching aid within that category. Although we do not use every topic heading in each Helping Hand, we use the list as a guide in considering content elements. Under each topic subheading, we have listed considerations of care that a patient/family might encounter. The framework for each topic category is presented to be used as a reference when developing your teaching aids. The framework elements included in the frameworks are discussed in detail in the following section (pages 85-93).

WRITING ABOUT DISEASES AND CONDITIONS

When developing teaching aids about diseases and conditions, many factors need to be considered. Is this a chronic, short-term, or terminal disease/condition? How much do the patients/families need to know? If the condition is a long-term one, such as diabetes or scoliosis, the instruction will be quite detailed and more complex than the average teaching aid (Fig. 4.6). But, if the condition is a short-term one, such as head lice or diaper rash, the instructions are not as all encompassing and focus on care and prevention rather than on discussion of related topics such as nutrition and anatomy.

We use the following framework for developing Helping Hands about diseases and conditions.

DISEASES/CONDITIONS FRAMEWORK

Definition/Explanation
Cause of disease/condition; part of the body affected or being treated; preventive measures

Emotional Care
Psychological preparation; maintaining trust; how to deal with feelings/frustration

Preventive Care
Prevention of cross-infection; prevention of pain and injury; prevention of recurrence of disease/condition

Equipment/Supplies
Equipment needed; where to purchase; care of; use of

Procedure/Treatment
How to do; when to repeat

Medication
Use of; care of; safety

Nutrition
Foods to eat or not to eat; fluids

Activity
Restrictions; limitation; continuing life activities; school; sports; fun things to do

Personal Care
Dental; skin care; hygiene; clothing

Environment
Maintaining cleanliness; preparation of environment to prevent disease/condition

Safety
Prevention of accidents

Communications
Patient; physician; nurse; where to call if have questions

Follow-up Care
Appointments; why important to keep appointments

Space for Additional Information
Blank space

WRITING ABOUT SURGERY

Going to a hospital for surgery can be a frightening event for patients and families. We try to eliminate misconceptions and to reduce anxiety when possible by giving careful explanation of what will take place. Since ours is a teaching hospital, it is considered the responsibility of the surgeon or his resident to initially explain the type of operation and the expected results. This information is reinforced and supplemented by the nurse in preparing the patient/family for the surgery. As you can see in the following framework, information about the preparation before surgery and care after surgery is stressed. Other information such as how to get to the hospital and what will happen there is also discussed briefly. (See also Figure 4.7, *Having a T & A.*)

SURGERY FRAMEWORK

Definition/Explanation
Explanation/purpose of surgery; part of body affected

Preparation for Surgery
Directions for Admission Date; time; where to report; phone numbers
At Home Diet; medications; explanation of surgery; personal care
In the Hospital Medications; diet; fluid restrictions; emotional support

Emotional Care
Support to child; explanation of surgery

Environment
Description of operating room; recovery room

Equipment/Supplies
Equipment needed before or after surgery

Procedure/Treatment
Care of incision; care of appliance or prosthesis

Activity
Restrictions; allowances; when to return to school; safety

Personal Care
Skin care; clothing after surgery

Nutrition
Special diet after surgery; restrictions

Medications
Medications needed before and after surgery

Communications
When to call the doctor; where to call if questions arise

Follow-up Care
Appointments—dates; place; importance of keeping

HELPING HAND
Homegoing Education
and Literature Program

Let's talk about...

Scoliosis

Scoliosis means an unnatural curve in the spine. The cause is usually not known. Different types of braces are worn to prevent more curving. If the braces are worn as directed, operations on the spine can sometimes be avoided.

PREPARING YOURSELF MENTALLY TO WEAR THE BRACE

It takes a lot of spunk to stick with wearing the brace. The first 2 weeks are the hardest time. After that, the brace becomes more familiar, and it won't bother you as much to wear it.

When the brace is first put on, you will have feelings that you "can't stand it." But keep it on as long as you can. If you feel you can't go through with it, take it off for a while. When you can get yourself together, put it on and try again. You may cry at times because you feel trapped, but stick with it. In a short time you will feel better and will be doing most of the things you did before.

The feeling that the brace is "too long" will decrease with time. It is important to keep the brace snug.

CARE OF THE BRACE

Wash the brace daily with a wash cloth and mild soap. Rinse with wash cloth and clear water and wipe dry. Do not put any part of the brace into water.

SKIN CARE

Wash and rinse your body thoroughly every day. Apply rubbing alcohol to toughen the skin. After it dries, dust lightly with corn starch to help prevent friction spots from forming where the brace might rub.

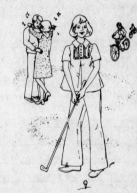

Check your skin for red spots. If necessary, use a mirror to see all areas.

The skin will itch a lot when the brace is first removed. Apply rubbing alcohol to the skin. It will help stop the itching in a little while.

SPORTS AND OTHER ACTIVITIES

It is important to get plenty of exercise. You can continue most sports and activities such as swimming, volleyball, biking, and golf. You should wear your brace for all these sports, except swimming. Do not go horseback riding because the jarring is uncomfortable. Do not play football or other contact sports.

Your doctor will advise you when you can return to school and continue activities.

Labels (left margin):
- Definition/ Explanation
- Emotional Care
- Equipment
- Personal Care & Preventive Care
- Activity

FIGURE 4.6 Example of Helping Hand on diseases and conditions

DIET

A well-balanced diet will help to keep you healthy. It will also help the treatment to be a success. If nausea (feeling "sick to your stomach") occurs, eat smaller amounts of food and liquids more often.

Nutrition

DENTAL CARE

Consult your dentist about how often you should have a dental check-up.

CLOTHING

Wear a cotton sleeveless undershirt under the brace. Buy one size larger than normally worn. Make sure it is 2 or 3 inches below the end of the brace. Smock-like tops are easy to get into. Shift-type dresses make the brace less noticeable. Buy jeans or slacks a size larger than you usually wear.

Personal Care

SPECIAL TIPS

· When you have to be some place at a certain time, allow yourself more time to get ready. Don't hurry getting into a car. You might tilt back and cause the brace to hurt you.
· Raise the height of the table or desk for eating and studying. A portable tilt table may help. Microscopes can be slanted or can be put on a higher level. Prism glasses can be worn for reading. Wedge-shaped pillows can help to maintain the desired position.
· A special toilet seat can be purchased at a hospital supply company. This will raise the height of the toilet and will make it easier to use.
· Try to sleep on the side that is curved out, as often as possible.
· Try to resume your normal activities as soon as possible. Don't lie around and feel sorry for yourself. Let your close friends know you are wearing a brace. They can help you be less self-conscious about "being different".

Environment

WHEN TO CALL YOUR BRACE SPECIALIST (Phone: _____)

· If there are any breaks in the brace
· If the brace feels too tight
· If there are any pressure areas on your skin

You will have appointments to see the brace specialist about every 6 weeks.

Appointments

WHEN TO CALL YOUR DOCTOR (Phone: _____)

_____

_____

WHEN TO CALL YOUR ORTHOPEDIC NURSE (Phone: _____)

_____

_____

Communications

FOLLOW-UP APPOINTMENTS

Be sure to keep the appointment with your doctor as scheduled.

Follow-up Care

FIGURE 4.6 (Continued)

Having a T&A

A "T & A" is having tonsils and adenoids taken out.

Your child is scheduled for surgery on (date): _____. You will be told the time of surgery when you come to the hospital.

PREPARING FOR SURGERY

- If your child develops a cough or fever before coming to the hospital, call the Ear, Nose, and Throat Clinic (E.N.T.) at _____, or call your doctor (phone: _____).
- Explain to your child what will happen at the hospital. You may tell your child that he is going to have two little lumps taken out of the back of his mouth. He will be taken to a big room. Then he will be given some sweet smelling air to make him sleep for a while. When he is asleep, the doctor will take out his tonsils. After his tonsils are out, he will go back to his room and will be awake.
- Your child can bring his favorite toy from home.

THE EVENING BEFORE SURGERY

Please <u>do not</u> give your child any food to eat or liquids to drink after midnight the evening before surgery. <u>This is very important.</u>

The child should have nothing to eat or to drink the night before surgery, so he won't choke while under anesthesia.

ON THE DAY OF SURGERY

- Bring your child to the Patient Services office in the main lobby at 8:00 A.M. The main lobby is at the entrance to the new building that faces Parsons Avenue (Picture 1). At this office you will be interviewed. Then you will be taken to the nursing unit by a volunteer.
- If you have hospital insurance, please bring the forms with you.
- Please do not bring any children that are not having surgery.

Picture 1 How to get to Children's Hospital

Definition

Appointment

Explanation & Emotional Care

Preparation for Surgery

ON THE NURSING UNIT

- Your child will have a medical examination. Parents - <u>please remain on the unit until you have talked with the doctor.</u>
- A parent may stay overnight with the child. Most children go home the next morning.
- A supervised playroom is available for older children to enjoy.

WHAT TO EXPECT AFTER SURGERY

- Your child may have a temperature of 100-102° for 1-7 days. If it is higher than that, call the E.N.T. Clinic (phone: _____).
- Pain in the ears may last as long as 2 weeks. These pains are usually worse in the morning but decrease during the day. Swallowing is painful. Have the child take the prescribed medication as directed to ease the pain.
- Raw white areas will appear where tonsils were removed. These will disappear in about 2 weeks.
- Occasionally, children will bleed from the nose or mouth, even 1 week after the operation. This bleeding is rarely serious, but we want to see your child if it happens. Call the E.N.T. Clinic (_____), your private physician (phone: _____), or the Emergency Room (_____), and take your child to the Emergency Room.

DIET AFTER SURGERY

Your child may eat or drink whatever he wishes. Food will not injure his throat. If he does not want food, be sure he drinks plenty of liquids (Picture 3). This will keep his fever down and keep his nose and throat from feeling dry.

ACTIVITY AFTER SURGERY

- Get your child up and about, do not keep him from playing (Picture 4). He may play outside.
- He may return to school 7 days after the operation.
- No swimming is allowed for 2 weeks after the operation.

FOLLOW-UP APPOINTMENT

Please bring your child to the E.N.T. Clinic in 3 weeks. An appointment slip will be mailed to you.

If you have any questions, please call _____.

Picture 3 Give plenty of liquids.

Picture 4 Your child may play outside.

Medication

Observation

Communication

Nutrition

Activity

Follow-up Care

FIGURE 4.7 Example of Helping Hand for Surgery

WRITING ABOUT PROCEDURES

When writing procedures for patients/families, remember they do not know all the principles of nursing and medical techniques. The instructions should be all-inclusive and clearcut. In some of the complicated procedures, such as *Your Child's Urinary Diversion,* we have arranged the procedural steps in frames, comic strip fashion (page 293). The frame consists of the illustration and corresponding directions. If one of the steps is difficult to perform and requires repeated practice, the instructions are right there in the same frame. The user need not reread the whole teaching aid or hunt for the guide to that step.

For less complicated procedures such as *How to Reduce a Fever,* the steps are listed in consecutive order with a number designating each step. The pictures emphasize the most important points of the teaching aid, rather than illustrating the step-by-step procedure (Fig. 4.8).

There are several procedures that require in-depth knowledge and preparation on the part of the family; one such topic is the *Care of a Child with a Tracheostomy.* This Helping Hand is quite lengthy and includes most information the patient/family would need regarding this care. In this Helping Hand, we arranged the information in segments. We know that relief people may occasionally substitute for parents and probably will not be as familiar with the child's care. We recognize that these people (as well as the family) may not be mentally prepared to cope with an emergency. So we not only arranged emergency procedures in separate segments but also wrote them on separate facing pages, so these instructions could be permanently placed in a logical place for quick reference (page 290 and 291).

PROCEDURE FRAMEWORK

Name of Child/Date

Definition/Explanation
Explanation of procedure; part of the body being treated; purpose; what we expect to accomplish; what we want to prevent

Emotional Care
Of patient; of family

Equipment/Supplies
What to obtain; where to obtain; preparation; cleaning and sterilization

Medication
Topical medications; irrigating solutions

Procedure
Method of performing; safety; prevention of contamination or cross-infection; observation; positioning; prevention of pain or injury

Observation
Change in appearance; odor; bleeding; symptoms

Personal Care
Hygiene; skin care; dental care

Nutrition
Diet; fluids

Activity
Limitations; restrictions; precautions

Safety
Prevention of injury; prevention of poisoning

Communication
When to call the doctor, nurse; where to call if questions arise

Follow-up Care
Appointments

Space for Additional Information
Blank space

WRITING ABOUT DIAGNOSTIC TESTS

The explanation of each diagnostic test must be given careful thought. The name of the test as well as what will happen can be formidable to many patients. Families also become apprehensive because they don't know exactly what to expect. Their apprehension may be transmitted to the patient and may heighten his anxiety, which can lead to lack of cooperation or extreme fear during the test. Therefore, we have focused on giving clear, accurate information supplemented with illustration of the test environment. Patients/families appreciate that many of their questions are answered beforehand.

In writing a teaching aid for diagnostic tests, it is important to consider the patients'/families' perspective, and to direct the content toward their point of view. For example, it may be anxiety reducing for the patient/family to see the drawing of the patient having an E.E.G. (Fig. 4.9).

Where possible, include sensory explanations about the test; explain the feelings that will occur during or after the test.

HELPING HAND
Homegoing Education
and Literature Program

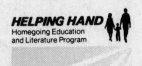

Let's talk about...

How to Reduce a Fever

Definition/ Explanation

A fever is a rise in body temperature above normal. If your child looks flushed, his skin is hot, and he is restless, he may have a fever. Take your child's temperature. If the temperature is above 103° by rectum, the temperature must be lowered to normal. One way to help the fever to come down is to give the child a sponge bath in a tub. The child will cry and will not want you to sponge him. But, continue the sponging because it is important to bring down the fever.

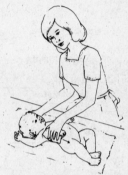

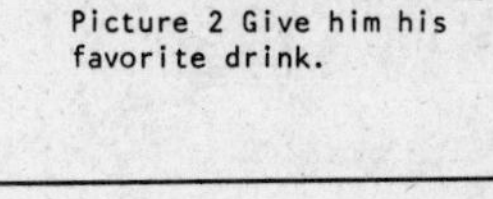

Picture 1 Gently stroke child's skin.

YOU WILL NEED

Equipment

Child's bath tub for infant
Regular bath tub for older child
Clean wash cloths
Towels

Safety

WHAT TO DO

Procedure

1. Fill the bath tub with 2 inches of water that is warm to your wrist.
2. Remove the child's clothing. Place child in tub or on a padded surface.
3. Wet and partially wring out a wash cloth.
4. Sponge child's body with the wash cloth. Use long soothing strokes over face, neck, arms, chest, back, and legs. Rub slightly. Sponge water on chest and back. (Picture 1).
5. Sponge child for 20 minutes.
6. Remove child from tub and cover him with a light blanket.
7. Wait 30 minutes.
8. Take child's temperature. (Observation)
9. If the temperature is still high, repeat sponging until the temperature is 101° rectally.
10. If child starts to shiver, stop sponging. When shivering stops, warm the water and put child back in tub or on padded surface. (Safety)
11. Dress your child so he is comfortable for the temperature of the home.
12. NEVER LEAVE CHILD ALONE WHEN TAKING TEMPERATURE OR REDUCING FEVER.

OTHER INFORMATION

- To help to keep the temperature normal, give clear liquids. Have the child drink as much water and juice as he will take. (Nutrition)
- Your child may have ________ aspirin, every _____ hours or __________ every _____ hours. Give this only as directed by a doctor. (Medication)
- Call your doctor or the Emergency Room if the temperature remains over_______° by rectum or _______° by mouth. (Communication)
- Call your doctor or the Emergency Room if he vomits medicine or fluids _______ times.

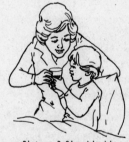

Picture 2 Give him his favorite drink.

FIGURE 4.8 Example of Procedure

Name of child

Appointment

Definition/
Explanation

Preparation
for the Test

Environment &
Equipment

Communication

HELPING HAND
Homegoing Education
and Literature Program

Let's talk about...

Having an E.E.G.

The electroencephalogram (e-lek-tro-en-SEF-ah-lo-gram) or E.E.G. is a recording of the electrical activity of the brain. It records your child's brain waves. The E.E.G. is painless and safe.

TO PREPARE THE CHILD FOR THE TEST
1. Explain the test to the child.
2. Shampoo the child's hair well.
3. Comb and brush the hair neatly. If hair is long, put it into a ponytail or tie it back.
4. Do not use any hair spray or hair dressing.
5. Do not tease the hair.

THE TEST
Your child will be shown what will happen. Moist discs (called electrodes) are placed on areas of the child's head. Cotton balls hold the electrodes and wires in place. The child is asked to lie very still with his eyes closed and try to relax. The machine records the faint electrical impulses of the brain on the graph paper. This test takes about 45-50 minutes.

AFTER THE TEST
A doctor will read the graph (or tracing). His report will be sent to your doctor or clinic.

If you cannot keep the appointment, or if you have any questions, please call the E.E.G. laboratory (_____).

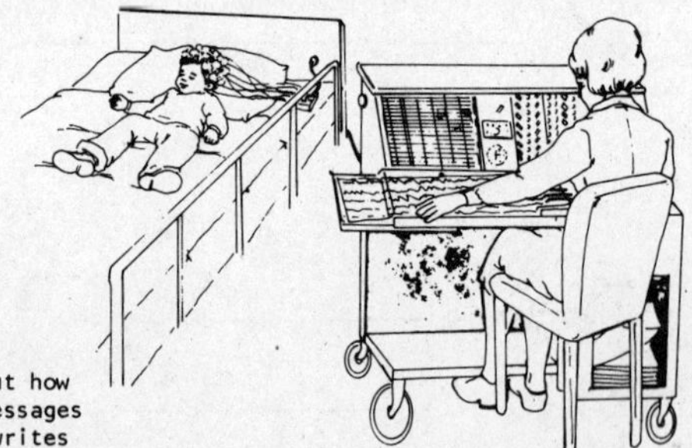

Child's Name: _____
Appointment:
Date: _____
Time: _____
Please bring your child to:
☐ Line 5 at Clinic Registration Desk (first floor)
☐ Emergency Room Desk

The discs pick up messages about how your brain is working. These messages are sent to the machine which writes them down.

FIGURE 4.9 Example of Diagnostic Test

DIAGNOSTIC TEST FRAMEWORK

Name of Child/Date

Definition/Explanation
Explanation and purpose of test

Preparation for the Test
Appointments Date, time; where to report; phone numbers
At Home (Before the test) Diet; medications; fluids; explanation of test to child
In the Hospital Medications; diet; fluids; explanation of test to the child

Environment
Description of test area; "what you will see, hear, and feel"

Equipment
Description of equipment used for test

Procedure
Preparation; how equipment is used

Emotional Care
Before and after test; during test

Activity
Activity after test; restrictions; when to resume activity

Nutrition
After the test; prior to test

Safety
Caution regarding care of medications used in preparing for test

Communication
Phone numbers if questions or a need to reschedule appointment arises

Follow-up Care
Appointments

Space for Additional Information
Blank space

WRITING ABOUT CHILD CARE/HEALTH INFORMATION

At our health center, preventive health information is not secondary to the treatment of disease. We do more than treat disease or conditions; we provide preventive health care as part of a total plan of patient care. We believe the health professional must provide preventive health information if we are to promote comprehensive health care systems. For example, childhood immunizations is a preventive measure that may be overlooked or ignored by parents. Our schedule for immunizations serves as a re-minder for parents; it helps them keep track of immunization requirements for their child which promotes the parents' active participation in their child's health care (Fig. 4.10).

The child care/health information category includes a list of topics ranging from bathing a baby to immunizations (Fig. 4.10). The elements of care which parents will encounter during their child's formative years, such as general care of the infant, growth and development, and dental care are included in this section. This category also includes teaching aids which do not logically fit into the other categories, such as the *Pediatric Nurse Associate* and *Going to University Hospital*. The framework for this section is fairly general, although each framework element is considered when a topic is developed.

CHILD CARE/HEALTH INFORMATION FRAMEWORK

Definition/Explanation
Explanation or purpose of information

Equipment/Supplies
Equipment needed; availability; preparation for use; cleaning

Procedure
Method of performing; observations

Emotional Care
Preparation of child; psychological aspects

Nutrition
Basic diet; fluid needs; restrictions

Personal Care
Hygiene; skin care; dental care

Activity
Restrictions; school

Medications
Type; how and when to give; storage; record keeping

Environment
Special considerations

Safety
Related to topic

Preventive Care

Communications
When to call doctor; where to call for more information or if questions arise

Follow-up Care
Appointments

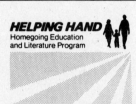

Let's talk about...

Immunizations

Definition/
Explanation

Immunizations (im-mu-ni-ZA-shuns) are medicines given to protect your child against certain harmful diseases. Immunizations are given by mouth or by injections (shots).

NAMES OF IMMUNIZATIONS	DISEASES IMMUNIZATIONS PROTECT AGAINST
DPT	Diphtheria (a bacterial infection that causes a membrane to form in the throat)
	Pertussis (whooping cough)
	Tetanus (lock jaw)
Trivalent Sabin (oral polio) (OPV)	Polio
Rubella vaccine	3-Day German measles
Measles vaccine (rubeola)	2-Week measles (hard measles)
Tuberculin skin test	This is a test to see if your child has Tuberculosis (TB). It is not an immunization.

Immunizations are usually given according to a special schedule. Ages when healthy infants and children should receive immunizations are:

Schedule

AGE*	TYPE OF IMMUNIZATION GIVEN
2 months	DPT and polio
4 months	DPT and polio
6 months	DPT and polio
15 months	Measles, rubella, mumps
18 months	DPT and polio booster
4-5 years	DPT and polio booster
14-16 years	DT (adult) booster and then every 10 years
Yearly	Tuberculin skin test

*The ages when immunizations are given may vary with each doctor.

FIGURE 4.10 Example of Child Care/Health Information

<u>WHAT TO EXPECT AFTER AN IMMUNIZATION IS</u>
<u>GIVEN</u>

Immunizations can cause your child to have
a fever. If his temperature is 101°
(rectally) or more, give (name of medication):
amount: _____. You may repeat
this one time 3-4 hours later.

Call the clinic (phone: _____) if the
fever lasts longer than 24-48 hours.

<u>YOUR CHILD'S IMMUNIZATION RECORD</u>

You will be given an immunization record
for your child. When each immunization is
given, your doctor or nurse will write the
date on this card. It is important that you
keep this record in a safe place.

You will need to take this record with you:

· When the child returns for medical
  check-ups
· When your child enrolls in school
· If your child is injured and has an open
  cut
· If you move to a new area and place of
  medical care

<u>OTHER INFORMATION</u>

German measles vaccine (rubella) should be given to girls before child-bearing age.
If a pregnant woman gets German measles early in her pregnancy, her baby can have
birth defects.

If you have any questions, please call _____.

Your child needs your protection.

Observation &
Medication

Communication

Record Keeping

Safety

FIGURE 4.10 (Continued)

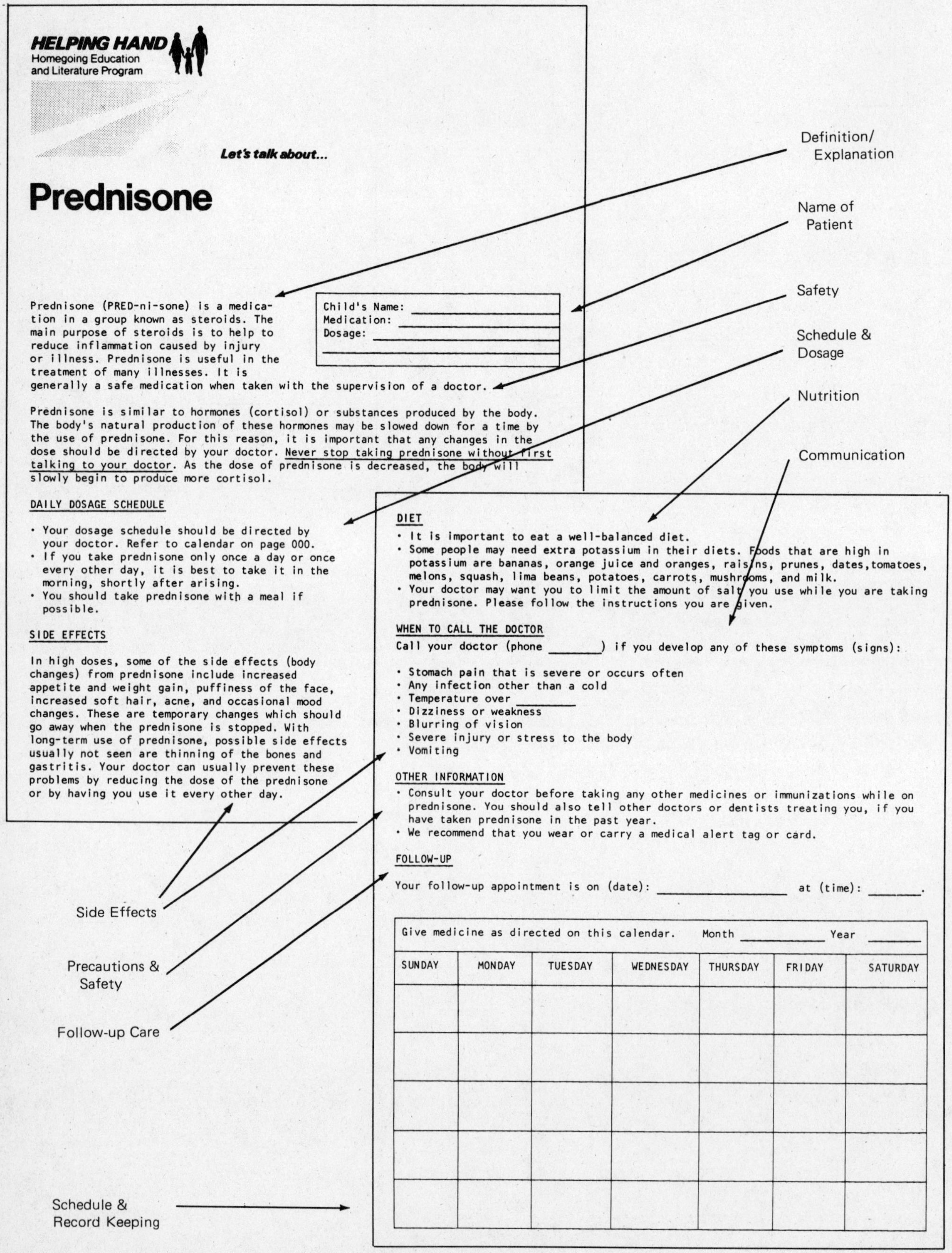

Definition/
Explanation

Name of
Patient

Safety

Schedule &
Dosage

Nutrition

Communication

HELPING HAND
Homegoing Education
and Literature Program

Let's talk about...

Prednisone

Prednisone (PRED-ni-sone) is a medication in a group known as steroids. The
main purpose of steroids is to help to
reduce inflammation caused by injury
or illness. Prednisone is useful in the
treatment of many illnesses. It is
generally a safe medication when taken with the supervision of a doctor.

Child's Name: _____
Medication: _____
Dosage: _____

Prednisone is similar to hormones (cortisol) or substances produced by the body.
The body's natural production of these hormones may be slowed down for a time by
the use of prednisone. For this reason, it is important that any changes in the
dose should be directed by your doctor. Never stop taking prednisone without first
talking to your doctor. As the dose of prednisone is decreased, the body will
slowly begin to produce more cortisol.

DAILY DOSAGE SCHEDULE

· Your dosage schedule should be directed by
  your doctor. Refer to calendar on page 000.
· If you take prednisone only once a day or once
  every other day, it is best to take it in the
  morning, shortly after arising.
· You should take prednisone with a meal if
  possible.

SIDE EFFECTS

In high doses, some of the side effects (body
changes) from prednisone include increased
appetite and weight gain, puffiness of the face,
increased soft hair, acne, and occasional mood
changes. These are temporary changes which should
go away when the prednisone is stopped. With
long-term use of prednisone, possible side effects
usually not seen are thinning of the bones and
gastritis. Your doctor can usually prevent these
problems by reducing the dose of the prednisone
or by having you use it every other day.

DIET

· It is important to eat a well-balanced diet.
· Some people may need extra potassium in their diets. Foods that are high in
  potassium are bananas, orange juice and oranges, raisins, prunes, dates, tomatoes,
  melons, squash, lima beans, potatoes, carrots, mushrooms, and milk.
· Your doctor may want you to limit the amount of salt you use while you are taking
  prednisone. Please follow the instructions you are given.

WHEN TO CALL THE DOCTOR

Call your doctor (phone _____) if you develop any of these symptoms (signs):

· Stomach pain that is severe or occurs often
· Any infection other than a cold
· Temperature over _____
· Dizziness or weakness
· Blurring of vision
· Severe injury or stress to the body
· Vomiting

OTHER INFORMATION

· Consult your doctor before taking any other medicines or immunizations while on
  prednisone. You should also tell other doctors or dentists treating you, if you
  have taken prednisone in the past year.
· We recommend that you wear or carry a medical alert tag or card.

FOLLOW-UP

Your follow-up appointment is on (date): _____ at (time): _____.

Give medicine as directed on this calendar.   Month _____   Year _____

SUNDAY	MONDAY	TUESDAY	WEDNESDAY	THURSDAY	FRIDAY	SATURDAY

Side Effects

Precautions &
Safety

Follow-up Care

Schedule &
Record Keeping

FIGURE 4.11 Example of Medications

WRITING ABOUT MEDICATIONS

In writing about medication, we must overcome the prevailing casual attitude toward the giving or taking of drugs. This is a serious responsibility since parents need certain information to follow the physician's prescribed regime with safety. Giving medications to children is even more serious because a child's body can react differently to medications than an adult's.

In the past, patients were given a prescription and told to have it filled and "take as directed." They had little knowledge about expected results or possible side effects. In some settings, nurses were not permitted to explain the purpose of the medication given to the patient. Some parents knew they were giving their child a "little white pill," but that was the extent of their knowledge. Through patient education and the Helping Hands we have tried to lift this "shroud of secrecy" (Fig. 4.11).

Currently, few Helping Hands are available on medications; however, we are presently collaborating with our pharmacy department to develop and provide more instructions about the general administration of medicine, as well as about specific medications.

MEDICATION FRAMEWORK

Name of Child/Date

Definition/Explanation
Name of medication; purpose; reason for administering

Medication
Administration How to prepare and give; reading label
Schedule and Dosage When to give; when to discontinue; how much to give
Side Effects Expected; abnormal
Storage Where and how to store
Record Keeping How to record medicine administration

Equipment/Supplies
Equipment needed; prescriptions—purchase and refill

Safety and Precautions
"Store out of reach of children"; how to dispose of equipment or outdated drugs; drugs to avoid; cautions against injury related to medication—driving cars, etc.

Communications
When to call the doctor; where to call if questions arise; contacting school nurse, teacher, and community health nurse; pharmacist

Activity
Restrictions; limitations related to medication

Nutrition
Diet and fluid intake related to medication

Personal Care
Dental care; skin care related to medication; appliances

Follow-up Care
Appointments

Space for Additional Information
Blank space

THE FRAMEWORK ELEMENTS

In this section you will find detailed explanations about each element mentioned in the preceding frameworks. This information should be used primarily for reference as you develop your teaching aids. For this purpose the elements are arranged in alphabetical order; the list below can serve as a quick reference for topic and page number.

FRAMEWORK ELEMENTS

ACTIVITY

Activity and play should be considered regardless of the subject of your teaching aid. Often, it is the first concern of a patient or family following surgery, a test, or a procedure. "Can I go out and play?", asks the child after T & A surgery. "Will the condition affect my personal life?", asks the man recovering from a heart attack. "Will she ever be able to do the things other children are doing?", asks a concerned parent about her diabetic daughter.

People should be instructed about activity *restrictions, limitations,* and *allowances* from the start. Don't wait until the child with a broken arm comes back with a disintegrated cast after splashing in the bathtub. The family and child should both know that "It may be easier for your child to have a sponge bath while the cast is on" (*Cast Care*). After a child has a T & A, it is helpful for the parents to read, "Get your child up and about, do not keep the child from playing" (*Having a T & A*). Instructions should be clearcut. It is more helpful to state, "swimming is not allowed for 2 weeks after the operation" than to make vague statements such as, "swimming is not allowed."

When procedures require an extended period of time, we often point out some activity that can still be done. "You will be able to sit up and do things with your other hand while you have an I.V." (*Having an I.V.*). Parents and children fear having a "trach" will prevent them from having outdoor activity. So, we let them know that outdoor play is permitted, "Outdoor play is fun for the child too. You must cover the trach to prevent cold air and dust from entering the lungs" (*Care of a Child With a Tracheostomy*).

In most cases, activity is not restricted after a test. However, following a cardiac catheterization, there is danger of bleeding from the site where the catheter was inserted. We state: "After the test, you *must* stay in bed for 24 hours. This allows time for the place in your groin to start healing. You will use the bed pan or urinal in bed instead of walking to the bathroom" (*Cardiac Catheterization*). Firm, unqualified statements are needed when there can be no exceptions to the rule.

Returning to school is one activity which children may not be so eager to resume. To assist parents, specific guidelines are offered. In *Having a T & A* instructions, we state, "He may return to school 7 days after the operation." In cases where return to school may differ, depending on the age or condition of the child or the opinion of the physician, specific dates may be indicated in the blank: "Child may return to school _____."

In writing about activity allowances and restrictions, be sure to consider the question of "sexism." No longer does the world of sports belong strictly to the male, nor are activities such as crocheting and rug making strictly for the female. In fact, it would be wise in many situations to encourage the obese girl to join in active sports, and the man recovering from a heart attack to take up weaving or sewing.

COMMUNICATIONS

Open communication is always important, but when illness is present the necessity of good communication becomes paramount. Communications provide the link from health professional to patient and from patient to health professional. Knowing when to call the doctor, who to contact in the community, and where to call if questions arise is extremely important for the patient's ongoing care.

Patients and families often have difficulty deciding *when to call the physician.* We have tried to overcome this by listing symptoms that can develop and asking them to call the physician if these occur. This relieves the parent who is concerned about "bothering" the physician needlessly (See "When to call the Doctor," *Aspirin Ingestion*).

When there are many variables in age, condition of patient, or preferences of a physician, we leave blank spaces to be filled in. For example, in treating scoliosis, the orthopedic nurse knows what problems may arise with the individual patient, and she indicates when the parent should call her (*Scoliosis*). If it is a medical problem she indicates that the parent should call the physician.

Blank spaces are also left so the physician's or nurse's phone number can be written in. Emergency phone numbers are listed when there is a possibility of an emergency (refer to *Care of a Child With a Tracheostomy*). Department telephone numbers are listed in case an appointment has to be changed or if there are questions. We encourage the parents to call the department if they are detained and may be late. To encourage communication, we also add a last statement on all Helping Hands: "If you have any questions, please call _____."

Communication with community professionals is also emphasized. If a child is on medication or treatment programs which might affect the child at school or elsewhere in the community, the school nurse and school teacher should be informed. Patients and parents may not think to inform other persons involved with the child's care; it's important to include this type of information in the teaching aid under "Other Information" or "Follow-up Care."

DEFINITION AND EXPLANATION

As with activity, definition and explanation of a procedure, test, medication, or surgery should be discussed. It is well-documented that compliance is greater when the patient/family knows the reasons for the medical treatment or the consequences of noncompliance. For example, if the parent is told only to "give the child penicillin four times a day," the child may soon return with the same infection. The physician may not understand why the medication was ineffective. The parent may have given the antibiotic until the child appeared well. But what the doctor failed to explain or what the parent did not hear was that "the full 10-day dose must be taken for the medicine to get rid of all the infection." With this explanation the parent would most likely have complied.

Definition and explanation also helps the patient/family to understand a certain test or disease process. The child who must have a "brain wave test" (E.E.G.) may be terrified because he thinks the people will be able to "read his mind," or will "electrocute" him. An explanation of the test, reinforced by an appropriate illustration, can assist in calming the patient by easing his fear of the unknown (*Having an E.E.G.*).

There are a few tips to remember concerning definition or explanation. Avoid overburdening the patient/family with information he does not need to know. For example, the Helping Hand *Impetigo* states, "Impetigo is a skin infection." It is not necessary to state that the causative organisms may be staphylococci or streptococci; remember, you are talking to the average lay person, not one who has had a course in bacteriology. The teaching aid should focus on what to do for the child now that he *has* impetigo. Later, the parents can find out more information from the health professional if they need or want to know.

EMOTIONAL CARE

Considering the patient's emotional needs may be as important as providing for his physical health. The parents need to know how their child is likely to react and how to deal with their own reactions to function and to be of help.

Feelings of *frustration* are hard enough to handle for those who are well. But imagine, for example, how you would feel if you had scoliosis and were required to wear a brace; feelings are magnified and frustrations intensify these feelings. With this in mind, we state, "When the brace is first put on, you will have feelings that you 'can't stand it'. But keep it on as long as you can. If you feel you can't go through with it, take it off for a while. When you can get yourself together, put it on and try again" (*Scoliosis*). We try to help alleviate some of the frustration by stating, "In a short time you will feel better and will be doing most

of the things you did before." The illustration (riding a bike, dancing with a boyfriend) helps support this thought.

Helping parents cope with *fear* is an area needing special attention. For example, parents have told us repeatedly that caring for a child with croup is one of the most frightening experiences they have ever had. So, in preparing the Helping Hand, *Croup*, we acknowledged that parents will be frightened, and indicated what will happen if they show signs of fear. We state, "Parents can help relieve croup by being calm themselves, which helps to quiet the child. This relieves the tightness of the larynx and allows the child to breathe easier." This statement is also followed by specific information about what actions to take.

Giving parents specific things to do helps alleviate fear. In the past our family doctors probably practiced this psychological strategy at the birth of a baby. Invariably in stories, the anxious father was told "to go put some water on to boil." Did medical history ever reveal what the doctor did with the boiling water? But it's safe to assume that the boiling water helped alleviate fear in the father by keeping him busy.

Many parents are afraid they might hurt their child when performing a procedure or treatment. We let them know that fear is expected and help them overcome it so they can function. For instance, "You may feel afraid when you first start doing the suctioning. This is normal. Try to remember you are not hurting your child, you are helping him to breathe," and if the trach tube comes out, "Try to keep your mind on what you are doing, rather than how he is acting. Each time it will become easier for you to do" (*Care of a Child With a Tracheostomy*).

In dealing with a child, honesty is always of utmost importance, especially when it is necessary to perform procedures that may be painful; if the procedure will hurt, we state this. When we prepare a child for having an I.V., we state, "It will stick a little and hurt at first, but if you hold still, it won't take very long." Then we tell the child what it will feel like when the tape is removed; "Taking off the tape will feel like taking off a Band-Aid" (*Having an I.V.*).

It is very easy for parents to be "overprotective" of their child if his condition requires extra attention. The child may become demanding and dependent. It is difficult not to show pity in some situations. We warn the parents about this to prevent them from falling into a trap. "It is important not to overprotect him, or treat him like he is sick. If you do, the child will feel different than other children, and may become over-demanding" (*Care of a Child With a Tracheostomy*).

Care is taken in the wording of the instructions to make it clear that both parents, not just the mother, are involved in doing the procedures. We feel it is necessary to include the father in the instructions and let him know the care of the child is a joint responsibility.

ENVIRONMENT

Although it seems trite, it's true that no matter where we are or what we are doing, the environment has some effect on us—physically and/or psychologically. Consider this heading in writing each teaching aid. How will the hospital or home environment affect, or be affected by, the patient/family? Is this topic a new, possibly anxiety-producing situation? Are there special measures the patients/families need to take regarding the environment?

Environmental factors sometimes cause or spread disease. For instance, in discussing hepatitis, we help the patient/family understand what they are dealing with by stating how hepatitis is spread. "It is spread by contact with urine, feces (bowel movements), water, or milk that has the virus in it" (*Hepatitis*). To prevent the spread of hepatitis, cleanliness in the environment is necessary. "Good hand-washing by all members of the family must be done: before meals, after using the bathroom, and before preparing or serving food." How does the family maintain cleanliness in the area where the contaminate is likely to be? We instruct the parents to make sure the home is free of rodents and insects. We also explain how to handle eating utensils, how to clean the bathroom sink and toilet bowl, and how to discard or treat toilet tissue, urine, and feces.

In some situations, precautionary treatment of the environment can prevent undesirable consequences. For example, allergy to dust affects a large segment of our population. To help parents cope with this problem, our Helping Hand *Dust Allergies* tells how to clean and dust-proof their child's bedroom, how to select the type of materials permitted in the bedroom environment, how to dust-proof a car, and other information.

While most areas in a hospital or clinic may be familiar and comfortable for us, these strange, secret places are an alien environment to the inexperienced patient and family. A series of tests can provoke anxiety reactions in young and old. Visiting the test environment or looking at a picture of it (like those in the Helping Hands) alleviates much of this anxiety. If we tell a child he is going to have an x-ray picture taken and he arrives in the department and sees a sign "Radiology", he may think, "Somebody lied to me. They are going to radiate me and I don't like it." Care must be taken in the preparatory explanation and instruction.

EQUIPMENT AND SUPPLIES

A chain is only as strong as its weakest link, and sometimes the equipment is the weak link. The suction machine won't suction if it is not properly set up, nor will it function during a power outage. What happens if the family's back-up electrical supply goes out? If the child's life depends on a suction machine, a generator is needed and plans for its use must be made.

There are several aspects to consider in regard to equipment: acquiring or purchasing equipment; preparing and assembling it; and using and caring for it. Before parents can begin to gather and to purchase equipment, they must know what those supplies are. All supplies and equipment needed are listed near the beginning of the teaching aid under the heading, *"You Will Need."* If the list is lengthy, we make a list of supplies with check boxes. Using this, parents and staff easily know when all necessary supplies have been obtained. When possible, we encourage the use of household articles rather than expensive hospital supplies: jars and bottles rather than hospital containers; measuring cups and spoons rather than graduated dispensers; wash cloths rather than 2″ × 2″ gauze pads.

The patient/family should also be given the information needed to purchase the appropriate supplies. For example, explain that by using a bulb syringe with a wide end, rather than standard end, nasal injury can be prevented (refer to *Suctioning the Nose With a Bulb Syringe*), and discuss the importance of using a graduated medicine dropper or spoon (available at most pharmacies) rather than a regular teaspoon in dispensing medications.

We suggest that the equipment be prepared and assembled before approaching the child to perform the procedure. If the child is anxious, this will reduce the time he has to worry about what is going to happen. We remind the parent of an infant never to leave the child unguarded while getting equipment.

After the equipment is purchased, instructions are given about how to *use* it. For example, a newly diagnosed diabetic patient is given step-by-step directions for preparing mixed insulin dosage and giving the injections. We also explain how to dispose of the syringe legally.

The patient/family is taught to clean, to sterilize, and to store equipment. Techniques for sterilizing reusable supplies are described. Instructions should be given for care of all equipment used, but particularly for expensive or special-order equipment. For instance, in the teaching aid *Scoliosis,* we state, "Wash the brace daily with a wash cloth and mild soap. Rinse with wash cloth and clear water and wipe dry. Do not put any part of the brace into water."

FOLLOW-UP CARE

Follow-up care is stressed in the teaching aid for more than one reason. Parents sometimes think that once the symptoms of disease are alleviated, it is not necessary to continue a medication. They may not realize that, without follow-up care, other complications can develop, such as hearing loss following an ear infection, or a heart condition following a "Beta Strep" infection.

Many times well-intentioned friends and relatives offer advice which the parents follow, instead of returning for follow-up care. In other cases, parents may continue a harmful procedure, such as applying a nonprescribed topical ointment to a burned area; the growing child could be developing contractures which the parents may not be aware of—follow-up care is important.

In the Helping Hands, we strongly support keeping appointments with the physician or other health professional. The specific dates for return vary with each, so we leave a space for the appropriate time to be written in. For diagnostic tests, the date and time of the appointment is listed and the phone numbers to call if they are detained or the test has to be rescheduled.

When possible, special consideration is given to parents who must travel a distance for an appointment. Maps to the hospital and the check-in location are included. A map has proven helpful for our oncology patients who receive their radiation therapy at a hospital across town. Until the map was developed, parents spent money on daily cab fare because they feared getting lost in an unfamiliar city (*Going to University Hospital*).

MEDICATIONS

"Medications" is one of the five major categories in our Helping Hand system, as well as a separate element in most frameworks. As a framework element, and therefore a subheading of a teaching aid, the discussion of medications is usually fairly general and brief. If extensive information is needed about the medication, a separate teaching aid is developed.

Administration

There are several factors to consider when writing about the administration of medication. Reading the medication label is extremely important; the label should be read when the drug is taken from the shelf, when preparing the drug, and again, when replacing medication on the shelf. Parents are cautioned to be fully awake and alert before dispensing medications. How many times have you heard of people spraying their hair with deodorant before they were fully awake? Or how many times has a sleepy parent reached for and given the wrong drug, only to discover afterward that an error was made. Parents are also cautioned to avoid distractions, such as other children interrupting or people talking. We stress the same rules for preparing medication at home as those used in the hospital medication room.

Studies have shown that writing a prescription does not necessarily mean it is going to be given or even filled. It is apparent to us that the patient/family needs help and reinforcement in this area. Providing parents with a medications schedule helps increase compliance (*Prednisone*, Fig. 4.11). Having the family keep these records assists the physician and nurse and involves the patient in his own care.

When giving medication to a child, cooperation needs to be established at the beginning. The purpose of the medication is explained to a child who is old enough to under-

stand. We encourage a firm, but kind approach on the part of the parents and suggest that they praise the child after the medication is taken, whether he has been cooperative or difficult.

In administration of medications, the equipment used is also a consideration. Supplies used to dispense drugs should be graduated to give accurate measurement, since the patient will not receive the correct dosage of medicine if the equipment is not accurate. Graduated devices are available in pharmacies. If medications are ordered to be given in teaspoons we advise the parents to use cooking measuring spoons that are used in preparing food because they do not vary in size as much as ordinary teaspoons used for dining.

Schedule and Dosage

When possible, medication schedules should be planned to coincide with the most convenient times for the patient and his family. The Helping Hand *When to Give Medications* (Fig. 4.12) helps the patient/family understand directions that may be confusing. If the patient is told to "take 1 teaspoonful four times a day," does he take 4 teaspoonfuls in 24 hours, or only during waking hours? Or does he take one-fourth teaspoon each time? By circling the hours when medication is to be taken, the physician or nurse can illustrate the times of day for taking the medication.

We emphasize that the entire amount of the prescription should be taken. The exact amount of each dose is written in the blank space provided.

Purchasing medications can be very expensive, so we advise parents to "shop around" before having a prescription filled to get the best buy. If a child will need several refills of the medication, we suggest that parents have the prescription refilled before it runs out. Sometimes some pharmacies do not stock all medications and require time for ordering unstocked medications.

Side Effects

Some normal side effects may be expected when a medication is first taken; other side effects are serious and abnormal. The patient and family should be told which symptoms are normal and which ones require the prompt attention of a physician. In the directions for taking birth control pills, we state, "During your first two packages of 28 pills, you may develop common side effects, such as breast tenderness, upset stomach, mild headache, small weight gain or a small amount of bleeding (spotting) between periods. If these side effects continue during your third package of pills, please call the clinic but do not stop taking your pills" (*Birth Control Pills*). Examples of serious or abnormal side effects when taking birth control pills are also given. The patient is advised to call the physician immediately if these side effects occur.

HELPING HAND
Homegoing Education
and Literature Program

Let's talk about...

When to Give Medications

Child's Name: ____________________
Age: ____________________
Medication: ____________________
Dose (Amount): ____________________

Give this medicine ________ times a day at the times circled on the picture.

HOW TO GIVE THE MEDICATION

- ☐ Take ____________ (time) before meals
- ☐ Take with meals
- ☐ Take after meals

THIS DRUG IS USED FOR

____

____

CAUTION

- Store all medicine out of children's reach.
- Store in locked cupboard when possible.
- Give medicine only as ordered by your doctor.
- When medicine is no longer needed, flush it down the toilet.
- If a child accidentally takes too much of this medicine, it can make him very sick. Call your doctor (phone: ________), the Poison Control Center (________), or the Emergency Room (________) if this happens.

WHEN TO CALL THE DOCTOR

Call your doctor (phone: ________) if any of the following symptoms (signs) occur.

1. ____________________
2. ____________________
3. ____________________

FIGURE 4.12 When to Give Medications

Patients may be allergic to certain medications or have diseases or conditions which preclude taking some medications. Children with glucose dehydrogenase deficiency should not take certain drugs. A list of drugs to avoid is given to the parents, and they are instructed to keep this list for reference if the child becomes ill and needs medical treatment. Other prohibited drugs can be listed in blank spaces (*G6PD Deficiency*).

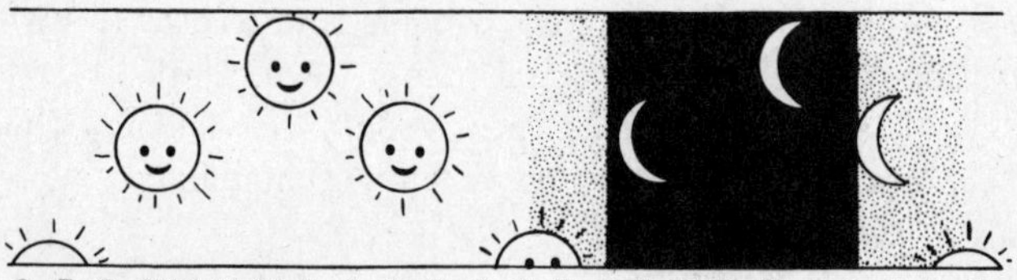

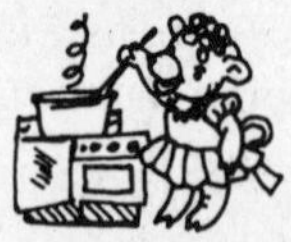

If sedatives are ordered, families are told that the child will be drowsy and should be protected from falls or injury while in bed or walking. Patients are cautioned against driving cars or riding bikes while taking sedatives, anticonvulsants, or tranquilizers. While taking these medications, lawn mowers, electric saws, and other power tools should not be used unless approved by the physician. Some medications, such as anticonvulsants may alter behavior, and families should be advised that the patient may act differently until stabilized.

Precautions

Contamination of topical medication must be guarded against to prevent infection of the injured area. Prevention of contamination is also stressed when repeated treatment with ointment is prescribed. We instruct the parents, "with a clean knife, remove only enough ointment for one treatment."

Safe *disposal* of unused drugs and supplies is emphasized. The patient/family is cautioned against using drugs if there is a change in color. For example, "Clinitest tablets will turn from white with blue specks to dark blue if they are too old for use. Replace old tablets with new ones, and flush old ones down the toilet" (*Urine Testing*). The presence of a precipitate also indicates the drug should not be used. Dangerous drugs should be disposed of as soon as the need is over. In the instructions *Atropine Drops For Eye Examination* we state, "Throw the unused medicine away by pouring them down the sink when the 3 days are over." If it is impossible to read the label, the drug should be discarded and replaced. Families/patients are reminded to check expiration dates and to dispose of medications if the date has passed.

Unused drugs should not be thrown in the trash because children or animals might ingest them. In the instructions *How to Give an Injection* we caution: "The law states that the syringe must be 'rendered inoperable.' This means the needle must be broken off and the plunger taken out. This will keep anyone from reusing a disposable syringe."

Proper storage conditions are also important. Some medications need to be refrigerated, and others kept at room temperature. Some medications are damaged by heat, light, or moisture; these statements are included in the teaching aid.

People must be reminded to store medication out of children's reach. This applies to all medications, those for adults as well as those for the child. A firm warning statement regarding the storage and disposal of pharmaceuticals is included in all medication Helping Hands. We use the words "caution" or "warning" in capital letters and set off the warning statement from the rest of the text with an outlined rectangle (Fig. 4.12).

NAME OF PATIENT AND DATE

In several of the Helping Hands, especially those about diagnostic tests or medications, we have included write-in blanks for the name of the patient and the date the Helping Hand is given. These are helpful for several reasons: (1) the child can relate to the instructions, since "these are for me," (2) the parent is assisted with medical record keeping, (3) the health professional can insure that the instructions are given to the right patient or family, and (4) if the Helping Hand is lost, the owner can be identified.

NUTRITION AND DIET

Good nutrition is an important factor for normal growth, development, and health of a patient. If it is suspected that the family has poor dietary habits, a teaching aid on the four basic food groups can be included in the home-going instructions. Parents are encouraged to follow the basic diet and avoid "junk foods" which contain empty calories. Proper selection of foods is a more significant factor than the amount of money the family has to spend for groceries. We discourage the selection of foods with high sugar content (such as pre-sweetened cereals) and sugary drinks.

Special attention is given to the diet and nutrition of children with allergies or other chronic conditions. If children are allergic to certain materials, such as Karaya gum, we give them a list of foods and products containing Karaya or India gum and instruct them to read labels carefully. If foods contain Karaya gum, other foods should be substituted (*Karaya or India Gum Allergies*).

For those patients taking prednisone, a list of foods rich in potassium is included since prednisone can cause potassium loss. For patients with iron deficiency anemia, a list of foods high in iron is provided, and excessive intake of milk is discouraged since children will not receive adequate iron-rich food if they continue to drink only milk.

Fluids to avoid are listed when appropriate. For example, patients who have a urinary diversion should not drink carbonated beverages because they are high in soda bicarbonate; this prevents the urine from remaining acidic (*Your Child's Urinary Diversion*).

Specific instructions about diet are included when preparing for a diagnostic test or surgery. For example, we tell patients exactly what to eat before having a gallbladder test. In preparing a child for surgery, we tell the parents the exact time food should be discontinued. Explicit instructions for infants state: "Give the 2 A.M. formula and nothing but water until the test is over." Nourishment is resumed following surgery as soon as fluids are tolerated. Maintaining adequate fluids is one of the main concerns in pediatrics. Because of the child's small size, dehydration can take place rapidly and must be prevented.

OBSERVATION

When performing a procedure, giving medications, or preparing for a diagnostic test, there are usually observations which the patient/family are asked to make. These statements are usually included under the appropriate subheading, rather than labeling one "Observation." For example, when changing a wet-to-dry dressing, we ask the parents to look for change in the color or odor of the wound, and to call the physician if "the drainage increases." We also tell them how the healing process takes place, "The wound should heal from the deepest part" (*Changing a Gauze Bandage*).

PERSONAL CARE

Discussing personal care can sometimes be a delicate subject. But as it relates to the condition, diagnostic test, or medication, the care of the body should be and is discussed. In *Care of an Artificial Eye* we instruct the patient to "Gently wash around the eye with a soft clean wash cloth and warm water. Make sure the lashes are clean. Pat dry." Colds and allergies increase the amount of drainage from the eye socket; so we instruct the patient to "Wipe this drainage away with a tissue. Start at the inside of the eye (next to the nose) and wipe toward his ear." At times, attention to personal hygiene extends to other family members. We ask the patient and family to bathe with pHisoDerm soap 3 days before a scheduled surgery date, to reduce the number of skin bacteria and prevent secondary incision infections.

Skin care is given special attention when decubitus ulcers could result. In the instructions for cast care and in those for wearing a brace we teach the patients to check for reddened areas daily. They are instructed to use alcohol to toughen the skin. If the reddened areas do not improve, they should consult their physician for advice and adjustment of the cast or brace. Protection of the skin for patients with ostomies is heavily emphasized in the instructions for urinary diversion.

Dental care is also considered in the total care of a patient. We try to send dental care instructions home with all patients, regardless of their diagnoses (*Cleaning the Teeth and Gums*). We encourage daily mouth hygiene when appropriate even though it is not the primary subject of the teaching aid. Some medications cause changes in the oral tissues. We encourage the parents of children who are taking certain drugs to maintain good oral hygiene to prevent irritation of the mouth.

Clothing is a factor to consider when caring for active children. Parents are advised to clothe children in loose-fitting clothing following an umbilical hernia repair. Tight clothing can produce skin friction and can cause the incision to become irritated. Suggested types of clothing are also indicated for patients wearing a brace or for those wearing ostomy appliances (*Umbilical Hernia Repair, Scoliosis, Your Child's Urinary Diversion*).

Care of bed linens and clothing is detailed in the teaching aids about scabies and head lice. Parents are advised to wash all clothing in hot water or have clothes dry cleaned following the application of lotion for either condition. If the clothing is not thoroughly cleaned the condition will recur. We place strong emphasis on proper care of clothing because either of these conditions can reach epidemic proportions if precautions are not taken (*Scabies, Head Lice*).

PREPARATION FOR DIAGNOSTIC TESTS

Often tests have to be cancelled due to misinformation or lack of preparation. The patient/family should have specific details when preparing for a diagnostic test; in the Helping Hands on diagnostic tests, we try to include as much information as possible.

For each diagnostic test teaching aid, a space is provided to designate the date, time, and location of the appointment. A phone number is also given in case the person must cancel the appointment.

If there are diet and fluid restrictions before a diagnostic test, the instructions must be very clear. For example, "Give your child a light supper between 4:00 and 6:00 the evening before the x-ray. We suggest fruit, fruit juice, vegetables (canned without fat or butter), and bread with jelly only. *Give no milk.* Your child should *not* have fatty foods like potato chips, meat, or fried foods" (*Having A Gallbladder Test*).

We believe psychological preparation is extremely important; especially if the tests are lengthy, if the child's eyes will be covered, or if the procedure causes pain or other sensations. We explain what the child will see, hear, and feel. For an example of such a test, see *Cardiac Catheterization*.

PREPARATION FOR SURGERY

Most Helping Hands on surgical procedures include the date and time the patient is to come to the hospital. In several cases, specific directions to the hospital and unit are given. Preparation of the child should be discussed in the teaching aid. Is a regular diet all right, or should the child have "nothing to eat or drink after midnight?" Can an infant have a 6:00 A.M. bottle? Is there any particular personal care the child should have at home (bath, hairwashing)?

Emotional preparation is also important. Explanations should be given to a patient about what is going to happen; the time to explain depends on the age of the patient. The main thing we stress is honesty. For example: if a child is going to have a T & A, we state: "You may tell your child that he is going to have two little lumps taken out of the back of his mouth. He will be taken to a big room. Then he will be given some sweet smelling air to make him sleep for a while. When he is asleep, the doctor will take out his tonsils. After his tonsils are out, he will go back to his room and be awake" (*Having a T & A*).

What will happen in the hospital is also discussed in the Helping Hands. This information may include facts about medications, diet and fluid allowances, what to expect after surgery, and additional instructions about the nursing unit (such as where the parents may wait during surgery).

PREVENTIVE CARE

Some aspects of preventive care have been discussed under Environment, Medications, Nutrition, and Personal Care. But because preventive care cannot be overemphasized, we include it as a separate element of every framework and consider it in writing each teaching aid.

The prevention of pain and injury is a high priority when treating a patient. You will notice that we use the word "gently" whenever rough handling could cause pain. For example, the diabetic instructions tell the best way to give an injection to make it less painful (*Giving an Insulin Injection*).

Recurrence of a disease or condition can be prevented if the cause is known and steps are taken to eradicate it. In some areas, scabies still plagues people for long periods of time because steps to prevent recurrence are not known or are not taken. Our Helping Hand *Scabies* states: "Family members should be examined and treated if they have signs of scabies on their skin. If you know where your child got the scabies, have the child avoid contact with that person until the person is treated and well."

PROCEDURES/TREATMENTS

Procedures and treatment methods are usually unfamiliar to the average patient or family. Therefore, you must take great care to accurately state all the steps in that method. Points to consider when writing a procedure are: the reason for the procedure, the equipment needed ("You Will Need"), the method ("What To Do"), handwashing, and safety.

When the reasons for the procedure and instruction are given, it is easier for the person to comprehend and to comply. For instance, when teaching *Crutch Walking,* we don't just say, "Never lean on underarm pieces". We add the reason, "This can cause nerve damage." We further state how to keep the body weight off the underarm pieces: "Always push down with hands."

Note the equipment and supplies needed to carry out the procedure/treatment. A list, separated from the rest of the text, lends easy access to the information and can also serve as a checklist (refer to Equipment, p. 88).

We have found that the easiest way to write procedures/treatments is in list form, using numbers to designate the steps. For example, to treat *Amblyopia,* the eye patch must be applied correctly.

"1. Remove the gauze backing. (The side that goes next to the skin will be sticky.)

2. Have the child close his eye.

3. Gently place the narrow end of the patch toward the child's nose (Picture 1). (If the child wears glasses, apply the patch directly over the eye and wear glasses over the patch.)

4. Put patch on _____ eye _____ day.

5. Remove the patch at bedtime."

We always stress safety and prevention of injury and infection when carrying out procedures. An example of preventing injury is pointed out in the instructions, *Caring for the Child With a Tracheostomy:* when suctioning, we instruct the parent to "Twirl catheter between thumb and index finger to keep catheter from sticking to the trachea."

An example of prevention of infection is: "Keep the bandage clean, dry, and in place until the doctor removes it. DO NOT take off the bandage. You may put more tape over the bandage to keep it on. If the bandage comes off or gets wet, call the doctor or clinic for advice" (*Umbilical Hernia Repair*).

SAFETY

Accidents and injury are best prevented when we educate patients and families about safe practices and give them reasonable explanations of what may occur if recommended practices are ignored. For the most part, safety tips are not listed separately under a safety heading, rather, they are incorporated into the appropriate section. For example, if the patient/family is using drugs or equipment we state, "Store out of children's reach." When instructing about the use of a thermometer, we state, "You are placing a piece of glass in your child's body. *Never leave child alone while taking his temperature"* (*Taking a Temperature*).

Warnings are given throughout the instructions whenever factors exist that could prove harmful. In the instructions for treating scabies, we state, "If any of the lotion happens to get into the eyes, wash the eyes with cool water" (*Scabies*). Another example is found in *Hydrocarbon Ingestion:* "Warning. Children who drink harmful products once, are likely to do it again. Children are naturally curious. *Keep all harmful substances out of the reach of children."*

SPACES FOR ADDITIONAL INFORMATION

In several Helping Hands, blank lines are provided for insertion of handwritten material; this serves to promote and to maintain individualized care of the patient. If there are several variables to be considered in preparing for the test, blank spaces are included. The physician can fill these in on an individual basis. For example, in *Having a Barium Enema* there are so many age groups who have this test that it is difficult to state the diet required, so space is left for this to be completed.

WRITING STYLE: SENSE AND SENSITIVITY

It is hoped that you now have much of the information needed to develop a system for creating your teaching aids. But one more area remains for discussion—how to put the words together. Authorities on writing styles differ in their advice to authors. Some, like Rudolph Flesch, advise to "write the way you talk." Other, more formal stylists, guide you in the "proper" way of writing.

For our teaching aids, we have chosen the informal style of presentation. We want patients and families to feel comfortable while reading the Helping Hands and, more importantly, we want them to *understand* the information. We also want the families to sense that we are discussing the information *with* them, so we begin each Helping Hand with "Let's Talk About . . . . "

The information in this part of the chapter will assist you in writing teaching aids in an informal, conversational tone. For many of you, this will be just a review or a refresher, but for others, it may be the most important part of the chapter. The following sections include discussion of grammar, punctuation, and style; a method for computing language level; and considerations about word choice.

GRAMMAR AND STYLE

In elementary school, we learned the correct method of constructing sentences and the proper use of words and punctuation. Hopefully, we have retained most practical applications of this knowledge. But, if some of us were asked to diagram a sentence or identify a dangling participle, we would be at a loss without our trusty English grammar book. Fortunately, it is a bit easier, and somewhat more automatic to construct simple sentences and list step-by-step procedures for a Helping Hand.

In writing our teaching aids, use of the "Fog Index" helps to eliminate the long, trailing, complicated sentences; use of the style guide and word lists assist in stating the information in the most understandable way.

We use our style guide to insure consistency in the use of grammar and punctuation, particularly in cases where correct usage may be arbitrary (Fig. 4.13). It also lists rules of form and style, such as paragraph indentation, use of phonetic spelling, use of headings and subheadings, and so on. You may use our style guide as a model in formulating your own guide.

GRAMMAR AND GENDER

TENSE

- Use whatever tense is appropriate in the information.
- Definition and explanation—present tense
- Body of instructions—present tense
- Things to be expected—future tense
- Actual past occurrences—past tense

PERSON

- In general, use second person "you," "your child."
- Third person can also be used.

GENDER

- Be cognizant of representing race and sex fairly.
- Speak directly to the parents or to the child: "your child," "the child," "you."
- Use either "he" or "she," but not he/she or s/he.

HEADINGS AND SUBHEADINGS

TITLES

- Use Prestype for all titles.
- Use Prestype within the text for emphasis if the material is lengthy.

FIRST LEVEL SUBHEADS

- Capitalize all letters in the subheading.
- Underline the subhead.
- Begin type two spaces below the subhead.

FIGURE 4.13 Our Helping Hand Style Guide

- Subhead should be flush with left margin.
- All text is flush with the margin.

MEDICATIONS

Your doctor may have given you a prescription for drugs or ointment. Use these medications as directed.

SECOND LEVEL SUBHEADS

- Capitalize the first letter of each major word.
- Underline the subheading.
- Subheading should be flush with the left margin.

KARAYA GUM IS FOUND IN

Candy and Gum

- Gum drops
- Jelly beans
- Kraft caramels
- Most chewy candies

THIRD LEVEL SUBHEADS

- Capitalize the first letter of each major word and underline.
- Indent this subhead under preceding heading.
- Text follows immediately after a dash.

LISTS OF INFORMATION

BULLETS (DOTS)

- Use dots to emphasize important points within the text.
- When dots are used for listing unrelated points under one heading, the first line is indented, all others are flush with the margin.

SPECIAL TIPS

- When you have to be some place at a certain time, allow yourself more time to get ready. Don't hurry getting into a car. You might tilt back and cause the brace to hurt you.

- When dots are used for material that is listed, all lines of type are flush.

FURNISHINGS IN THE CHILD'S ROOM

- Bed—Beds in the child's room should have wooden or metal frames. Do not use a couch, sofa, or hide-a-bed.
- Mattress—Place the mattress in a vinyl (soft plastic) cover which has a zipper. If a box spring is used, it must have a plastic cover, too.

FIGURE 4.13 (Continued)

STEPS

- Use numbers for designating steps in a procedure.
- Place numbers flush with the margin.
- For steps with 2 or more lines of type, indent material under first line of typing.

WHAT YOU SHOULD DO

1. Stay calm.
2. Take your child to the bathroom and shut the door. Turn on the shower and hot water faucets to make steam. Be careful to keep away from the hot water (Picture 1).
3. Sit with the child and let him breathe in the steam.

CHECK BOXES

- Check boxes are used to emphasize equipment needed, important procedures, or information to parents.
- The first line of type is indented 4 or 5 spaces, all lines to follow are also indented.
- Double space between each statement if space allows.

THE DOCTOR'S ORDER

☐ Change bandage and clean wound with _____ solution _____ times per day.
☐ Change soiled bandage. Do not clean the wound.
☐ Do not remove bandage. If bandage is soiled, apply sterile gauze bandage on top of the bandage that is on the wound.

PARAGRAPHS

- Begin all paragraphs flush with the left margin.
- Leave one space between paragraphs.

PHONE NUMBERS

- If a phone number follows the location, put it in parentheses.

Call the Emergency Room (123-4567).

- If a blank line is left for phone numbers, enclose it in parentheses: with "phone".

Call your doctor (phone:_____).

FIGURE 4.13 (Continued)

PHONETIC SPELLING

- Spell a word phonetically if the word is long and/or if it is unfamiliar to patient/family.
- Enclose phonetically spelled word in parentheses:

`Electrocardiogram (e-lek-tro-CAR-dee-oh-gram)`

- Do not use the dictionary pronunciation symbols.

PICTURE AND PAGE IDENTIFICATION

REFERENCE TO PICTURES

- Use the word "Picture" rather than "Figure."
- Spell out "Picture" in text; say (Picture 1).
- In general, include "(Picture 1)" as part of the sentence rather than placing it outside sentence.

`Put jars in the pan (Picture 1).`

CAPTIONS

- Emphasize the most important point in instructions and/or illustration.
- Keep captions brief.
- If caption is a complete sentence use a period; if it is a phrase, do not use a period.
- Spell out "Picture" in the caption: Picture 1.

PAGE IDENTIFICATION

- Page numbers are usually placed in the upper right corner.
- Type title of Helping Hand before page number.
- Type "(continued)" or "OVER" on the bottom right hand corner of all pages except the last.

PUNCTUATION

APOSTROPHE

- Indicates ownership or a relationship analogous to ownership. The apostrophe precedes the "s", except in the plural possessive and in the possessive of "it" (its').

COLON

- Introduces material that follows immediately.
- Use before the enumeration of items.

FIGURE 4.13 (Continued)

COMMA

- Use to set off sentence elements.
- Use to separate words; place the comma before the conjunction in a series of two or more items: knives, forks, and spoons.
- Omit commas in short sentences.

HYPHEN

- Use to join words combined into a single adjective modifier: fine-toothed comb, well-balanced diet.
- Use for separating phonetic syllables of words not common to the lay person: gastrostomy (gas-TRAH-sto-me).

PERIOD

- Use after complete sentences.
- Do not use periods after incomplete sentences, such as those found in lists or those following a statement using a colon.
- Place period *inside* parentheses when they enclose a complete sentence.
- Place period *outside* parentheses when one part of the sentence is enclosed.

PARENTHESES

- Use to set off explanatory matter or abbreviated words which follow a technical term: intrauterine device (IUD).
- Use to set off phonetic spelling of words.

QUOTATION MARKS

- Use to set off words commonly used, but not technically correct: Hepatitis is often called "yellow jaundice."
- Use to set off an abbreviated form of a medical word: Tracheostomy, "Trach." Then, use the shortened word *without* quotation marks, throughout the teaching aid.

SEMICOLON

- Use between two related statements joined together without a conjunction.

FIGURE 4.13 (Continued)

LANGUAGE LEVEL

The Helping Hands address people from all walks of life and many age groups. For this reason we have chosen to write our instructions at a sixth to eighth grade reading level. To stay within this range, we use a formula developed by Robert Gunning, a communications expert. The Gunning formula enables us to arrive at what he calls the "Fog Index." The higher the index the more "fog" exists in the written material, the lower the number, the less fog. Gunning's formula offers a quick way to compute the reading level of written instructions. This is how it is done:

1. Count off 100 words in the written material you want to test. Do not use a larger sample than this, because the formula does not work otherwise. Make a mark at the end of the hundredth word. If the material is lengthy, you should take several samples, say at every tenth page or hundredth page.

2. Figure the average length of sentences in the 100 word sample. Stop with the sentence that ends nearest (either before or after) the 100-word mark. For example, if two sentences make up 104 words, then the average sentence length would be 52 words. If

there are 10 sentences in 96 words, the average length is 96 divided by 10 or 9.6 words.

3. Next, find the percentage of difficult words. To do this, count the number of "hard words" in the sample. These are words of three syllables or more. Divide this number of difficult words by the total number of words in the sample. (In a 100-word sample, the number of hard words can be used directly as the percentage figure.) Do not count compound words that are a combination of short easy words (like bookkeeper or white-collar). And do not count words in which a third syllable is formed by adding "ed" or "es" (for example, expected or assesses).

4. Last, add the percentage of hard words to the average sentence length. Then multiply the sum by 0.4. This will give you the Fog Index. (Gunning, p. 35-39). The answer indicates the school grade reading level necessary to read the passage easily. (The reading level of college graduates is 17.) A sample calculation follows:

$$14.3 \text{ Average words per sentence}$$
$$+7.0 \text{ Percentage of hard words}$$
$$\overline{21.3}$$
$$\times 0.4$$
$$\overline{8.52} \text{ Fog Index (8th grade level)}$$

It may seem that a Fog Index of 6.0–8.0 is too low, since most of our readers are adults. But it must be remembered that the stress of an illness or medical condition interferes with a person's ability to comprehend what he is reading. In addition, many medical terms are not merely "hard words"; they may be completely unfamiliar terms. To allow for these factors, and to make reading comfortable for a school age patient, we keep the Fog Index low.

WORDS, WORDS, WORDS

The careful use of words in a pediatric or any health care setting cannot be emphasized enough. Young children interpret things literally. They also have difficulty grasping the meaning of subtleties and abstractions. For these reasons, some adults have difficulty communicating with children. For example, a nurse might say to a child, "You are on strict bed rest." To a youngster or even an adult this might mean "lie perfectly still for a while before you get up." Therefore, the vocabulary used in writing instructions must be clear and concise. There are three main categories of words to consider; these are medical jargon, common words, and slang terms.

Medical Jargon

The medical jargon used in our everyday conversation must be carefully monitored in our writing. We cannot write exactly the way we talk, because the words we use in the hospital setting can have a different meaning to the lay person or child. For example, a child thought he was going to "die" when he was told, "I am going to inject the dye for the test." In writing the Helping Hand, *Cardiac Catheterization,* we carefully chose the words to describe the test procedure and avoided the use of the word "dye." "A solution is then put into the tube, and it flows into the heart. This shows a picture of your heart on a screen like a TV screen."

We should be constantly aware of what our words mean to others. Casual use of clinical words and abbreviations in conversing with patients usually confuses them and often causes them undue uncertainty and anxiety about their hospital stay.

Some clinical words such as hematocrit, impaction, reflux, and hemorrhage are simply not part of a person's vocabulary. Others, such as elimination, culture, scrub, stool, traction, and sterile, mean one thing to the health professional and quite another to most patients/families. We believe health professionals who use clinical language without consideration of the patient's possible misunderstanding or misinterpretation add to the communication gap between staff and patients and also increase the chance for errors.

For our use in writing the Helping Hands, we have compiled a word list of medical terms and abbreviations used in our setting. In the list, the alphabetized words are those commonly used in medical terminology, the words and phrases in parentheses are suggested ways of stating the previous term. A few of the words are: ambulate (walk); bacteria (germs); CBC (count the cells in your blood); discharge (go home from the hospital); decubitus (sore, bedsore, scab); fracture (broken bone); force fluids (drink lots of water or juice); NPO (nothing to eat or drink). These words serve as a reference guide and reminder as we write our teaching aids; they also promote a consistent use of words.

Common Words

Even nonclinical terms may cause difficulties. In the course of our professional education we learned to write "utilization" when we meant "use," "facilitate" for "make easier," "objectives" for "goals," "examination" for "test," and so on. But in writing instructions for patients, it is imperative that we un-learn this approach to word usage. We have to make a conscious concerted effort to substitute the simple common word when one can be found with the same meaning. A thesaurus is an indispensable aid in finding understandable synonyms. Another useful reference is a dictionary written for school-age children. You may wish to compile a list of commonly used words; the list serves as a quick and ready reference which provides consistency in word usage.

One language scholar has estimated that for the 500 most commonly used English words, there are fourteen thousand meanings. It's amazing that people, especially children, are able to make sense out of most language!

Slang Terms

Slang terms and colloquialisms are woven into the fiber of our culture and language. But each subculture has its own set of slang terms and may resent their use by persons who do not belong to their group. When a slang term becomes widespread in usage, it is usually abandoned by the group who originated it. Consider the demise of the term "groovy." When teenagers, who first used the term, began hearing it from the lips of their parents and stodgy news commentators, they branded the word "old-fashioned," clearly "out-of-it"!

So slang has two major drawbacks in written communication. If you use the term and do not belong to your readers' subculture it will be resented and most slang terms are quickly outdated. So, if you use them in your teaching aids, you will either have to revise the instructions when the term is no longer popular, or suffer the embarrassment of being out of tune with the times. It is far safer and more practical to avoid slang terms altogether.

As you can see, the words you use determine the readability, interest and information-sharing ability of your teaching aids. Words are wonderful, but they must be used carefully and with thought. Don't be too disappointed if your first attempts at wielding the written word are not the success you desired. It takes time. Practice helps—and so will our Helping Hands. Feel free to use our Helping Hands in writing your teaching aids; if you can use them verbatim, that's just fine, but you will probably need to modify the information slightly to meet the needs of your setting and patient population. The Helping Hands are presented in Part 2 of this book for your information and use: we hope they will Help you in this challenging and rewarding endeavor.

USING HELPING HANDS: A REWARDING EXPERIENCE

A 13-year-old girl was admitted to our hospital with a possible diagnosis of lymphoma. Her abdomen was distended with some type of solid mass; she was extremely tired and uncomfortable. That night after all the patients were asleep, the nurse discovered the young girl wide awake and very "anxious." She sat down to talk with her to find out the reason she couldn't sleep.

After some time the girl finally revealed that she was frightened about what was going to happen to her. She had been told she was going to have a bone marrow test the following day, and since she really didn't know what

that meant, she had concluded that they were going to take out a piece of bone.

The nurse, concerned that the girl had not been given an adequate explanation, proceeded to tell her about the test. The nurse also gave her the Helping Hand to read to reinforce what they had discussed.

After asking several questions, the girl told the nurse she "felt lots better." She hadn't understood that, "they were going to take a little blood" and not, "a piece of bone." Nor did she know they were going to use "numbing medicine."

The nurse told the girl that she had to leave to check in on some of the other children, but that she would come back in a little while to see if she had any further questions. Later, when she went back to see her, the young girl was fast asleep.

The following night, the nurse made a point to stop in and ask how she was feeling. The young girl replied, "Even though the bone marrow test hurt a little, I could take it because I knew what was happening. The Helping Hand really helped! I hope you have instructions like that for the other tests I have to take."

Stories such as this one continue to provide the incentive for directing our energies to patient education. The development of each Helping Hand potentially bridges another gap of misunderstanding or lack of communication. *Patients and families must have information to understand, and must have information they understand to ask questions.*

Have you ever observed two people who speak different languages trying to converse? They may spend much time attempting to overcome the language barrier with the few words they each know. They struggle. They pause. They gesture. Then suddenly smiles appear and the anxiety is gone. They have communicated—and they understand.

This is the feeling you will experience with your patients and families when you overcome the language barrier of that "foreign language" of medicine. By providing understandable instructions and written reinforcement, patients are able to understand: and that's what the Helping Hands are all about. Good luck and good writing!

SELECTED READINGS

Berrey, Lester V., *Roget's International Thesaurus.* Rev. ed. New York: Thomas Y. Crowell Co., 1962.

Chinn, Peggy. *Child Health Maintenance in Family Centered Care.* St. Louis: C.V. Mosby Co., 1974.

Flesch, Rudolph. *Say What You Mean.* New York: Harper & Row, 1972.

Gunning, Robert. *The Technique of Clear Writing.* New York: McGraw-Hill Book Co., 1968.

Hilt, Nancy and Schmidt, E. William, Jr. *Pediatric Orthopedic Nursing*. St. Louis: C.V. Mosby Co., 1975.

Klinzing, Dennis R. and Klinzing, Dene G. *The Hospitalized Child: Communication Techniques for Health Personnel*. Englewood Cliffs, N.J.: Prentice-Hall, 1977.

Larson, Carroll and Gould, Marjorie. *Orthopedic Nursing*. 7th ed. St. Louis: C.V. Mosby Co., 1970.

Leiffer, Gloria. *Principles and Techniques in Pediatric Nursing*. 2d ed. Philadelphia: W.B. Saunders Co., 1977.

Loebl, Suzanne; Heckheimer, Estelle; Spratto, George; and Wit, Andrew; *The Nurse's Drug Handbook*. New York: John Wiley & Sons, 1977.

Marlow, Dorothy R. *Textbook of Pediatric Nursing*. 3d ed. Philadelphia: W.B. Saunders Co., 1973.

Petrillo, Madeline and Sanger, Sirgay. *Emotional Care of Hospitalized Children: An Environmental Approach*. Philadelphia: J.B. Lippincott Co., 1972.

chapter 5

Pictures and Print: Putting It All Together

Jenene De Mars Warmbier

"The artist does not express his own feelings, but what he knows about human feelings. The images formed by the artist extend the limits of a child's experience . . . and the frontiers of human knowledge."

Susan Langer

A story is often told about the great master, Michaelangelo. Admiring onlookers visited daily to check the progress of his magnificent fresco on the ceiling of the Sistine Chapel. Each day for years Michaelangelo lay on his back atop a tower of scaffolding and unfolded with his brush the majesty of the "Creation of Man." One day an admirer stopped the Master as he was finishing a day's work. "Ah, to have been born with such great talent! God has truly blessed you!" The artist reflected on his years of pains-taking, punishing labor. "My friend," he said, "talent is only 1% inspiration. But it is 99% perspiration."

You can probably recall experiences in your own life when you have envied artistic talent. Remember the time in third grade when you drew a Nativity scene for Christmas open house? Can you ever forget your embarrassment when your teacher thought your St. Joseph was one of the brown cows in the stable? There was probably a smug little boy or girl in your class whose cows *always* looked exactly like cows. This child was the one chosen by the teacher to spend class time decorating bulletin boards and painting the safety contest posters. And you decided that artists are born, not made, and were so relieved when art was no longer a required school subject.

But now you're faced with the problem of illustrating your teaching aids, and that old bugaboo, artistic talent, comes back to haunt you.

WHAT TO ILLUSTRATE AND WHY

If, until now, your training and experience has been concentrated in the health care field, you probably have had little exposure to the world of graphics and printing. The abundance of unfamiliar terms and techniques discussed in this chapter may be a bit overwhelming at first. That's understandable. But we hope these "thumbnail sketches" of graphic media and methods will help you in developing your teaching aids.

We like to think of this information as a kind of cook-book for the new bride. We have included several "recipes" here and have tried to explain how to use and to combine "ingredients." While the new bride may take a simple recipe and follow it to the letter on her first culinary adventure, in time she will gain confidence and skill. Eventually, she will add her own creative touch, substituting a pinch of this or adding a dash of that, perhaps producing a gourmet's delight that clearly outshines the original recipe in quality and uniqueness.

When you first set out to produce your own teaching aids, you may be more comfortable in following our "recipes" to the letter. But in time, you will probably feel sufficiently confident to experiment—to try varied approaches to solving a problem and to formulate new techniques for creating your own pièce de résistance.

Creative graphics, like creative cookery, cannot be neatly summarized and contained in a precise recipe. There are *few* firm rules to follow—only guidelines, hints, suggestions, and a healthy mixture of instinct and intuition. And, like culinary art, developing visual graphics that are appealing and impressive takes time and practice.

The information in this chapter should be referred to as one would consult a cookbook. It's not necessary to memorize the recipes or to know all the definitions of terms at the outset. It's not even a requisite to have all the tools on hand before you can begin. You may find that you don't need some of these devices, or you may discover useful graphic aids that have not been included here. As you deal with printers and graphic arts suppliers you will hear new terms that are part of the jargon of the trade, and you may not find them discussed in these pages. To define all the terms would fill a tome the size of the original Gutenberg bible, but many of these terms are either too technical or too uncommon to be included here.

You may be expecting to find a "recipe" here that teaches you how to draw. But lessons in drawing and illustrating are not within the scope of this chapter. Nevertheless, we *do* offer a guide to determining what to illustrate, idea sources for illustrations, criteria for judging quality of the finished artwork, information on printing processes, and guides to using graphic materials and techniques. There are a number of suggested readings at the end of this chapter which offer a wealth of reference material about drawing and illustrating technique. In addition, some useful crutches are provided in this book; the illustrations in the Helping Hands and the body outlines of children and adults may be traced or copied for use in your teaching aids.

WHY ILLUSTRATE?

"Why not just skip the illustrations?" you might ask. Who is going to miss the illustrations if the teaching aids are well-written and to the point? Well, think for a moment about your earliest learning experiences as a child. Remember picture storybooks? Did you ever make up your own story by simply "reading" the pictures? Think about how much *information* the pictures gave you. You knew a teddy bear was fat, soft, brown, fuzzy, and small enough to cuddle under your arm by just looking at the picture. You didn't need to read to learn this.

Most adults have not unlearned the habit of looking at a picture for information. If you open a Sunday newspaper and turn first to the editorial page, you're a rare bird. Most people look first at the comics, the pictorial magazine section, or the richly illustrated department store ads. Now obviously, a picture is rarely enough to give you all the information you need. And it does you little good to be captivated by an advertisement for a shiny new sports coupe if the ad doesn't tell you how much it will cost and where you can buy it. But the picture alone can tell you a lot of what you want to know, and it can attract your interest and make you want to read what is written about the picture.

Some investigators claim that learning is nearly 80% visual. The percentage may vary with a person's age, cultural background, or education. But it's interesting to note that a study conducted by the Communications Research Center of Boston University offered these conclusions about the highly visual medium of comic strips: (1) comic strip readership is widespread among various age, education, and occupational levels and (2) as one progresses from grade school through college, the percentage of regular readers of comics increases (by a factor of almost two); highly educated persons are favorably inclined toward the medium (Brown et al, p. 426–427).

The attention-getting feature of illustrations cannot be lightly dismissed. When we began sending the drafts of Helping Hands to staff members for their review and comments, we supplied only the written copy. Illustrations were added later. The edited papers trailed back to us with all the speed of a snail going to an escargot party. It wasn't that our reviewers were not enthusiastic about the program or did not recognize the need for patient teaching aids. But with the monotonous appearance of double-spaced typed drafts, the proposed Helping Hands became hopelessly mingled with other mountains of words-on-paper that heaped the desks and "In" baskets of our reviewers. When we added illustrations and prepared the papers in semifinal layout form, the time for papers to be returned was reduced by nearly half.

The need for attention-getting illustrations is even more important when the users of the teaching aids are young patients and their families. Much of the printed material available to patients assumes that most people like to read, and that everyone reads well. In Chapter 4, we've talked about how our Helping Hands contain language that is readable for the majority of our patients. Pictures that patients can also "read" enhance the meaning of the written word. Before a Helping Hand is printed, we share it with patients and families for their critique and comments. In most cases, they study the pictures first. Then they read the text to see what story it tells about the pictures. Less often do we see them read the text first, and then study the pictures for more information.

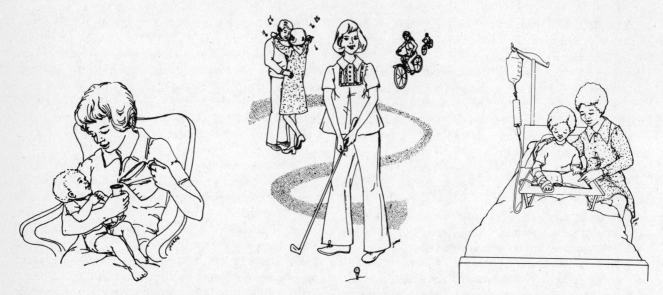

FIGURE 5.1 Pictures give the reader a powerful psychological suggestion to imitate the behavior that is illustrated.

Even when the information is clearly and logically written, steps in a procedure can be confusing to a patient. But art is a universal medium that can be used effectively to relate complex medical concepts to patients who are not familiar with medical practices and terminology. If you have ever tried to *tell* a child how to tie his shoe laces without actually showing him how to do it, you know that words alone do not convey to a child what is, for him, a complicated procedure. When teaching a patient a procedure, such as how to change a dressing, you would first demonstrate the procedure before sending the patient home with written instructions. But once at home, the patient does not have you beside him to refresh his memory of steps in the procedure that he has forgotten. Illustrations of these steps can "stand in" for you and can clarify the written instructions since you cannot be there to demonstrate again or to answer questions.

Are you still unconvinced about using illustrations in your teaching aids? Then perhaps you can take a lesson from Uncle Sam. He's the fellow with the white hair, goatee, top hat, and red, white, and blue vested suit, who has become a symbol of our country. During the World War II, few people could resist being stirred by feelings of national pride and patriotic duty when confronted by the "Uncle Sam Wants You" poster. The intense expression on his face, the index finger pointing a command, challenged every American to serve his country. But how do we know Uncle Sam looks like that? He exists only through the creative imagery of an illustrator. Imagine the poster without the picture. How much emotional impact would the words have by themselves?

When you illustrate your teaching aids, you can convey love, warmth, acceptance, confidence, trust, and a whole rainbow of positive feelings. You will influence the patient or parent to identify with the emotional tone set by the pictures. For example, in Figure 5.1, the mother in the

picture is cuddling her baby in her arms while she feeds him through his G-tube. The picture gives the reader a powerful psychological suggestion to do likewise. The child who has an I.V. in his arm turns the pages of a book with his free hand, while mother smiles approvingly (Fig. 5.1). This picture also conveys a psychological message. The child says to himself: "That kid in the picture has an I.V. just like me. If he can use his other hand to do things,

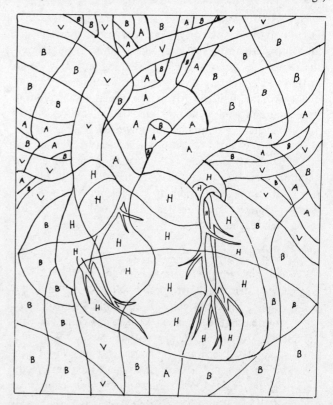

FIGURE 5.2 Instructional games invite the reader to participate physically as well as intellectually in the learning process.

so can I." A girl with scoliosis is pictured enjoying golf, biking, and dancing while wearing her brace under a stylish, loose-fitting blouse (Fig. 5.1). The message for the patient is clear: "I don't have to act like an invalid just because I'm wearing a brace."

Some types of pictures can invite the patient to become involved physically as well as emotionally in the content of the paper. Instructional games or puzzles (such as cross-words or connect-the-dots), as well as coloring pages for younger children, can aid in the retention of material the patient has learned. For our Helping Hand *Cardiac Catheterization*, we devised a "color by number" type of picture (Fig. 5.2). When the child has finished coloring, he has a picture of how his heart looks inside his body. We also designed a crossword puzzle (Fig. 5.3) for diabetic children. This puzzle entertainingly tests their knowledge

Insulin Crossword Puzzle

ACROSS

1. One treatment for _____ is insulin.
5. Another word for Mom
7. Be sure to _____ injection sites.
9. _____, two, three!
10. If blood appears in syringe, start _____.
11. Opposite of Jr.
12. NPH and Lente are _____ insulins.
15. Use a new _____ and syringe for each injection.
16. A preposition
19. There should be _____ air bubbles in the syringe.
20. Short way of saying advertisement.
22. Many years _____, insulin was discovered.
23. _____ up the area before injection.
26. Cloudy and clear insulin in the syringe is a _____ dose.
28. _____ of injection means changing injection sites daily.
30. Amounts of medicines are called _____.
32. "_____ unto others. . . ."
33. For a _____ dose, you use one type of insulin.
35. "_____ frog" (game).
36. _____ the syringe to get rid of air bubbles.
37. Wash your _____ before preparing insulin.

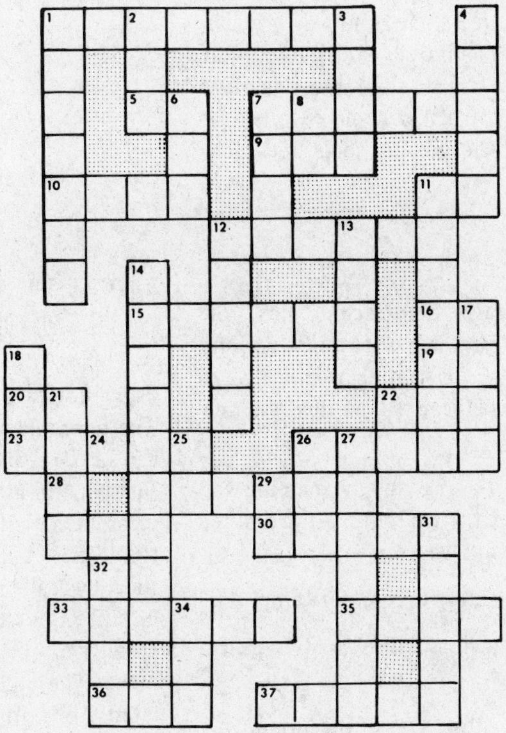

DOWN

1. _____ of all used syringes.
2. There are injection sites on the _____.
3. The place for an injection is called a _____.
4. _____ insulin can be mixed with cloudy.
6. _____ must be put in the bottle before insulin can come out.
7. _____ the bottle of cloudy insulin between the hands.
8. Opposite of Off.
11. A _____ is used to inject insulin.
12. _____ the injection site with an alcohol swab.
13. Dispose of all _____ syringes and needles.
14. Giving medicine with a syringe and needle is called an _____.
17. Eating proper _____ is important.
18. The syringe _____ protects the needle.
21. Mud; soil.
22. A chopping tool.
24. Opposite of Yes.
25. Laughing sound.
26. Sound a cow makes.
27. Your medicine is called _____.
29. Short for "I would."
31. _____ are another name for cotton balls.
32. A well-balanced _____ is important for health.
34. A space between things.

ACROSS: 1. Diabetes, 5. Ma, 7. Rotate, 9. One, 10. Over, 11. Sr., 12. Cloudy, 15. Needle, 16. If, 19. No, 20. Ad, 22. Ago, 23. Pinch, 26. Mixed, 28. Rotation, 30. Doses, 32. Do, 33. Single, 35. Leap, 36. Tap, 37. Hands. DOWN: 1. Dispose, 2. Arm, 3. Site, 4. Clear, 6. Air, 7. Roll, 8. On, 11. Syringe, 12. Clean, 13. Used, 14. Injection, 17. Food, 18. Cap, 21. Dirt, 22. Ax, 24. No, 25. Ha, 26. Moo, 27. Insulin, 29. I'd, 31. Swabs, 32. Diet, 34. Gap.

FIGURE 5.3 Insulin crossword puzzle.

of diabetes and administration of single and mixed-dose insulin.

Hopefully the preceding examples and arguments have convinced you of the advantages of illustrated teaching aids. But an equally important question is still unanswered: *who* is going to do the illustrating? You were conditioned in elementary school to think that you "can't draw a straight line without a ruler." So to have illustrated teaching aids, it appears that you'll have to commission a freelance artist or medical illustrator, or you'll have to do the illustrations yourself. You may feel there is no way you can turn out professional looking illustrations yourself without extensive art training. But the truth—a carefully guarded secret—is that even the nonartist can become surprisingly adept at illustration by using the graphic tools and techniques described in this chapter.

WHAT TO ILLUSTRATE

Once you've decided to illustrate your teaching aids, you must determine which parts of the written instructions should be pictured. The "right" illustration is not always the obvious one. Read through the draft of the teaching aid and look for these features:

- The degree of difficulty the patient or parent will have in visualizing a part of the anatomy, a procedure, or medical equipment and supplies

- Psychological and cultural factors that require emphasis

- Attitudes and concepts, such as safety and hygiene, that should be stressed

- Aspects of the topic that involve "fear of the unknown"

Difficulty in Visualizing Anatomy, Procedures, and Equipment

Let's take an example, "tracheostomy care," and see how the first item in this list applies. Are the patient and parent able to visualize how the unseen part of the trach tube fits inside the trachea? Do they understand where the trachea is located and its relationship to the larynx and lungs? It's easy to assume that a family knows more about anatomy than they actually do. Many people are embarrassed to admit their ignorance of anatomy and are reluctant to ask questions about things they don't understand. A simplified anatomical drawing will provide the needed information before they have to ask, thus saving them from embarrassment (Fig. 5.4). Procedures like suctioning may also be hard to visualize. Illustrations can show how to hold the catheter, how to use the Y-connector, and how to twirl the catheter. If you have instructed the mother in the child's care and have given her an illustrated teaching aid, she can use the pictures to explain procedures to the child's father or to others who may be involved in his care.

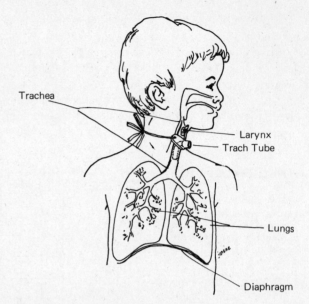

FIGURE 5.4 Simple anatomical drawing of the respiratory system shows how the trach tube fits inside the trachea.

Psychological and Cultural Factors

The psychological impact of a disease or chronic condition can be far-reaching for a young child. A picture may show the patient at home with family and friends, engaged in pleasant activities that are suitable for his age and condition. There are several psychosocial messages here. Despite the physical limitations imposed by the child's condition, he still enjoys, and is enjoyed by, his family and friends. His growth and development are given emphasis and encouragement. The child, although ill or incapacitated, is not isolated from other family members, nor is he overprotected by them.

Just as the patient needs to identify psychologically with your illustrations, he should also be able to find cultural similarities. People of different racial and ethnic groups should be depicted. In the real world all children are not blue-eyed blond boys. Black, Chicano, and Oriental children should be able to find representative models in your illustrations. Both girls and boys should see women doctors and fathers who cuddle their babies. It's not necessary to have one white, one black, and one Oriental child in every picture that depicts three children. Nor do you need to show one female doctor for every male. This kind of "equalizing" can look stilted and artificial. But if your patient population is predominantly black, it only makes sense to have more black children than others in your illustrations.

Attitudes and Concepts Requiring Emphasis

Attitudes and concepts may be difficult to illustrate because they are abstract. But they require emphasis because a patient will not be inclined to change ingrained habits, in such areas as safety or personal hygiene, unless you can foster a change in attitude. But how do you illustrate "clean" or "safe"? We use a handwashing picture in many of our Helping Hands (Fig. 5.5). The sometimes complicated cleaning or sterilizing procedures are also illustrated in great detail.

Safety is a more difficult problem. To illustrate the danger of aspirin ingestion, you can show a child climbing up into the medicine cabinet; but for the child who sees the picture, it may look like an example of what he *should* do. Forceful captions such as DANGER and WARNING: KEEP OUT OF CHILDREN'S REACH will solve the problem to some degree. Another alternative is to show some positive action, such as a parent installing a lock on the medicine cabinet. Whenever feasible, the illustration should be an example of recommended or acceptable behavior, since the visual image may remain in the reader's memory longer than the caption beneath it.

Fear of the Unknown

Another area that may need graphic emphasis concerns the patient's fear of the unknown. When a child is being prepared for surgery, he is often shown the anesthesia mask, the recovery room, and even the intensive care unit. Seeing the rooms and equipment beforehand can reduce his anxiety (Fig. 5.6). Even for a simple diagnostic test, such as a routine x-ray, a child may conjure up many frightful fantasies about what he expects to see in Radiology. When the child cannot be given a "sneak preview" of what he will see, you can show him a *picture* of the diagnostic equipment to help dispel these fantasies and fears. To give the patient a realistic picture of the room and equipment, you may use photos, drawings, or a combination of the two called photo-sketching.

So, in deciding what parts of the teaching aid should be

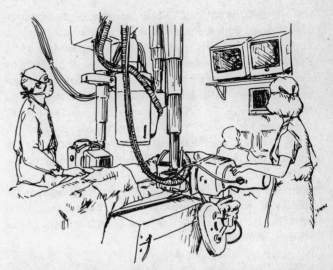

FIGURE 5.6 Cardiac catheterization: The heart lab. Showing a patient a picture of what he will see and experience helps to dispel fears and fantasies.

illustrated, look beyond the obvious subject matter. Think of all the messages that a good illustration can convey. Since most diseases and conditions affect the *total* patient, each illustration should also reflect a multitude of the patient's concerns and needs.

FUNNY YOU SHOULD ASK

Through illustration you can make learning fun for the patient. You can invite his participation in the learning process and can help him to retain what he's learned. But should you use cartoons, humorous captions, and "cute" little characters to achieve these goals? It's necessary to place yourself in the patient's shoes to answer this question. If you've ever been hospitalized, you probably received a good many humorous "Get Well" cards. How did you feel about the humor in them? Some cards probably brightened your day, making you chuckle enough to strain your stitches. But some of the humor probably seemed "sicker" than you were. You may have felt that "bedpan jokes" were no longer funny when you had to use that cold metal throne six times a day. Humor can sometimes backfire.

If used properly, humor can delight, amuse, and inform the patient. But laughter is not the best medicine if it is meted out in doses which ridicule, embarrass, or offend. If a young girl sees a picture of an impish raccoon smiling cheerily while having a bone marrow test, she is not likely to trust you again after she has had *her* bone marrow test. The experience was anything but "fun and games" for her and the light-hearted illustration represents a kind of dishonesty to which children are very sensitive. But a picture of a bunny rabbit enjoying breakfast in bed may delight a youngster without destroying your credibility. The key to tasteful, effective use of humor lies in being sensitive to the patient's needs and fears. You must respect

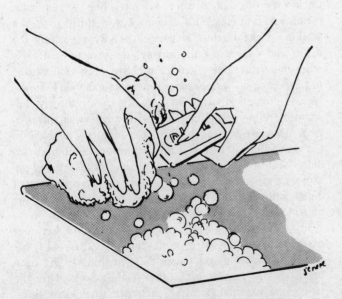

FIGURE 5.5 Illustrating correct habits, such as personal hygiene, can foster a change in attitude.

his integrity if you want to earn his trust. So humor must always begin with the patient's frame of reference. Remember that the patient is in an unfamiliar situation—one which can produce much anxiety. Don't compound his fears by use of threatening images, such as huge syringes or exaggerated body casts and traction equipment, even if *you* think it's funny.

Because humor can be such a double-edged sword, we rarely use humorous drawings or cartoon characters in our Helping Hands. *Amblyopia* represents an uncommon departure from this general rule. While amblyopia is a condition that requires medical attention, we believed that the subject of wearing an eyepatch could be treated in a lighter vein. In this instance, we made an exception to our usual policy (*Amblyopia*).

A "HOARSE" OF A DIFFERENT COLOR

A common pitfall in illustrating teaching materials is the failure to understand how the patient perceives his world. We may intend to communicate the message *figuratively*, but the patient may interpret our statement or illustration quite *literally*. While young children are the most prone to literal interpretations, many adults retain this childlike characteristic. For instance, some adults cannot be dissuaded from their belief that heaven *literally* has pearly gates!

In representing human anatomy, care should be taken to avoid figurative images that may mislead the patient. For example, one small patient became anxious when her father told her he was "a little hoarse today." The child expected that at any minute daddy would sprout hooves, silken mane, and flowing tail, and would gallop around her room like an unbridled colt. When Scott was told that his intestines were something like a garden hose coiled up inside his tummy, he immediately wanted to know if his sister had a "hose" too. On being assured that she also had a hose, he became puzzled. "Well, if Michelle has a hose," he asked, "how come she doesn't have a nozzle?"

Children may actually expect to get a peek at the "frog" in mother's throat, or may wonder why their knee "hinge" doesn't rust when it gets wet. You may be successful in convincing a child that his heart doesn't really look like a valentine, but you may find yourself substituting one confusing metaphor for another. If you tell him his heart is like a pump, he may wonder if it looks like the sump pump in the basement of his home or the pump at the well on Aunt Matilda's farm! What is even worse is to draw a picture of a child's chest with a pump in the center of it. The young patient is sure to wonder what he is going to do when "the well runs dry".

In a misguided attempt to draw understandable analogies, illustrators have depicted sinuses that drip like faucets, "spare tire" waistline flab, brains that contain pounding hammers, toes sprouting edible "ears of corns", and a host of other visual malapropisms too numerous to mention. It is not, however, the use of analogies that causes difficulty; it is the comparison of two things which have *more differences than similarities*. When used correctly, verbal and visual analogies can increase the patient's understanding, since people learn most easily when they are able to relate new concepts to familiar ideas or experiences. For example, it is perfectly acceptable to illustrate an aneurism by drawing a small bubble. (An aneurism looks very much like a bubble and can be expected to behave like one.) But it would be misleading to represent the circulatory system as the "body expressway system"—complete with overpasses, road signs, and traffic jams. While there are many similar aspects to these two transportation networks, there are far too many dissimilarities, and a literal interpretation of the "expressway" could lead to many false conclusions.

Just as figurative visual images may cause confusion, too much abstraction will also mislead the patient. A sketch of bodily organs should generally include enough of the body outline to let the patient know where those organs are located. Pictures of the urinary system or reproductive system, for example, should not appear suspended in space without familiar "benchmarks." (Many young teenage girls believe their stomach and uterus are the same thing, or at least are located in precisely the same area of the abdomen.) For sketches of the torso, familiar, visible benchmarks include the waistline, navel, and nipples. Most people can relate the placement of unseen interior organs to these exterior parts of the body.

The use of cross-sections is another area that requires particular attention. Without modifications, cross-sections may also be too abstract for the lay person. In our Helping Hands on postural drainage, we show a diagram of "a look inside the airways." This cross-section drawing of the trachea was originally pictured as a circle lined with mucous membranes and cilia. This drawing was modified to show a section of the trachea in perspective. By suggesting the depth and volume of the airway, we gave the patient a more understandable visual picture. The cross-section used in *Gastrostomy Tube Feeding* is another example of how a typical medical drawing was modified. Our surgery and anatomy reference books gave far too much visual information. While we wanted to show the inflated "bubble" on the tip of the catheter as it appears inside the stomach, we didn't feel it was necessary to diagram all the layers of the skin and abdominal cavity. In this case, we *subtracted* detail without *abstracting* the drawing so much that the patient might be confused.

So, in illustrating your teaching aids, remember that oversimplifying can be as misleading as undersimplifying. Avoid figurative images unless the two things being compared closely parallel each other in most ways. Give the patient an external point of reference when drawing internal organs. Avoid abstractions, such as cross-sections, unless you can show a direct correlation to a familiar part of the anatomy. In short, give enough information to make the picture clear, but not so much that you overwhelm.

Pictures, like words, are merely symbols. Because they are symbols, they have no meaning apart from the experiences of the people who see and interpret them. Therefore, the more clearly the picture is drawn from a patient's point of view, the more effectively your meaning will be communicated.

ILLUSTRATIONS: FROM INSPIRATION TO EVALUATION

If your experience resembles ours, the ink will scarcely be dry on your first few illustrations when you will begin to think about revising and improving them. At first, you may be unable to pinpoint the reasons for your disappointment with the finished products. Perhaps the illustrations seem trite, prosaic, or lacking in sparkle and originality. As time goes on, these early errors may be compounded, and you may find yourself repeating the same mistakes over and over. Without the stimulus of fresh, creative ideas, and without specific criteria for evaluating your work, your budding efforts may wither on the vine. For this reason, we offer some "first aid" suggestions for flagging inspiration, and some criteria that serve as "last aid" for evaluating the finished designs.

IDEAS FOR ILLUSTRATION

Trying to generate original ideas for illustration may be the most vexing problem you will face. While some ideas spring quite naturally and effortlessly from the text of the teaching aids, others have to be extracted almost as painfully and laboriously as an impacted tooth. You may sit at your drawing table, reading the text for the tenth time, without a glimmer of an idea on what or how to illustrate. The fact is that ideas have to come from somewhere, and their origin is not always the fertile field of your imagination. But don't despair! There are few truly original ideas in the world; most "novel" ideas are old ones that have been remodeled, reshaped, and recombined.

Sources of Ideas

If you look around your office right now, you're likely to see countless printed materials that can become the "seed" of an idea. Newspapers, catalogs, news magazines, health organization pamphlets, nursing journals, children's books, textbooks, greeting cards, travel brochures, wrapping paper, posters, and even junk mail all hold possibilities for the germination of a "new" idea for an illustration. We discovered a goldmine in the dime or quarter children's books offered in a library discard sale; at this price, we felt no compunction about cutting up these discarded books for our resource file. Catalogs, whether they display medical supplies or mail-order household goods, are an especially fruitful source.

From one source may come the idea for how to pose a pair of human figures—perhaps a nurse and a patient. From a second source comes the styles of clothing worn by the subjects. Still other sources may give ideas for the arrangement of the composition or for household goods and other accessories that you want to depict in the illustration. For example, the illustrations in our Helping Hand on hepatitis were inspired by several supermarket newspaper ads that displayed fruits, vegetables, and other foodstuffs. The idea for the four-leaf clover was plucked from a greeting card. The result was a "lucky combination" for the Basic Four food groups.

The problem of how to illustrate range-of-motion exercises was solved when we saw a series of pictures on weight reduction exercises. Motion of the arms and legs was indicated by the dotted outline of the extremities. We borrowed this technique and applied it to our own original drawings.

Of course these illustration sources are only the springboard for ideas; they are never the actual illustrations you will use. Tracing or copying the published work of another artist is strictly taboo. Plagiarism of artwork is as much an offense as the pirating of written composition. There is one notable exception to this rule. Most materials published by the Government Printing Office are not copyrighted and belong in the public domain. Therefore, the illustrations may be copied, traced, or used "as is" without danger of violating a copyright.

Resource File

To be most beneficial to you, illustration ideas should be catalogued and filed by subject matter. The selection of subject categories is completely arbitrary; it is based on how you will be most likely to think of the subject matter. For example, you may have a picture of a child in bed with a thermometer in her mouth and may think that the picture would be useful for a future teaching aid on fever reduction. But the picture might also have possibilities for teaching aids on strep infection, colds and flu, chicken pox, and on a host of other health subjects. So how should the picture be filed? In our resource file, this picture is filed under "Children, Resting," since we would be inclined to look for pictures of resting children for any of the health topics mentioned above. If the picture were placed in a folder labeled "Chicken Pox" it would probably be overlooked when seeking ideas on any one of the other topics. Here is a sampling of some of our subject categories; you will certainly want to add others as the need arises:

- Anatomy
- Children, Action Play
- Children, Resting

- Furniture and Furnishings
- Hands and Faces
- Infants and Toddlers
- Medical Instruments and Supplies
- Orthopedic Equipment
- Surgery
- Toys, Games, and Animals

Your filing system may be as simple or as elaborate as your needs, inclinations, and imagination dictate. But these subject categories are probably sufficient to get you started. Since catalogues are usually indexed by subject matter, there is usually no need to cut them apart; they may be filed separately in your resource file.

On the back of any picture selected for your resource file, write the title of the subject file in which the item belongs. This will simplify refiling when the pictures have been removed from the file.

CRITERIA FOR JUDGING ILLUSTRATIONS

Your first attempts at illustration may fall below your expectations. But you need not be ashamed of your efforts unless you repeatedly make the same errors. To ward off a repetition of errors, some criteria for evaluating your work may be helpful. We suggest that you use the criteria outlined here as a checklist to judge each illustrated teaching aid.

General considerations. Have parts of the anatomy, procedures, and medical equipment that are hard to visualize been pictured? Have major psychological and cultural factors been emphasized? Have positive health habits and concepts been stressed? Have aspects of the topic involving "fear of the unknown" been represented?

Aptness. Is the illustration *appropriate* to the content of the teaching aid? Does it portray the *essence* of the subject, the heart of the message? Does the illustration appeal to the age, sex, race, and other cultural and social aspects of the intended patient audience?

Accuracy. The only thing worse than no information is *misinformation.* Does the illustration accurately represent the patient's own experience? Are medical supplies and equipment drawn with enough detail to make them recognizable to the patient? Are anatomical drawings sufficiently complete and correct? Do illustrations of procedures depict the steps in proper sequence?

Composition. How is the illustration "put together"? Do the parts of each drawing fit harmoniously together or do they seem unrelated? Does the composition draw the reader into the text or does it lead him off the page?

Contrast and balance. Are the light and dark areas well balanced? Is there adequate contrast, or are all the elements in the drawing of equal value? Are curved lines contrasted with angular ones; softness balanced with firmness?

Clarity. How *clear* are the illustrations? Is there unnecessary detail, line-work, or decoration which distracts from the message? Is the pose or the angle from which the subjects are drawn the *clearest* way to portray the scene? Is the type (if any) sufficiently readable and legible? Is the meaning of the picture immediately apparent and understandable? Does the illustration present the subject from a patient's frame of reference?

Proportion and perspective. Are human figures drawn with correct proportions? Are head sizes, length of arms and legs, sizes of hands and feet correct? How accurate is the perspective? Is there a feeling of distance and space? Is each illustration the proper size for the page and for its relative importance to the text?

Number. Are there too few illustrations, or are there too many? Can two illustrations be combined for greater impact and space economy? Is there another important point that should be illustrated?

Caption identification. Does the illustration require a caption? Or does the illustration make a strong enough statement that a caption is unnecessary? Does the caption reinforce the message of the text? Is it brief and to the point? If the illustration is referred to in the text, does the caption identify the corresponding picture or figure number? Is the caption a part of the illustration unit?

Logical flow. Are illustrations placed as closely as possible to the explanatory information in the text? Are they arranged in logical sequence?

Style and tone. Do the illustrations reflect empathy with the patient without being overly sentimental? Do they convey warmth and concern? Are they honest and straightforward? Are they too clinical? Too simplistic? Too negative in attitude? Is there rhythm, spontaneity, and movement?

Meeting these criteria is quite a challenge, but by using the tools and techniques described in the following sections of this chapter, you will be well on your way to reaching these goals.

SELECTING A PRINTING PROCESS

The tools and techniques for creating visual images have come a long way since the days of Michaelangelo. When Renaissance artists were painting their frescoes, the tools of their trade consisted of rather primitive paints and brushes and some makeshift scaffolding. It is little wonder that Michaelangelo saw his craft as "99% perspiration." But with modern graphic aids and techniques, the person without training in drawing can create effective graphics with far less "perspiration." It takes a working knowledge of some of these techniques, combined with an awareness of the materials and supplies available. The greater your knowledge of these media and the methods for using them, the more flexibility and success you will have in expressing your ideas.

FACTORS TO CONSIDER

Before deciding what materials and supplies you will need, you should determine how your teaching aids will be printed. A number of printing or copying processes may be considered. Consider the factors listed below; then select the process which best meets your needs.

Availability and Convenience

If your hospital or clinic is large enough to have its own in-house printing department, you may find this is the most practical choice, provided it can meet your other requirements.

Cost

Even with an in-house printing operation, you will probably be billed an interdepartmental charge for each printing job. You should compare the cost and services of private printers with departmental charges, provided your hospital policy allows you to contract with outside vendors.

Size of Run

A *run* is the number of copies made at any one time from an original plate or duplicating master. You should estimate the size of your average run, since some processes are best suited to very small runs, while others are designed for runs in the hundreds or thousands.

Size of Page

Your printed page will probably be 8½" × 11", but there may be times when a larger size is desired. For example, our Helping Hand on postural drainage is printed on 11" × 17" paper so we can have a fold-out presentation that parents can post on a wall above the child's treatment area. While the printing or copying process you select may not always meet all possible size specifications, it should at least accommodate the largest size you expect to print *most* of the time.

Typesetting

For most of the commonly used printing or duplicating processes, printing can be done directly from your typewritten page or typed master. It is enough to say here that the decision to use typewritten versus typeset copy will influence (and possibly restrict) your selection of a printing or copying process. Typesetting is discussed in detail later in this chapter (see Hot and Cold Type).

Color

Many small printing companies have significantly higher prices for printing in more than one color or in any color other than black. Often they rely on a fast, volume business, and it is not economical for them to scrub down the printing press to remove black ink so a colored ink can be used. You also pay a premium in time. The promise of "same day printing" does not usually apply to jobs using colored ink. If you would like to use a second color (in addition to black), you might consider ordering a large run of your letterhead in color. Teaching aids may then be printed on the letterhead paper, thus eliminating the cost of a two-color run each time.

Quality

The teaching aids you produce represent you and your health care facility to your patients. You want to be proud of them. Somewhere between instructions scribbled on a napkin with a purple crayon and an engraved missive from the White House there's a happy medium of acceptable quality. The quality of your printed materials should reflect the high level of respect and concern that you have for your patients. Copies that are faded, blurred, too black, or too grey will not be read as willingly and may be seen by the patient as an indication of lack of regard for him.

DUPLICATING AND PRINTING PROCESSES

To insure obtaining the highest quality for the lowest cost, you will want to become familiar with the capabilities and limitations of whatever duplicating or printing process you select. The descriptions that follow won't explain everything you will need to know about printing, any more than a medical dictionary explains everything a health professional should know about medicine. Printers, like other specialists, spend years learning their trade, and much of their terminology and techniques may mystify and confuse the average layman.

You may be inclined to think there is no reason to learn so much about the technical aspect of printing. After all, isn't it the printer's job to figure out how to prepare your teaching aids from the copy and illustration you give him? Of course it's his job! But he can't do his job unless you have adequate communication with each other.

You're likely to feel that you've crossed an invisible border into a foreign land where the language is incomprehensible when the printer points out that your photo needs a 120-line screen, that you didn't allow for "bleed," or that your illustration cannot be reduced to the size and proportions indicated in your "mechanical." As a result, you may be charged for services you don't really need, and have printing done which far exceeds (or falls well below) the quality of work you expect. So it's a good idea to get to know your printer and the language of his trade. The information here is only an outline of basic knowledge; the suggested readings at the end of the chapter supply more detailed information on the tools, techniques, and terminology used in the printing industry.

A few methods of duplication are simple enough that you can operate the equipment yourself without the services of a printer. These include thermography, electrophotography, stencil, and spirit duplication, among others. Most commercial printing is done by letterpress or offset lithography. The following is a brief description of the processes you may consider using:

Duplicating Processes

Thermography Thermography is copying by heat. This type of copying prints only black images on white coated paper. While the cost is low, and the quality of reproduction is fairly good, it is not generally suited to large runs.

Electrophotography Many office copiers, such as Xerox, operate on the electrophotographic principle. An electrostatically charged material, called a toner, is used in creating the image. Depending on the model of the copier, there are many advantages, including enlargement or reduction, color copying, collating, copy feeding, and automatic counting. A few models are capable of producing halftones (as in photographs); but if you use this method, the quality of reproduction may suffer if your teaching aid includes photographs (see Photographs, page 117). For runs of twenty-five copies or more, it is probably less costly to use another method.

Stencil duplicators Stencil duplicators (mimeograph) can be relatively inexpensive to purchase and to operate. For these duplicators, the stencil is "cut" by typing directly onto the stencil master. When the master is attached to the machine's cylinder, ink is forced through the stencil onto the printed page. While you can produce a greater number of readable copies with a stencil duplicator than with a spirit duplicator, it is harder to execute a refined or detailed illustration on a stencil master. Also, this method cannot be used if you have the type set commercially.

Spirit duplicators These duplicators use a specially treated carbon paper and make possible the use of more than one color on a single master. The drawing or typing surface of the master can be backed with colored carbons and a colored image is impressed on the reverse side of the master. You can add a second or third color by backing a part of the design with a different colored carbon. During the copying process, a wetting solution softens the resin on the master and a small amount of "ink" is transferred

to the duplicator paper. While this method has the advantage of color printing, only about one hundred clear copies can be reproduced from a single master, and the master cannot be reused.

Printing Processes

Letterpress The earliest form of printing using movable type was based on the letterpress process. Letterpress printing uses the relief principle and is the only form of printing that can be done directly from type. If you own a rubber stamp, you have a crude form of letterpress based on the relief principle. Letterpress is still widely used for very large or very long runs consisting mostly of reading matter. Its versatility is a bit more restricted when a great number of illustrations or photographs are used. Letterpresses are generally larger and more costly than offset presses, making them prohibitive for use by small printing businesses, so your institution's print shop or small local printer will probably not be using letterpress. It is also unlikely that you will select the letterpress process if you plan to use many illustrations, or if your teaching aids are prepared from typewritten, rather than typeset copy (see What Type of Type? page 120).

Offset lithography Of the two major forms of commercial printing—offset lithography and letterpress—offset printing has gained measurable popularity in recent years. Your hospital printing department and neighborhood print shop probably use offset presses. The term "offset" simply refers to the fact that ink is *offset* from the plate to a rubber-surfaced fabric, called a blanket, and onto the paper. This is done by means of rotating cylinders in the printing press (Fig. 5.7). Offset lithography is planographic, which means that all parts of the printing plate are level. The part of the plate that carries the design attracts the ink and the rest of the plate is pretreated to repel ink. There is offset equipment designed for short, medium, and very long runs of 10,000 copies or more. You will find variations from printer to printer in the prices quoted for a job. The printer's skill certainly affects the quality of offset reproduction you receive, but the major difference among offset printers is in the type of plate (or master) used to produce a print.

Our hospital printing department uses an electrophotographic copier to make a "paper plate," which can then be used to print the desired number of copies. A paper plate produces satisfactory line drawings and type, but cannot accommodate photographs or other halftones. The most commonly used type of offset plate is made by a photomechanical process. A specially coated metal plate is exposed to a film negative of your original work. The negative or plate can be "touched up" by the printer. Lines, shadows, spots, and other imperfections in your pasted-up page can often be opaqued on the negative so

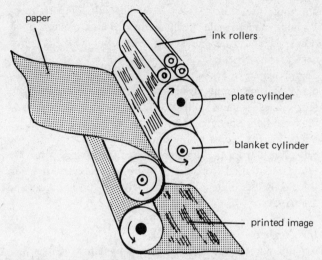

FIGURE 5.7 Principles of offset lithography. Ink is *offset* from plate to rubber blanket and then from blanket to paper by means of rotating cylinders in the printing press.

that they will not appear on the printed page. The result is often a cleaner, sharper looking copy than can be obtained from a paper plate. Photographs and other halftones can also be used. However, the cost of making the plate is generally higher and more time is required to complete the job.

Our experience The Helping Hands we produce are typed on an IBM Selectric typewriter and are illustrated with black and white line drawings. This eliminates the need for typesetting, halftone screening, and color printing. Our hospital printing department can produce as many or as few copies as we need on its offset press using a paper plate. For us, this was the most practical choice when we considered availability, convenience, cost, size of run, average page size, and overall quality.

You may decide to use another process in printing your teaching aids. But, since we have found black and white offset reproduction to be the most practical solution to our needs, we will concentrate on discussing the kinds of materials and supplies needed for this type of graphic preparation.

MATERIALS AND SUPPLIES FOR ILLUSTRATION

An illustrator without good graphic aids is like a nurse or physician without a good stethoscope and watch. No amount of effort or expertise can compensate for a lack of proper tools. Some of the items you will need to produce quality illustrations are listed here. Most are available at commercial art supply houses or at engineering and drafting supply companies.

BASIC DRAWING TOOLS

High quality pens, ink, pencils, and papers should be among your first investments. Without them it will be much more difficult to produce satisfactory line drawings (Fig. 5.8).

Pens

Many cartoonists and other illustrators use felt tip markers exclusively. Although it is a matter of individual preference, felt tip markers do have certain drawbacks. If you use a nonrefillable felt tip pen you may get a line that becomes grey, fuzzy, or "mushy" as the ink is depleted.

There are, however, a number of technical ruling pens that give a clean, even-flowing, consistently black line. Fountain pens, such as the Koh-i-noor Rapidograph, Speedball, or Castell writing instruments, are filled with India ink, and with proper care will not clog or skip. We use Castell pens because they are easily cleaned with water. These pens come in a range of line widths from very fine to very wide and bold.

Crow quill pens, which are dipped in India ink, may be used for fine lines. The width of the line may be varied by changing the angle at which the pen is held, the amount of ink used, and the amount of pressure applied. Be sure to select pens that give you a bold enough line that will not "break up" and disappear when the artwork is printed.

Ink

Black India ink may be used in most technical fountain pens. Be sure to use only the type of ink recommended by the manufacturer.

Pencils

Keep a supply of standard No. 2 pencils on hand for rendering preliminary pencil sketches. Charcoal pencils

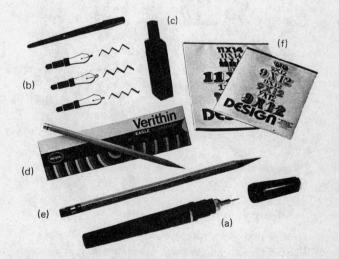

FIGURE 5.8 Basic materials: (a) ruling pen, (b) crow quill pen, (c) India ink, (d) nonreproducing pencil, (e) No. 2 pencil, (f) 100% rag layout paper.

may be used for finished art work if the lines are kept very distinct and black, without shading effects or grey areas. If you want to suggest shaded areas with charcoal pencils, use them only with coarsely textured paper; the areas that appear grey are actually specks of black that adhere to the raised parts of the paper's surface between the recessed white areas. Although the appearance of a charcoal drawing is different from a pure line drawing, it can be reproduced in the same manner as line art.

Nonreproducing pencils, which render a light blue line, are used when guidelines are needed on finished artwork. The light blue line does not reproduce when the art is photocopied.

Papers

Use standard artist's tracing paper for your preliminary sketches. Changes in the drawing can be made easily, since the paper is translucent and easily erasable. For finished artwork, use a high quality drawing paper. (If you try to scrimp and use typewriter bond or duplicator paper, you may have problems with lines that bleed, fuzz, or feather.) To insure sharp, clean lines, use 100% rag layout paper for final ink drawings. This paper is available in a variety of sizes and weights and is also semitranslucent for ease in tracing your pencil sketches.

USEFUL DRAWING AIDS AND DEVICES

A number of graphic tools and devices will help you to achieve professional results and save time as well (Fig. 5.9).

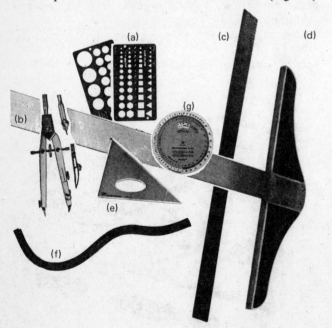

FIGURE 5.9 Aids and devices: (a) templates, (b) ink compass, (c) metal-edged ruler, (d) T-square, (e) triangle, (f) flexible curve ruler, (g) circular proportion scale.

The most useful devices are templates; ink compass; ruler, T-square, and triangle; flexible curve ruler; circular proportion scale; and pantograph.

Templates

Made of transparent plastic, templates aid in drawing perfect circles, squares, ellipses, and other forms. Each template contains openings in numerous sizes of the same form. By taping thin coins to the underside of the template, you can raise it from the drawing surface for inking. When the template is raised from the drawing surface in this manner, the inked line will not "bleed" between the template and the paper.

Ink Compass

An ink compass is useful for making circles larger than those found on your circle template. The writing tip of the compass is filled with the dropper from a bottle of India ink.

Ruler, T-Square, Triangle

Your ruler should have a raised metal edge for ruling, inking, or cutting along straight lines. A T-square will be needed for aligning your artwork for paste-up (see "The Work Surface" page 120). The T-square should be long enough to extend the length of your drawing surface. A triangle is used along with the T-square to make lines that are perpendicular to the T-square.

Flexible Curve Ruler

This plastic or metal device will hold nearly any curved shape when bent into the desired form. The raised lip edge allows you to guide your ruling pen along the edge for a perfect curved line. This device is especially useful for drawing IV tubing, hoses, or catheters.

Circular Proportion Scale

You may wish to have your illustrations reduced or enlarged. A circular proportion scale is a plastic or cardboard device which has an inner wheel and a larger outer wheel. Both wheels are marked in inches and fractions of an inch. By rotating the outer wheel, you can determine the percentage of reduction or enlargement you will need, as well as other possible proportions.

Pantograph

The pantograph may also aid in reducing or enlarging a drawing. This is a precision drawing instrument made of metal or wood bars with adjustable joints (Fig. 5.10). The pivot point of the device is clamped or thumbtacked to the drawing surface. A stylus held in one of the joints is guided over the picture that you want to reduce. Pencil lead, held in the tip of another bar, outlines the design and replicates the reduced picture on a second piece of paper.

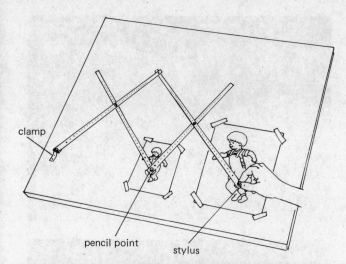

clamp

pencil point

stylus

FIGURE 5.10 Using the pantograph: The stylus is guided over the large drawing. A pencil point sketches the reduced drawing on a second sheet of paper. Positions of pencil point and stylus are reversed to produce enlargements.

To enlarge a drawing, the positions of the stylus and pencil are reversed. By adjusting the joints, you can achieve a wide range of reduction or enlargement proportions.

AIDS FOR PASTE-UP

A paste-up, sometimes called a *mechanical,* consists of all the elements of your page—the type, artwork, and/or photographs—which are assembled together on a piece of paper or artboard. The paste-up is *camera-ready,* which means it can be photographed directly to make a printing plate. Here are some of the materials you may want to use in assembling your paste-up.

Adhesives
Artwork is pasted up using rubber cement, "invisible" tape, or a wax coating machine. With rubber cement, the artwork can be removed and repositioned before the cement has dried. (If you use rubber cement, check your pasted up originals from time to time to see that the artwork has not come loose from the page.) All traces of rubber cement must be thoroughly cleaned from the master; otherwise, the residue will become dirty and leave a smudge or shadow on your printed pages. Because rubber cement can become dirty easily, some printers prefer that you lightly affix the artwork with a small piece of tape on the underside of the art. If pure white paper is used for both artwork and paste-up surface, there is little chance of a line or shadow around the artwork, even when the art is not permanently sealed to the page. Artwork can also be taped permanently in place with invisible tape which ordinarily does not show on the finished print.

The most versatile adhesive is wax. A coating machine heats the wax electrically, and a thin coating of melted wax is rolled onto the paste-up area or the back of the artwork that is being applied. Artwork can be lifted and repositioned easily.

Before selecting an adhesive, check with your printer to see which type is preferred.

Erasing and Opaquing Materials
A kneaded eraser is handy for removing pencil lines from the art. A white liquid opaquing solution (the kind often used by typists) is used to paint out areas on the original that you don't want to appear on the printed copy. And, if you use rubber cement, you will need a rubber cement pick-up to remove dried cement from the paste-up.

Cutting Tools
A frisket knife is a tool with a small, sharp pointed blade which is used for cutting shading film and assembling the paste-up. The knife blades can be replaced in the holder as they become dull. Single-edged razor blades may be used instead of a frisket knife, provided they are discarded as soon as the edges begin to dull.

Burnisher
This is a wood, metal, or plastic tool used to transfer lettering or shading film to the mounting surface.

PRINTED GRAPHIC AIDS

There are many graphic aids available which can greatly enhance the appearance of your final product; they add the "finishing touch" to the teaching aid and give a professional look with a minimum amount of effort. These include transfer shading film and lettering and ready-to-use art.

Transfer Shading Film and Lettering
A variety of patterns and designs may be added to your artwork to create shaded or textured areas. The effect is that of a halftone (a solid or gradated grey area), but your printer will not have to specially screen the artwork before it is printed. Lettering, symbols, and numerals are also available in a wide range of sizes and styles. Prestype, Chartpak, and Letraset are just a few of the suppliers who produce these graphic aids. Ask your commercial art supply house for a catalog of their products.

Adhesive-backed shading film By using these shading film sheets you can suggest, among other things, the rough texture of brick, the nubbiness of a wool sweater, or the grain of wood panelling. The pattern is printed on clear acetate and backed with an adhesive (Fig. 5.11).

To use a pattern or shading film sheet, place it over the area of the artwork to be decorated. Being careful not to cut through the backing sheet, use a frisket knife to cut a

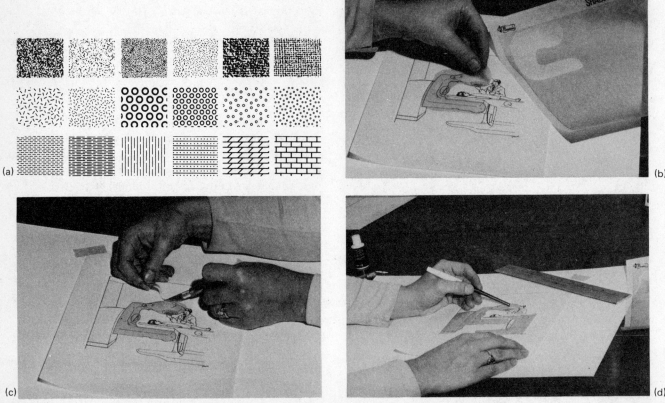

FIGURE 5.11 Adhesive-backed shading film is available in a variety of textures and patterns (*a*). (*b*) A section of the film is cut away from the backing with a frisket knife; (*c*) the excess film is cut away; (*d*) the surface is rubbed with a burnisher for good adhesion.

piece of film larger than needed. Peel the film from the backing sheet and place it on the drawing. Carefully cut away the excess film, leaving the film in place on the areas to be shaded. Rub the shaded areas with the burnisher to insure full adhesion.

Dry transfer shading, lettering, and symbol sheets Dry transfer shading and texture sheets are available in a lesser number of patterns. The pattern is printed on the underside of a transparent sheet. To use a dry transfer sheet, place it over the area to be shaded and rub with a burnisher; the pattern will be transferred to the artwork. Use a kneaded eraser or cellophane tape to remove any areas of the pattern that are inadvertently transferred.

Dry transfer lettering is available in numerous sizes and letter styles (Fig. 5.12). This lettering is applied in a manner similar to the texture and pattern sheets. Special tips and techniques for applying the letters are outlined in the suppliers' catalogues.

Dry transfer symbol sheets, figure silouettes, and decorative borders are particularly useful when the same design or symbol must be repeated many times. Symbols, such as stars, circles, squares, asterisks, and arrows are repeated numerous times on each sheet and often display a range of sizes for the same symbol. Small squares can be used as check boxes for a list of items. Arrows may be used to point out important parts of a diagram. These symbols may be transferred to the artwork very quickly and the results are consistently professional.

Ready-To-Use Art

While the previously-described graphic aids are used chiefly for creating original art, Clip Art and Modulart are two forms of ready-to-use visuals that require no artistic talent or drawing skill to apply.

Clip Art Clip Art, a terrific timesaver, is offered in booklets or separate sheets of designs covering a wide range of subject matter (Fig. 5.13). The ready-to-use line art illustrations may be cut out and pasted directly on your mechanical. Hands, faces, dogs, buildings, children, trees, and a vast number of other visuals can be adapted to your particular needs. For example, to illustrate a hand holding a syringe, you simply clip a picture from the Clip Art "hands" booklet. Choose a picture of a hand that is posed in the proper position, add your own drawing of a syringe,

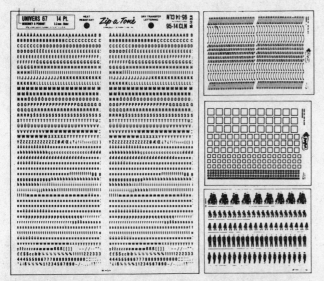

FIGURE 5.12 Dry transfer lettering and symbol sheets.

and your illustration is complete. An illustration of a child playing with a dog may be composed by combining a Clip Art figure of a child and one of a suitably posed dog. Clip Art is updated periodically with new designs. If you subscribe to the Clip Art service, you'll receive a steady flow of well-designed artwork. This line art is intended to be used for graphic reproduction, so there is no copyright on the materials, and you are free to use them as you wish.

Modulart   A variation of Clip Art is Modulart. As the name suggests, the images are printed in modular form on a transparent film base. For example, you may have a sheet of arms and legs, another sheet of the human torso, and still another having only facial features. A cartoon figure may be composed by selecting the facial features you want to use (eyes, nose, and mouth), and combining them with the Modulart head, torso, arms and legs, that are posed in the desired position. Each "module" is cut out, arranged in place, and then burnished to the artwork. The adhesive backing holds the composite form in place. You can draw directly on the Modulart visual to add your own pen and ink details and embellishments. If you're striving for realism in your illustration, Modulart has its limitations. The human figures depicted are highly stylized, and illustrations of realistic-looking people cannot be achieved. But Modulart does offer valuable creative possibilities when time is a major consideration, or when you are uncertain of your freehand drawing skills.

USE OF PHOTOGRAPHS

There may be times when you will want to use photographs in your teaching aids. But photographs require special handling for most types of offset printing. Areas of a photograph are neither solidly black nor completely white, but contain continuous or gradated tones.

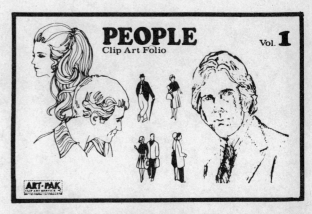

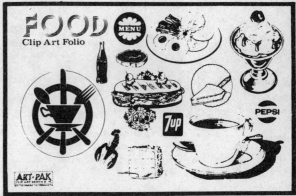

FIGURE 5.13 Ready-to-use art: Clip Art may be cut out and used on your paste-up.

To better understand what is meant by "continuous tone" or "middle value" try this experiment. Use a sheet of white paper, India ink, and a narrow brush. Paint a band of black ink across the top of the page. While the ink is still wet, blend in another stripe of ink beneath the first, but dilute the ink with a little water. Continue down the page, diluting the ink and lightening the shade a little more each time. The bottom stripe should be clear—the white of the paper. All the shades of grey in between are "middle values." If the entire paper were painted with any one of these grey tones, it would be a continuous tone.

Because the printer cannot reduce the amount of ink that is transferred to the page, he can print only the deepest value of whatever color ink is used. In offset printing, the middle values, or grey areas, cannot be printed without converting these continuous tones into *halftones*. The illusion of middle values must be created by converting these continuous tones into tiny dots. Large black dots spaced closely together will look like a darker value than small black dots spaced farther apart.

Changing the continuous tone into a dot pattern is done by using a *halftone screen* (Fig. 5.14). One type of screen is made of glass which has been ruled with very thin lines spaced evenly apart. A second sheet of glass ruled in the same way is cemented at right angles to the first glass. The

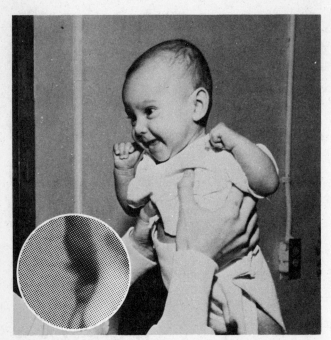

FIGURE 5.14 Halftones and continuous tones. Part of the photo has been magnified (inset) to show the dot pattern in the screened photo.

number of lines per inch determines how fine the dot pattern will be. (A 133-line screen would be one having 133 vertical and 133 horizontal lines per inch.) When the glass screen is placed in front of the camera film, the printer can re-photograph your picture through the screen. During exposure the screen acts as a mesh of tiny lenses to create a pin-point dot pattern on the negative. This negative is then used to prepare the printing plate. This same procedure is required to reproduce watercolor or charcoal drawings that have gradated or continuous tones.

Preparing Photographs for Paste-up

Before a plate can be made, photographs, line art, and type must be placed in proper position and photographed. Positioning this composite is called stripping. The stripper arranges all the negatives that will be used for a plate on a coated paper called a goldenrod mask. This mask is then photographically exposed to make a plate.

Stripping and platemaking is the only way that negatives of your photographs can be used. But there is a way to use actual prints of photographs that circumvents the added cost and time involved in stripping. You do this by making a paste-up using a PMT or Velox of your photo. The PMT, or photomechanical transfer, is a photo which has been converted to a halftone dot pattern. A positive print is made from the negative and the PMT can be used in your paste-up, just as you would use a line drawing. A Velox is another form of continuous tone photograph that has been converted into a halftone. The Velox is also treated exactly like line art during paste-up and plate-making. Parts of the photo may be removed with opaquing fluid, and transfer

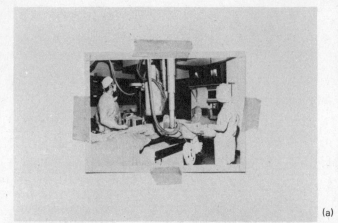

(a)

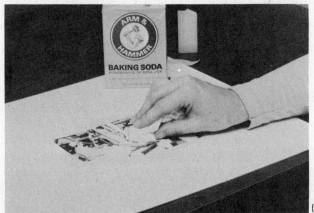

(b)

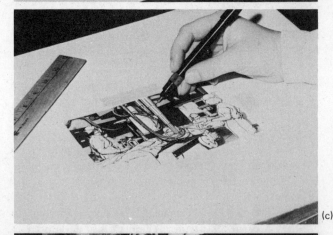

(c)

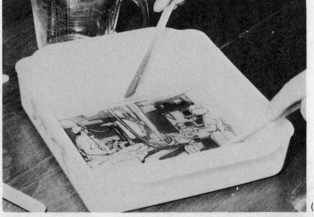

(d)

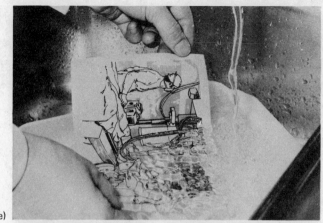

(e)

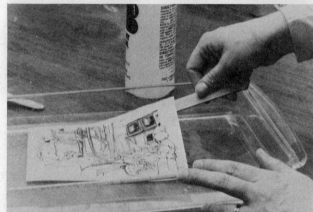

(f)

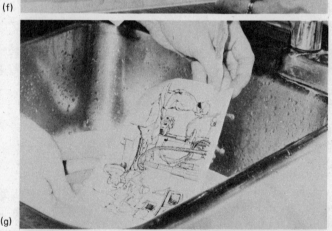

(g)

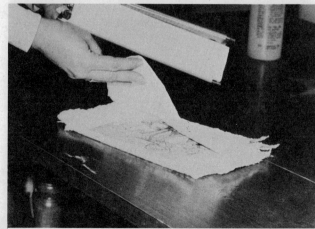

(h)

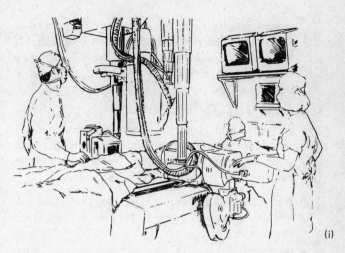

(i)

FIGURE 5.15 Photosketching: (*a*) the glossy photograph; (*b*) rubbing the surface with baking soda; (*c*) outlining the photo with waterproof ink; (*d*) bleaching in iodine solution; (*e*) rinsing the photo; (*f*) fixing the photosketch in hypo; (*g*) washing; (*h*) drying; (*i*) the completed photosketch.

lettering may be applied directly to the surface of the Velox if desired.

Photosketching

Photographs may also be used in a way that eliminates the need for halftone screening. The technique is called photosketching (Fig. 5.15).

1. Start with a photograph of your subject, preferably a nonglossy print. (If a glossy print is used, the surface should first be rubbed lightly with baking soda to reduce slickness and remove oil from fingerprints. This will cause the ink to adhere better to the surface.)

2. Draw directly on the photograph using waterproof India ink and pen or brush.

3. Outline only the parts of the photograph that are important, or make details more distinct which do not appear clear on the photo. Use as much or as little detail as you like. Correct any errors with white opaquing fluid.

4. Let the ink dry thoroughly. This will take at least 30 minutes. (Any ink that is not completely dry will wash off during the bleaching process.)

5. Mix ordinary iodine (purchased from the drugstore) with two or three parts water and pour into a shallow glass pan. Place the photo in the iodine bath, ink side up, being careful not to touch any of the inked area.

6. As the iodine bath removes the original photographic image, all the image except the black ink outlines will become a dark orange-brown. When all the back-

ground is dark orangish-brown, remove the photo-sketch from the pan and rinse it with cool water. If the India ink bleeds, you probably did not allow enough drying time before immersing the photo in the iodine bath.

7. Further bleaching is needed to give you a clear black and white print. Soak the photosketch in a chemical solution called a hypo, or photo-fixing bath (available at photography supply stores). This step removes all remaining yellowish stains left by the iodine.

8. Wash the photo under cool running water for 3-5 minutes. (You can put it in the sink and let water flow over it.)

9. Place the photosketch between sheets of blotter paper or absorbent cloth, and put a weight, such as a book, on top of it. This will absorb excess moisture and prevent curling.

10. When the photosketch is dry, it should look like a pen and ink drawing of your subject.

Photosketching is especially useful when complicated medical equipment or procedures must be illustrated. An actual photo may contain too many details or distracting background items. With photosketching, you can simplify the picture easily without worrying about the difficulties of perspective or proportions. If you have a medical photographer on the staff, he may be familiar with the technique and can do the actual processing for you.

THE WORK SURFACE

A hardwood drawing board and a light table make ideal work surfaces. The most commonly used drawing board has a hardwood surface and is supported by tubular steel or wood legs to form a table. The sides of the table top are at perfect right angles to the top and bottom. This precise alignment is essential for making guidelines on the paste-up that are exactly square. The board may be adjusted to the height and tilted to the angle most comfortable for the artist (Fig. 5.16).

It is advisable to protect the hardwood surface of the board with some kind of pad. You may purchase a commercially available pad or make your own. Several large sheets of plain newsprint held in place with push pins or masking tape provide a satisfactory padded work surface (Fig. 5.16).

A light table resembles a drawing table in construction except that the underside is illuminated with fluorescent lights and the table surface is made of frosted glass to prevent glare and eyestrain. Few hardwood drawing tables contain a built-in lighted area, so even with the drawing board, it's desirable to have some kind of underlighted work area for tracing, paste-up, and layout work. If a

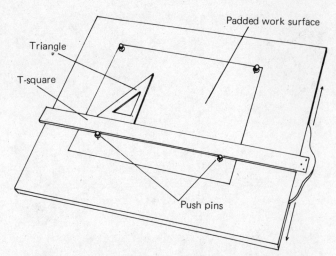

FIGURE 5.16 T-square slides along edge of drawing board for ruling horizontal lines. Push pins hold the T-square in place when using a triangle to draw vertical lines.

full-sized light table is not economically feasible, a light box may be improvised. An x-ray viewing box may be used if the sides are perfectly square. However, if the viewing surface of the box is made of plastic, the plastic should be replaced with a sheet of frosted glass. Glass is more resistant to the cuts and scratches of a frisket knife. Small, commercially produced light boxes, designed primarily for use with stencil masters, are also available.

WHAT TYPE OF TYPE?

By the time you read these words, you probably will have read millions of handwritten, typewritten, and typeset words on paper. Each person's handwriting has its own style, character, and personality, but did you realize that type also has a distinctive character and personality? Handwriting may consist of tiny, tightly-formed letters with very little spacing between the letters and lines, or it may flourish in a large bold scrawl. Like handwriting, type is expressive; it can be masculine or feminine, delicate or forceful, old-fashioned or modern. Even the characters on a typewriter can have personality. For example, if you compare two popular IBM type styles, Letter Gothic and Prestige Elite, you realize that even the names of the type have a distinctly different flavor. And for each of these styles, the appearance of the type is consistent with the name.

When we began to develop our Helping Hands, we naively assumed that type is type is type. We have since learned a lot about the features of type that contribute to the overall attractiveness and readability of our teaching aids. We got to know type "families" and "faces"; we studied their "point sizes" and contemplated caps, leading, letterspacing, word spacing, and serifs.

In becoming acquainted with type, we learned a new language, or jargon, in which words like "point," "bold," "condensed," and "lead" have particular meanings. Why did we bother? We knew that our patients would not say, "Ah, look! They've used a fourteen point boldface sans serif Helvetica type." Most people aren't consciously aware of why they want to read one piece of printed matter but don't want to read another one. They don't realize that the character of the type and its spacing affects them psychologically. Regardless of the quality of the message, if the reader is subconsciously turned off by the type, he probably will not read the material or assimilate it as he should.

So, to give your teaching aids the sort of character you want them to have and to insure that your patients will want to read what you've written, here are *some* of the type fundamentals which are helpful to know.

TYPESET VERSUS TYPEWRITTEN

The Helping Hands used at Children's Hospital are typewritten rather than typeset. The pages in Part 1 in this book have been typeset by the publisher; in Part 2 typewriter composition was used. Various methods are used to set type, from the cumbersome process of setting individual pieces of type by hand, to the faster and more versatile processes of machine and photographic composition. Typeset copy is more costly than typewritten copy. The typesetter bases his rate on the square inch or the length of a line, depending on the nature of the copy. But the advantages of typeset copy will become apparent as we look at some of the features of type in the following paragraphs.

(*Note:* If you decided to typewrite your teaching aids [as we have done], you may want to skim the following two sections—"Features of Type" and "Hot and Cold Type"— and continue with "Planning the Printed Page." These detailed discussions of type are mainly concerned with typeset copy, although some of the information applies to typewriting also.)

FEATURES OF TYPE

Many features of type contribute to the overall appearance, size, and shape. While typesetters could list numerous others, here are some of the more familiar terms used to describe type.

Type Face

Type is designed to give the letters particular shapes and characteristics resulting in a style of type called the "face." Artisan, Letter Gothic, and Prestige Elite are three kinds of *typewriter* "faces." Helvetica, Univers, and Times

HELVETICA LIGHT
HELVETICA LIGHT ITALIC
HELVETICA MEDIUM
HELVETICA MEDIUM ITALIC
HELVETICA BOLD
HELVETICA BOLD ITALIC
(a)

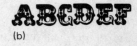
(b)

Franklin Gothic

Baskerville

Univers

Times New Roman
(c)

ARTISAN

Artisan

PRESTIGE ELITE

Prestige Elite

LETTER GOTHIC

Letter Gothic
(d)

FIGURE 5.17 Features of type: (*a*) a family of Helvetica type; (*b*) highly ornate type face reduces readability; (*c*) common typeset faces; (*d*) common typewriter faces.

Roman are names of commonly used *typeset* faces (Fig. 5.17).

Case

The layman distinguishes between small letters and capital letters. In type jargon, the small letters are called lower case and the capitals are upper case.

Points

The height of a letter is measured in *points* (Fig. 5.18). There are 72 points to an inch. To find the point size of a type face, the letters are measured from the top of the tallest upward strokes (ascenders) to the bottom of the longest downward strokes (descenders) in the alphabet of

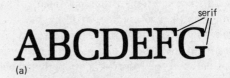
(a)

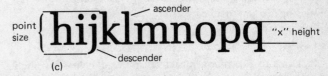
(b)

(c)

FIGURE 5.18 Sizes and styles of type (*a*) serif type, (*b*) sans serif, (*c*) ascenders, descenders, "x" height, and point size are indicated on these lower-case letters.

that type face. For example, if the difference between the top of the letter "d" and the bottom of the letter "p" is one-half inch, the type face would be 36 points. But the "true" size of a letter is its x-height—the height of the lower case "x". With 36 point type, the "x" height may only be 20 points. Typewriters can produce type ranging from 8 to 16 points. Typeset copy is available in a wide range of faces from 6 to 72 points, with some composition methods capable of producing even larger sizes of type.

Serifs

Some styles of type have thin crossbars called *serifs* at the tops and bottoms of the letter. Type faces without these crossbars are called *sans serif* (Fig. 5.18). Both are available in typewritten and typeset faces. There is much debate about the legibility of serif versus sans serif type styles. Those who favor serif type claim that people are accustomed to reading serif type in newspapers, magazines, and typed reports, and this familiarity makes serif type more desirable. Proponents of sans serif type claim that the absence of serifs gives the type a cleaner, uncluttered look that makes it more legible and modern. You may want to have a sample teaching aid prepared in both serif and sans serif type of the same size and see which is the most appealing and readable.

Word and Letter Spacing

On a standard electric typewriter, identical space is allowed for each letter. The upper case *M* is assigned the same amount of space as the lower case *i*. All spaces between words are equal in size and the spaces between the lines are constant (either single spaced or double spaced) unless the typewriter is adjusted manually. The right margin is uneven because ordinary typewritten copy cannot be justified. *Justification* refers to the adjustment of spacing between words and between letters so all lines in a column of type are of equal length. With great effort, a typist can simulate justified copy, but there may still be unnatural looking gaps between the words or improperly hyphenated words. With typewriters such as the IBM Executive, adjustments can be made in the spaces between words (word spacing) and between letters (letterspacing). By using the Executive, the skilled typist can produce justified copy, but the process is slower than ordinary typewriting. When type is set, letterspacing, word spacing, justification, and line spacing are all possible.

Leading

In terms of the visual impact on the reader, line spacing is probably the most important. The amount of space between lines of type is called leading (pronounced ledding) and is measured in points. When the type is set without leading, it is said to be "set solid." But, even without

leading between the lines there will be some space. This is because few letters in the alphabet occupy the entire amount of space indicated by the point size; most lower case letters are the "x" height. There is no fixed rule about the amount of leading that should be used. Judgment is based on the height of ascenders and descenders, the size and boldness of the type, the length of the line, and other factors. In general, common sense will dictate how much leading is needed for readability; too much may be as unwise as too little. If you decide to have your type set, the compositor (typesetter) can guide you in determining the amount of leading needed to give your teaching aids a pleasing appearance.

Other Features of Type

The terms light, medium, and bold are used to describe the thickness and blackness of type. While most typewriter faces are medium in boldness, a few faces are available in light type. Type that is truly bold cannot be produced on the typewriter, but is available in many point sizes and styles in type that is set. Condensed type, as the name suggests, is narrower than standard type of the same face, and occupies less linear space. Expanded type is wider and often thicker than the average. Italic type, as you may know, is slanted to the right. Script styles of type are designed to imitate handwriting. One style of script can be produced on the typewriter. Script and italic should be used sparingly, since they are not usually as legible as standard type.

Type Families

Remember that we said type can have personality? The design and general shape of the letters gives a type face its own particular style. In a family of type, these characteristics are always the same, but there may be other variations. For example, a "family" of News Gothic type may include italic, condensed, expanded, medium, light, or bold examples (Fig. 5.17). As in human families, some members may be fatter, thinner, or bolder than others, but there are certain traits that are common to all members of the family. Any one "family member" in the same face is called the *font*. Fourteen point Helvetica Bold Condensed would be one of perhaps a dozen fonts in the Helvetica family; other fonts might include 10 point Helvetica light or 8 point Helvetica italic.

HOT AND COLD TYPE

You've heard the expression, "hot off the press." This is probably a reference to the hot liquid metal that is poured into forms to produce slugs of type. The monotype machine produces individual slugs for each letter, whereas the linotype produces a full line of type in a single slug. One way to understand hot metal type is to visualize children's blocks with raised letters or figures. The slugs of type are arranged in justified lines, like placing blocks in a row, and all the lines of type needed for a page are "locked up" into a rectangular metal frame, called a chase. An individual letter or whole line of type may be removed and replaced without resetting the entire page. Letterpress printing could be done directly from this locked up form, although intermediate steps are usually taken to preserve the type for repeated use by making a printing plate. As with children's blocks, the raised or relief surface of the letter accepts the ink and is pressed to the page during printing. This kind of typesetting is used chiefly in letterpress. It can also be used in offset lithography after a print has been made of the type.

All other typesetting systems produce what is called *cold type*. Cold type is simply any type that is not set by hot metal composition. Except for typesetting designed for large display or headline lettering, the major forms of cold type composition consist of direct image typesetting and phototypesetting.

Direct Image Composition

The humble typewriter produces the simplest and least sophisticated form of direct image "strike on" composition. More versatile machines like the IBM Selectric Composer, the Varityper, and Justowriter have keyboards resembling a typewriter, but make use of a built-in mechanism which aids the operator in line justification. The Magnetic Tape Selectric Composer uses a cartridge of magnetic tape which is coded during the typing of unjustified copy on a machine resembling an ordinary Selectric typewriter. The tape is then "played out" on a Selectric Composer which uses a special type font, or element, containing the correct size and style of type.

Direct Image Transfer Type

As mentioned in "Printed Graphic Aids," you can "set" type by directly applying transfer lettering, such as Prestype. Dry transfer lettering is too slow, expensive, and cumbersome for practical use in text material but may be used to advantage in short headings, captions, and labels in a diagram. Moderate use of these letters "dresses up" a teaching aid and gives a polished look to typed pages (see Step-By-Step Layout and Paste-up, pages 134–135).

Phototypesetting

In phototypesetting, the characters are stored on a photo matrix which may be a disc, a drum, a film strip, or a grid. From a keyboard or tape the copy is put into the machine. The keyboard or tape selects reference marks which correspond to marks on the matrix. When the correct character has been selected, light is exposed through the matrix. The light is deflected by mirrors, prisms, and lenses to the proper position, and the image is created on photosensitive paper or other material.

Phototypesetting has the advantage of great speed and versatility. With some machines, type can be curved into a loop or wave, expanded or condensed, like a mirror image in a fun house. The cost varies with the amount of labor and the types of equipment involved.

Mechanical Lettering Aids

Except for typewriting and dry transfer lettering, all the methods described until now require the services of an experienced typesetter. But there are a number of mechanical lettering aids available that you can learn to use. If the text of your teaching aids is typewritten, you may want to use one of these mechanical tracing lettering sets for your captions, titles, and labels in a diagram.

Lettering systems by LeRoy, Letterguide, and Varigraph produce lettering and symbols in a surprising number of type faces, sizes, and styles (Fig. 5.19). A metal or plastic template, resembling a ruler, contains letters of the alphabet or other symbols. The template is used with a scriber, a device that holds a stylus, and a pen or pencil attachment. Using a T-square to hold the template in place, you guide the stylus around the letter on the template. As the stylus traces the letter, the pen or pencil in the scriber reproduces the letter in the desired position on the artwork. After moving the template for the next letter, the procedure is repeated. Since the tip of the ink pen does not touch the letter outline of the template, there is less chance of smearing the ink when the template is moved to the next position. With some lettering systems, the scriber may be adjusted to make outline and ornamental letters, italics, and letters that overlap or curve around an illustration. You do not need special skill or experience to use these

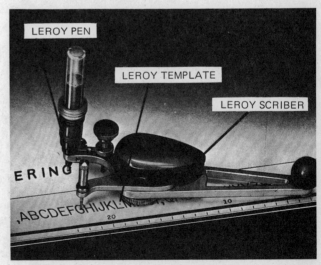

FIGURE 5.19 Components of a mechanical lettering system. Letterguide is placed against a T-square as the tracing pin is guided around the letter. When a letter is complete, the lettering guide is moved into position for the next letter.

lettering systems; professional results are possible with a little patience and practice. Engineering and drafting supply stores are the best source of lettering systems and accessories.

PLANNING THE PRINTED PAGE

Whenever you undertake a new project, you must have an overall plan of organization. If you wanted to build a house, you couldn't—or at least shouldn't—start digging the foundation until after you have a blueprint. A blueprint is a plan that arranges all the major elements in the design of the structure. It indicates the overall size, shape, and major dimensions of the building, but it doesn't specify such particular features as the color of walls or type of carpeting to be used in the home. In designing your patient education program, you also need a blueprint for the overall size, shape, appearance, and general makeup of your teaching aids. This blueprint, or general design, is called a *format*. It consists of all those elements of design that are common to every teaching aid.

Our Helping Hand format evolved through trial and error. In planning the design for our original Helping Hands, we made a number of format decisions. These included: the letterhead design; the width of the page margins; the size and style of type for the text, titles, and subheads; the placement on the page of form numbers, publication and revision dates, and copyright statement. A standard format insures a certain level of uniformity and consistency throughout all the Helping Hands; each teaching aid can be instantly recognized as a part of the overall program.

FACTORS TO CONSIDER

Some of the areas you should consider in designing your format include: letterhead, margins, size and style of type, readability and legibility, and title placement.

Letterheads
In planning your format, you may consider using a letterhead or other identifying symbol or design. The letterhead bears the name of your patient education program and the address and phone number of your institution. It need not be as formal as business letterhead; too much formality may seem pompous and inhibit the reader. But it should introduce your program to the reader and project the image you wish to convey. The informal style of type in our Helping Hand letterhead has a youthful flavor that accentuates our commitment to pediatrics. The letterhead is printed in blue ink on white paper to give color relief to an otherwise black and white page. (The added cost of colored ink was not a major consideration, since we had a very large run for the letterhead. All the Helping Hands are printed in regular black ink on letterhead paper.)

Margins
Initially, the format called for a left margin of 2¾ inches. All illustrations were placed inside this margin. As later Helping Hands were developed, we realized that the wide left margin did not always give us the flexibility we needed to include meaningful illustrations. For instance, on some papers, only one large illustration was desired, but the margin space was too narrow for this illustration. In other instances, a series of small illustrations showing steps in a procedure did not correlate well with the text when they were aligned vertically inside the left margin. So we decided to relax our somewhat rigid format specifications, and design individual page layouts to integrate illustrations of various sizes with the written material.

The size of margins should be standard throughout your teaching aids, but there is no infallible rule governing their size. Here are some guidelines that have evolved through time and experience:

- For an 8½″ × 11″ page, the gutter margin should be no narrower than ¾ inch. (The gutter is whichever side of the page would be bound in a book.)

- The margins at the top of the page and opposite the gutter margin should be the width of the gutter or more, and as much as twice the width of the gutter.

- The bottom margin should be at least as wide as the top margin.

Size and Style of Type
The style of type for the body copy has also undergone a "face lift." Originally body copy was typewritten in upper case Letter Gothic, a sans serif type face. We felt that if the text were typed completely in upper case (all capital letters), the papers would not have the ordinary, hum-drum appearance of the majority of printed materials that are set in lower case. Capital letters have an air of urgency and authority about them (most headlines are set in upper case). We learned, though, that it was difficult to emphasize the most important words or phrases in the text without using extensive underscoring. And there was another nagging problem with our choice of type style that was hard to pinpoint at first. The type was clean and legible, without ornamental serifs to "clutter up" the letters. But we finally realized that even though each individual letter was highly *legible,* a whole paragraph or more of this type style in upper case was not especially *readable* (Fig. 5.20).

Readability and Legibility
For most people the terms readability and legibility mean the same thing. But there's an important difference. A letter or type face is *legible* when it can be recognized quickly. (An Old English monogram initial heavily ornamented with scrolls and serifs, would be an extreme example of illegibility.) But written material is *readable* when several paragraphs or pages can be read comfortably

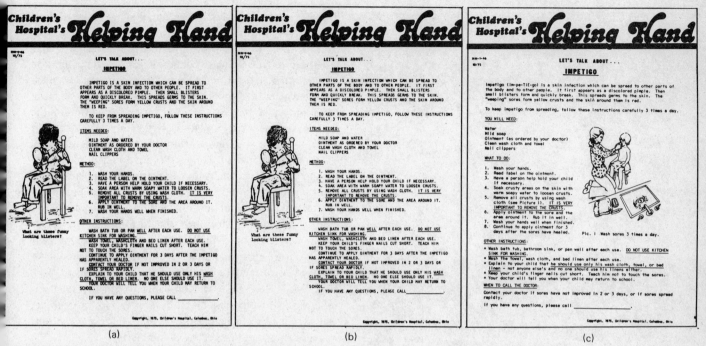

(a)   (b)   (c)

FIGURE 5.20 Evolution of a Helping Hand. (*a*) Earliest Helping Hand in upper-case Letter Gothic type; (*b*) modified teaching aid in upper-case Artisan; (*c*) current Helping Hand with revised layout, format, and lower-case type.

without strain. Text material that is printed in upper case is generally considered less *readable* than that printed in lower case type. In addition, the insufficient line spacing of the Letter Gothic upper case hindered readability. When we changed to upper case Artisan type style, the amount of line spacing was increased by two points per line. And with the addition of this very minute bit of white space between the lines, the text became more readable. We recently made a further change to lower case Artisan type—a somewhat reluctant concession to the typesetter's rule that "lower case type is more readable than upper case type" (Fig. 5.20).

Title Placement

On earlier Helping Hands, the title was set in dry transfer lettering centered below the letterhead. This type was bolder but only slightly larger than the body copy. We now use a larger and bolder condensed transfer type and have allowed more space between letterhead and title. These changes lessen the dominance of the letterhead and accentuate the importance of the title. Form numbers and dates are placed inside the margins. (The format of the Helping Hands in Part 2 of this book has been modified slightly by the publisher.)

Making the Format Template

The format template is nothing more than a guide to layout and paste-up. Use a sheet of grid paper or obtain a golden-rod mask from a printer's supply company. With a bold pen or marker, rule off the margins, letterhead, form

number, and title placement on the page (Fig. 5.21). Since the reverse side of the page will not carry the letterhead, the top margin for page two should also be indicated on the template. (An alternative is to make a separate template for reverse sides of the page.) Later, when you prepare the page layouts, the template is placed under the page, so that each layout conforms to the standard dimensions of the format. (See page 133 for suggestions on aligning the page on the work surface.)

LAYOUTS THAT WORK

We have compared the format design with a blueprint for a building. To pursue the analogy, we might compare the layout with a design for the furniture arrangement in one of the rooms of the building. The blueprint has already determined the general structural elements of the room (the length, height, width). But within the room, there are many design choices to be made. For a pleasing arrangement, the sizes, shapes, colors, and functions of furniture and accessories should be considered. All should fit together in a way that invites you into a room and makes you feel "at home."

A good layout works in the same way that pleasing interior design enhances the furnishings in a room. It balances visually heavy elements; it takes into account the function of illustrations, type, and text material; it highlights important items by making them focal points on the page. Try to imagine a living room decorated with stylish, attractive furniture that somehow doesn't "work." The room appears out of balance and lacking in harmony. Decorative elements compete for positions of importance,

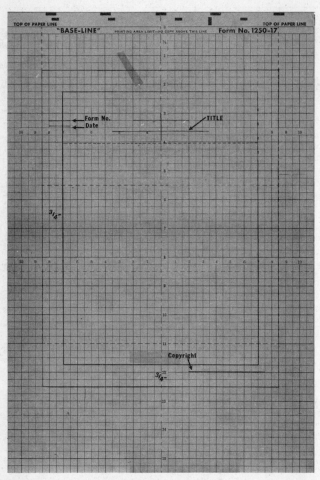

FIGURE 5.21 Format template drawn on a goldenrod mask. By conforming to a standard format for each teaching aid, we achieve consistency and uniformity for every paper.

patterns clash, colors fight, and textures vie for the attention of your senses. Although each piece of furniture or accessory may be lovely by itself, it has been combined with other pieces in a way that creates discord rather than harmony.

In a well-planned room, you may not be aware of everything the interior designer has done to create patterns that please the eye; you will only know that you are comfortable in the room. The same thing is true of a well-designed page layout. The planning isn't obvious, but the reader is pleased and comfortable with the look and "feel" of the teaching aid.

The layout arranges type, illustrations, photographs, and white space on a page in a pattern that promotes readability. To insure that your teaching aids are pleasant to read, the following features of the page layout should be considered: layout function, white space, balance, logical rhythm and flow, and mood.

Function

The art of layout design did not come about to make artists happy and keep designers out of unemployment lines. Layout has an important function—to make reading comfortable and satisfying. Most layout theory evolved from a need to create advertisements that arrested the attention of the buying public. In a magazine ad, for example, the message must immediately interest, engross, and convince the reader. And reading the message must be comfortable and satisfying or the reader will promptly flip to the next page. Although you are not designing advertisements, you cannot afford to disregard the function of layout. Your patient is not a "captive audience," and although you may not have to compete with other advertisements, you do have to contend with all the other sensate stimuli which surround him and vie for his attention.

So, as the saying goes, form should follow function. No design element should hinder reading speed or comprehension. A page that functions as a teaching aid should be designed to attract the interest of the learner and to meet his needs. The learner will probably not be attracted by solid blocks of type unrelieved by illustrations; instead, he will expect to see generous use of white space and captions under illustrations that restate text material.

White Space

The margin around a page provides a picture frame of white space that is essential to a good layout. Modern publications are generous with white space in other areas of the page as well. From 30% to 50% of the total page area is usually allocated for visual material (photos, illustration, headlines, quotes, and white space). The liberal use of white space avoids the cramped feeling of pages filled up with solid type. From a design standpoint, it's better to lengthen an article to another page than to sacrifice the "breathing room" of white space. How much space to allow is always a judgment call. With design requirements in "one corner of the ring" and economy in the number of typed pages in the "opposite corner," it is not always easy to referee these decisions.

Ordinarily, most of the copy and illustrations will be set inside the margins. At least one side of each illustration or block of type should be aligned with the invisible reference lines of the margin. In arranging blocks of type or illustrations on the page, be conscious of how the space is broken up. A general rule is that the space should never be divided into parts of equal size (Fig. 5.22). You should avoid using pictures or blocks of type that cut the page exactly into halves, quarters, or thirds. Exact divisions tend to separate the elements from each other. Allow enough space between illustration captions and the rest of the text. Captions should be treated as part of the illustration unit and should not visually merge with the copy.

Balance

All the graphic elements in your layout have visual weight, but some elements are heavier than others. Bold block letters are heavier than italic type of the same point size.

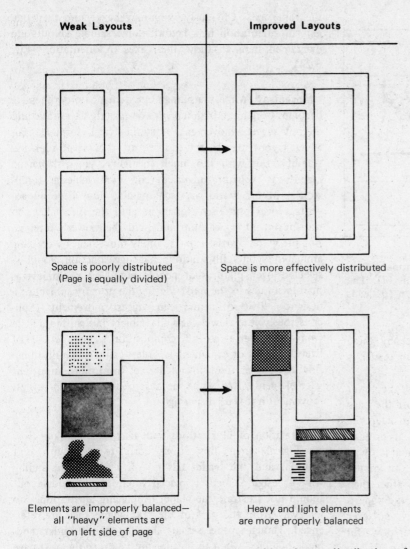

Weak Layouts | **Improved Layouts**

Space is poorly distributed
(Page is equally divided)

Space is more effectively distributed

Elements are improperly balanced—
all "heavy" elements are
on left side of page

Heavy and light elements
are more properly balanced

FIGURE 5.22 Weak layouts are revised to achieve better distribution of space and more effective balance of "heavy" and "light" elements.

Photographs and other illustrations are usually heavier than text. Dark colors are heavier than pastels. Your page layout will appear lopsided, and even seem to be leaning to the left or right, if heavy elements are not visually balanced with light ones (Fig. 5.22).

Balance can be achieved in a very formal manner by having the left side of the page contain exactly the same number and size of elements as the right. For example, engraved wedding invitations often use a formal layout style to achieve balance; each half of the page is a mirror image of the other. Formal balance may be compared to a balancing scale that has a 10-pound weight on either side. Informal balance, on the other hand, is achieved by equalizing the distribution of visual weight. We might place a 10-pound weight on one side of the visual scale and balance it with five 2-pound weights, or with three 2-pound weights and one 4-pound weight. Formal balance has an air of dignity, while informal balance conveys a feeling of spontaneity.

Logical Rhythm and Flow

A layout is a pattern of interlocking shapes and lines. The designer should plan the layout so the reader's eye is led from one dominant area to the next area of importance in logical order. To achieve this flow, you should be aware of these principles: primary optical area, axis of orientation, movement, correlation of illustrations with text, and focal point.

Primary optical area Contrary to popular belief, the eye does not scan a page from left to right, line for line. Instead, it takes a spiralling path from the upper left corner of the page to the lower right corner. The area in the path of this random spiral is called the *primary optical area* (Fig. 5.23). The upper right and lower left corners are called *fallow* corners, because without a strong visual magnet to attract the reader's attention, these areas will be ignored. For this reason, we often design layouts that have arresting illustrations placed in these two fallow corners. The eye of

fallow corner

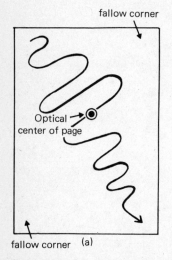

Optical center of page

fallow corner   (a)

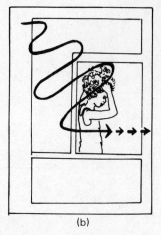

(b)

FIGURE 5.23 The primary optical area from upper left to lower right corner is shown in (a). The figure facing the outer margin in (b) leads the reader's eye off the page.

the reader is pulled off its instinctive course by these illustration magnets. The area scanned by the reader is thereby expanded to include the whole page.

Just as the eye is drawn irresistibly toward the lower right corner, it can be unwittingly led right off the page by a poorly planned layout. If your goal is to keep the attention of the reader until he has looked at or read everything on the page, you don't want to lose him halfway down with visual suggestions that carry him out of the composition. A hand pointing off the page (rather than into it), an arrow which moves the eye toward the paper's edge, the profile of a figure gazing into the Never-Never Land of the right margin all can be subtle, yet powerful influences that pull the eye of the reader right off the edge of the page (Fig. 5.23). The human eye is stubborn and lazy. Once it has been led away, it resists making the effort to venture back into the text again. So, as a rule of thumb, pictures and other design elements that suggest movement should always face into the page.

Axis of orientation Another peculiarity of human vision is its penchant for order and logic. Every graphic element must somehow be related to one or more of the other elements on the page. Perhaps the right side of an illustration aligns with the left margin of a block of type. Or possibly a photo centered at the bottom of the page is the same width as the title that is centered at the top of the page. However you achieve this organization, take care that no graphic element is left an "orphan." An orphan is a piece that seems unrelated to the rest of the composition. To avoid producing "orphans," be sure there is some *axis of orientation* for every element. This invisible axis may be horizontal or vertical (and in rare cases diagonal), but every piece should have a companion piece that is related along

the same axis. Obviously, you may have more than one axis of orientation in a layout. Some sample layouts are diagramed here to show their axes of orientation (Fig. 5.24).

Movement While the human eye demands orderliness, it becomes bored and irritated with designs that are static and do not suggest movement. A symmetrical, formally balanced layout may be the easiest way to achieve order and stability. But with too much formality, you risk having layouts as weighty, dignified, and immovable as tombstones. In the world of visual media, films have an advantage over printed materials because the filmmaker can use movement to capture and hold the viewer's interest. But the graphic artist can also imply movement by creating animated layouts. Illustrations that suggest action should be selected over pictures of people posed as motionless as marble statues in the park. Placing the primary subject of a design a little off-center can suggest movement. (Subconsciously, the viewer feels the subject has shifted a little from the center area of the composition.) The repetition of lively patterns or ornamental borders can create a rhythmic flow as long as they do not detract from more important page elements. Italic type, because of its slant, can suggest movement if it is used sparingly.

Correlation of illustrations with text Rhythm and flow are logical when illustrations correlate well with text material and the reader has no difficulty understanding why a design element is placed where it is. Good layout should not frustrate the reader by placing illustrations too far away from the part of the text where they are referenced. Thought processes are interrupted and understanding is hindered when the reader must turn to the next page to find the illustration referred to in the text. Likewise, if the first paragraph of the text refers to an illustration placed at the bottom of the page, the reader must make a visual leap to the picture. Whenever the reader is forced to make long jumps back and forth repeatedly from text to illustrations, he may lose his concentration, thought continuity, and interest. To overcome this problem, we sometimes design layouts that place the illustration in frames—comic strip fashion—with the text information in the same frame with the picture. This device is especially effective when a procedure consisting of numerous complex steps is illustrated (refer to *Diabetic Urine Testing*).

Focal point When you try to make every element in your layout equally important, the result is a page where nothing has much importance. Just as a well-designed room arrangement should have a focal point—an object of primary interest and importance—a well-planned layout should highlight one major element and play down the importance of all other elements. The optical center of a

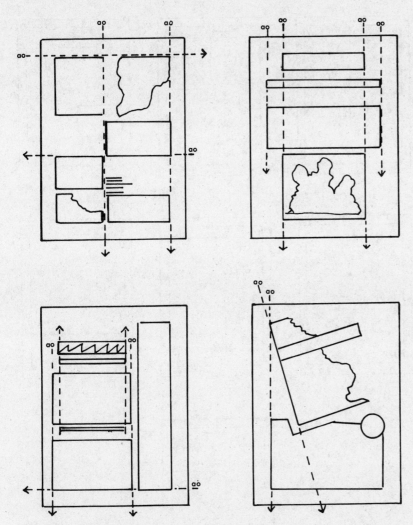

FIGURE 5.24 These layouts are diagramed to show axis of orientation (ao). No single element is left an "orphan."

page is about 10% above the mathematical center of the page (Fig. 5.23). The major element may be placed at the optical center, or this point can serve as a pivotal area. The eye of the reader may be led from this pivotal area into the next design element or block of type that you want him to read. The second element flows logically and graphically into the third area and so on, until the reader has scanned everything on the page in the appropriate sequence.

Mood

The cornerstone of a sound layout is simplicity. Often the novice designer is infatuated by the wide selection of graphic aids at his disposal. If he has ten sizes and styles of type on hand he may succumb to the temptation to use all of them on one page. He may be carried away with busy ornamental borders and other decorations that add nothing to the mood or message of the page. He may be flirting with disaster if he allows "fanciness" to overshadow function. Simple page designs set a relaxed mood, provide an uncluttered environment, and facilitate learning.

To insure simplicity in your layouts, it might be wise to remember the old journalists' maxim: "When in doubt, leave it out."

STANDARDIZED LAYOUTS

Planning individual layouts for each new page is a challenging but time-consuming, creative task. To speed up the production of our Helping Hands, we devised several standard layouts (Fig. 5.25). Illustrations are prepared with one of the standard layouts in mind. When the copy is completed, the page is typed and the illustrations pasted-up according to the pre-selected layout. This approach is only partially successful; the page elements rarely respond willingly to a pat formula.

Ideally, a layout design grows out of the individual requirements of the page. Trying to squeeze these elements into a predetermined mold is comparable to forcing toothpaste back into the tube. You may wish to adapt some of the suggested layouts shown here, but they should be used

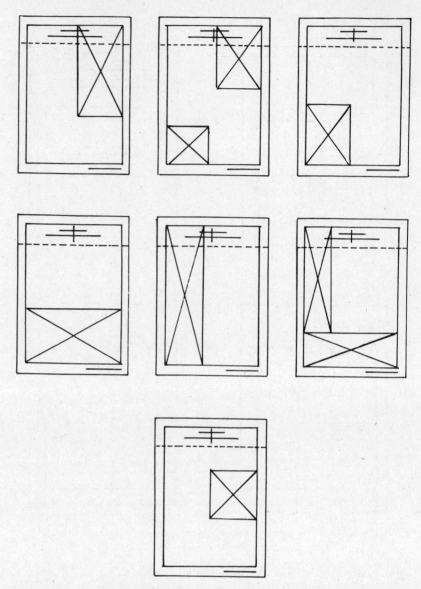

FIGURE 5.25 Sample layouts used for Helping Hands. These should be used as starting points only and should be modified to suit individual needs.

as starting points only. The layouts should be modified and reshaped as the individual needs of each teaching aid become apparent.

EXPANDED LAYOUTS

An expanded layout creates the illusion that the optical area is expanded beyond the limits of the page. Usually, a photograph or halftone color screen is extended to one or more edges of the page. The photo is said to *bleed* to the edge. Expanded layouts can be dramatic, but they present some production problems. The printer needs a gripper margin of at least 1/8 inch on the edges of the page. This is the area allowed for mechanical "fingers" to hold the paper as it passes through the press. When the page design

bleeds to the paper's edge, the printer must use paper larger than specified, and then trim away the excess. This extra operation adds cost to your printing job, so if you are watching your budget, it is best to stay away from layouts that bleed to the paper's edge.

FROM LAYOUT TO PASTE-UP

To paraphrase the question, "Which comes first, the chicken or the egg?" we might ask, "Which comes first, the illustrations or the type?" How can you design a layout without knowing the amount of space needed for the type? And how can you plan the size and number of illustrations and be sure they will fit on the page? The following discussion explains how to determine the amount of type that will fit, how to fit illustrations with typed material, and how to paste-up the page in accordance with the layout.

DETERMINING HOW MUCH TYPE WILL FIT

Since our Helping Hands are not typeset, we do not have to specify the type face, point size, and leading for each page. Thus, problems of copyfitting are greatly simplified. Copyfitting is the term for mathematically computing how much type (in a given face and size) can be fit into the page area designated for your copy. Just how much of the manuscript will fit into a particular area varies widely with the style and size of type used, the amount of leading, and other factors.

Typeset Copy

There are conversion charts and type books available which tell you how many characters of a given face will fit into a linear pica. (A pica is a typesetter's measurement equal to one sixth of an inch). If you plan to have your papers typeset, prepare the copy in manuscript form with wide margins and doublespaced lines. After looking over the manuscript, the typesetter will compute the number of lines of a given length that can be set in the type face you have chosen. If you have designed a layout that calls for a block of type 5 inches wide by 4 inches deep, you will know in advance if the copy will fit. Sometimes your layout may have to be adjusted to accommodate the block of type. As you become more familiar with the ratio of manuscript lines to lines of typeset copy, you will be able to judge more accurately how much space to allow on your layout.

Typewritten Copy

Once you become accustomed to the procedure, estimating the space needed for typewritten copy becomes a simple task with the aid of Charts A, B, and C. These charts are based on the fact that there are six single-spaced typewriter lines per vertical inch, regardless of whether pica or elite type is used. The elite chart (Chart B) is based on a character count of twelve characters per horizontal inch, and the pica chart (Chart C) on ten characters per horizontal inch. (We should stress here that a character is any letter, number, punctuation mark, or *space,* made by the typewriter.)

To calculate the amount of space needed for typewritten copy, follow these steps:

1. *Make a manuscript page typing guide.* First, measure and rule off 3/4-inch margins on all four page edges. Use a pen or marker to make thick black lines. Beginning with the first typing line beneath the top margin, type the number 1 just outside the left margin line. Double space, type the number 2, and continue down the page. You should finish with twenty-eight lines, double-spaced (see Step-by-Step Layout and Paste-up, Fig. 5.26).

2. *Have the text typed in manuscript form.* Before inserting paper in the typewriter, back each page with the typing guide (you should be able to see the margin lines and numbers through the paper). Or, you may prefer to type directly on a Xerox copy of the typing guide. Typing begins on line 1 and continues across to the right margin line. Care should be taken to type up to, but not more than a few characters beyond this margin. A full manuscript page will have twenty-eight 7-inch double-spaced lines. After the page is typed, if

CHART A
CHARACTER COUNT FOR MANUSCRIPT PAGES*

No. of Lines	Total Characters		No. of Lines	Total Characters		No. of Lines	Total Characters	
	Pica	Elite		Pica	Elite		Pica	Elite
1	70	84	11	770	924	21	1470	1764
2	140	168	12	840	1008	22	1540	1848
3	210	252	13	910	1092	23	1610	1932
4	280	336	14	980	1176	24	1680	2016
5	350	420	15	1050	1260	25	1750	2100
6	420	504	16	1120	1344	26	1820	2184
7	490	588	17	1190	1428	27	1890	2268
8	560	672	18	1260	1512	28	1960	2352
9	630	756	19	1330	1596	29	2030	2436
10	700	840	20	1400	1680	30	2100	2520

*Based on an average manuscript line length of seven inches.

CHART B
MANUSCRIPT CHARACTER COUNT CONVERSION

Elite Type

Depth of Typed Column (inches) Single-Spaced	Width of Typed Column (inches)										
	2	2-1/2	3	3-1/2	4	4-1/2	5	5-1/2	6	6-1/2	7
2	288	360	432	504	576	648	720	792	864	936	1008
2-1/2	360	450	540	630	720	810	900	990	1080	1170	1260
3	432	540	648	756	864	972	1080	1188	1296	1404	1512
3-1/2	504	630	756	882	1008	1134	1260	1386	1512	1638	1764
4	576	720	864	1008	1152	1296	1440	1584	1728	1872	2016
4-1/2	648	810	972	1134	1296	1458	1620	1782	1944	2106	2368
5	720	900	1080	1260	1440	1620	1800	1980	2160	2340	2520
5-1/2	792	990	1188	1386	1584	1782	1980	2178	2376	2574	2772
6	864	1080	1296	1512	1728	1944	2160	2376	2592	2808	3024
6-1/2	936	1170	1404	1638	1872	2106	2340	2574	2808	3042	3276
7	1008	1260	1512	1764	2016	2268	2520	2772	3024	3276	3578
7-1/2	1080	1350	1620	1890	2160	2430	2700	2970	3240	3510	3780
8	1152	1440	1728	2016	2304	2592	2880	3168	3456	3744	4032
8-1/2	1224	1530	1836	2142	2448	2754	3060	3366	3672	3978	4284
9	1296	1620	1944	2268	2592	2916	3240	3564	3888	4212	4536
9-1/2	1368	1710	2052	2394	2736	3078	3420	3762	4104	4446	4788

there are fewer than twenty-eight lines, the number will be indicated opposite the last line of type. Paragraphs should be indented the same number of spaces that will be required on the finished copy. Quadruple space between paragraphs and anyplace else where double-spacing will be required on the final page. Lists of items should have the same spacing between columns as you will want on the finished page. (Although at times you may decide to count two half lines as one full line, partial lines are usually counted as full lines.)

3. *Find the number of characters on the manuscript page.* Using Chart A, *Character Count for Manuscript Pages,* take the total number of lines and find the character count for the kind of type used (pica or elite). For example, if a page has twenty-nine manuscript lines, you will have a total of 2,436 elite characters.

4. *Determine how many characters will fit into the designated space.* Using your total character count, refer to Chart B for elite type or Chart C for pica type. (The figures at the top of each column represent the width of a block of type in inches. The figures down the side are vertical measurements in inches.) Now find a character count on the chart that is close to, *but not less than,* your character count. If, for example, your character count is 2,436 elite characters, the type would fit easily into a space 4 inches wide by 9 inches deep. Other possibilities are 5" × 7" or 6½" × 5½".

CHART C
MANUSCRIPT CHARACTER COUNT CONVERSION
Pica Type

Depth of Typed Column (inches) Single-Spaced	Width of Typed Column (inches)										
	2	2-1/2	3	3-1/2	4	4-1/2	5	5-1/2	6	6-1/2	7
2	240	300	360	420	480	540	600	660	720	780	840
2-1/2	300	375	450	525	600	675	750	825	900	975	1050
3	360	450	540	630	720	810	900	990	1080	1170	1260
3-1/2	420	525	630	735	840	945	1050	1155	1260	1365	1470
4	480	600	720	840	960	1080	1200	1320	1440	1560	1680
4-1/2	540	675	810	945	1080	1215	1350	1485	1620	1755	1890
5	600	750	900	1050	1200	1350	1500	1650	1800	1950	2100
5-1/2	660	825	990	1155	1320	1485	1650	1815	1980	2145	2310
6	720	900	1080	1260	1440	1620	1800	1980	2160	2340	2520
6-1/2	780	975	1170	1365	1560	1755	1950	2145	2340	2535	2730
7	840	1050	1260	1470	1680	1890	2100	2310	2520	2730	2940
7-1/2	900	1125	1350	1575	1800	2025	2250	2475	2700	2925	3150
8	960	1200	1440	1680	1920	2160	2400	2640	2880	3120	3360
8-1/2	1020	1275	1530	1785	2040	2295	2550	2805	3060	3315	3570
9	1080	1350	1620	1890	2160	2430	2700	2970	3240	3510	3780
9-1/2	1140	1425	1710	1995	2280	2565	2850	3135	3420	3705	3990

If you want to divide the type by paragraphs, the character count for each paragraph is taken, and the same procedure is followed.

FITTING ILLUSTRATIONS WITH TYPED COPY

A rough sketch of your layout determines the general number and placement of illustrations. Once you know how much space will be occupied by the copy, you can refine your layout. First compare a rough sketch of the layout with your calculations for the type. Will there be enough room for your illustrations? If not, you may decide to eliminate an illustration, reduce the size of one or more illustrations, change the line length of the copy, or move some of the copy to a second page (Fig. 5.26).

Aligning the Page

Before beginning your revised layout you must position the format template on the work surface. Place a sheet of high quality white paper squarely over the format template. The horizontal and vertical lines of the grid paper or goldenrod mask should show through the paper.

Hold the T-square firmly against the side of the drawing board, and slide it over the page until the upper edge of the T-square aligns with a horizontal line on the grid paper. Next, attach both pages to the work surface with push pins or tape. If you will be using a lettering guide or template, the T-square may be held in place by push pins inserted against the lower edge of the T-square. The T-square, triangle, and templates may be used with pencil or pen,

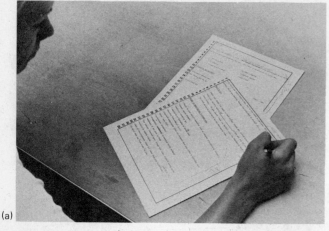

(a)

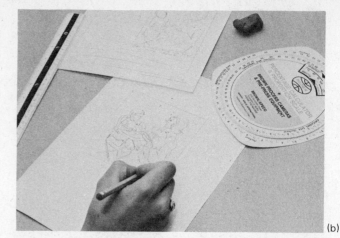

(b)

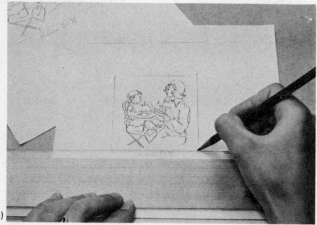

(c)

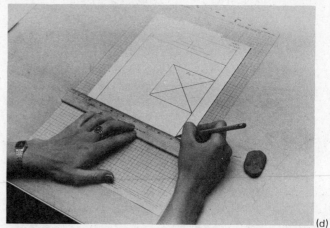

(d)

Your child has had a head injury, and is now ready to go home. For your child's safety, there are several things you will need to do at home.

WHAT TO DO:

1. Watch your child for signs of head injury (signs are listed below).
2. Call your child's doctor at _____ if you see any of the signs of head injury. (If you cannot reach the doctor, call the Emergency Room at 461-2500 or bring your child to the Emergency Room.)

SIGNS OF HEAD INJURY TO WATCH FOR:

- Change in your child's behavior such as extreme irritability (cross)
- Nausea (upset stomach)
- Vomiting (throwing up)
- Complaints of headache or stiff neck
- Bleeding from nose or ears
- Increased sleepiness (does not respond when you offer a favorite toy)
- Fever over 101°
- Convulsions (seizures)
- Staggering or swaying while walking
- Weakness of one side of body
- Eye changes (crossed eyes, droopy eye lids, trouble using eyes)
- Blurred or double vision
- Loss of consciousness (does not waken when you touch and talk to him)
- If child does not "look right" to you

ACTIVITY:

Your child may return to school. The child should avoid rough activities until after his follow up visit with the doctor. The types of activities to avoid are:

- Bike riding
- Swimming
- Skate board riding
- Tree climbing
- Contact sports
- Gym class

FOLLOW UP APPOINTMENT:

Your child should see the doctor 2 or 3 weeks after leaving the hospital. Call the doctor for an appointment if the appointment has not already been made.

If you have any questions, please call your doctor or _____.

(e)

(f)

(g)

134

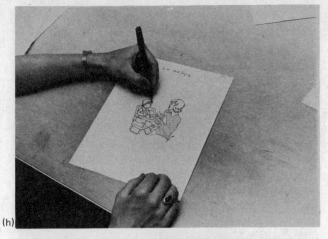

(h)

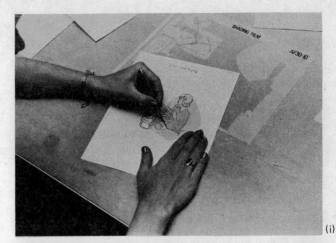

(i)

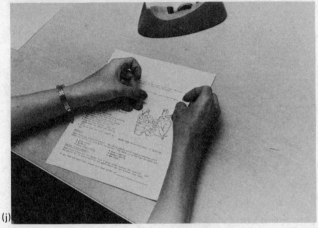

(j)

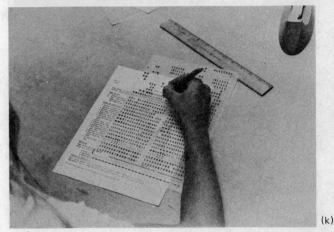

(k)

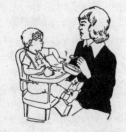
(l)

FIGURE 5.26 Step-by-step layout and paste-up: (*a*) The text of the teaching aid is typed in manuscript form and edited. The character count is computed. (*b*) Using the character count figures, a preliminary layout is prepared. Pencil sketches of illustrations are drawn proportionately larger than the desired finished size. (*c*) Pencil sketches are reduced to the size indicated in the layout and then photocopied. These copies of the illustrations are ruled and keyed to the layout. (*d*) Using a nonreproducing pencil and the format template, a refined layout page is prepared for the typist. (*e*) The teaching aid is typed, single-spaced, on the layout page. (*f*) Copies of pencil sketches are cut out and lightly taped to the typed page. The teaching aid is then photocopied for distribution to reviewers. (*g*) After reviewer's comments are compiled, the layout is revised and the teaching aid is retyped according to the new layout. (*h*) Pencil illustrations are revised (if necessary) and then traced in ink. (*i*) If transfer film is to be used, it is applied to final ink illustrations. (*j*) Photostats of ink illustrations are permanently pasted up. (*k*) Title, form numbers (if used), and major headings are applied to the final paste up, using transfer lettering. (*l*) The completed teaching aid is ready to be printed.

but they should never be used with a cutting tool that will damage the plastic edge.

Preparing the Copy and Illustrations

Using the T-square and a nonreproducing pencil, rule off the margins, letterhead, and title areas that appear on the format template. With pencil, define the areas designated for type, illustrations, titles, and captions. Rule the illustration areas with diagonal lines from corner to corner as shown in Figure 5.25, and identify each with a notation, such as "Picture 3." The ruled page is then given to the typist, who works from the manuscript copy and types directly onto this sheet. (If your type has been set, you would use *reproduction proofs* of the type, and paste them up in the designated areas.)

Once the page is typed and proofread, illustrations are prepared. Use the layout as a guide for the size and number of illustrations. When illustrations or photographs are used actual size, it is easier to visualize how the finished page will look. (There may be times, though, when you will want to prepare larger sketches and have the illustrations reduced later. In this event, use your circular proportion scale to compute the proportions of the enlarged sketch. An illustration with a finished size of $3'' \times 5''$, for instance, should be drawn *proportionately* larger. You can start out with a sketch $6'' \times 10''$ and have it reduced 50% to fit the layout. But an illustration of $6'' \times 8''$ will never reduce to $3'' \times 5''$, no matter what your reduction percentage is.) If you are using photographs, you should have a PMT or Velox made. These are pasted-up like line art.

We often use photocopies (Xerox) of pencil illustrations for the first paste-up. These copies are outlined in nonreproducing pencil to the exact dimensions indicated by the layout. Photos and line art are "keyed" on the reverse side with an identifying description, i.e., "Picture 3." Line art is then cut out and taped lightly to the typewritten page. Transfer lettering and shading film are not generally added at this point.

The pencil sketches reproduce well enough to give the reviewers an adequate idea of the look of the finished Helping Hand. They are invited to critique the illustrations, as well as the text, for accuracy and appropriateness. Changes are easily made on the pencil sketches before they are rendered in ink.

Once all the comments of the reviewers have been compiled, necessary changes are made in the illustrations, and the page is retyped. If there are extensive revisions, a new layout may be required. Corrected pencil illustrations may now be rendered in ink on good quality rag layout paper. Shading effects and transfer letters may be added if desired.

Using Photostats

Most paste-up artists use the original artwork for the paste-up. In our case, this is not practical, since the same drawing may be needed for a future teaching aid. We maintain a file of all original artwork for ready reference and re-use. To provide a clean, crisp copy of the finished artwork, we have *photostats* (or stats, for short) made of the work. Reductions of original artwork can be done in the same operation.[1] If there is a number of illustrations to be reduced and photostatted at the same time, they may be grouped, or *ganged* on the same board, provided the reduction percentage is the same for all. To gang illustrations, tape them lightly to a large white board. Since all the artwork is photographed at the same time, you pay only for the *reduced* size of the negative and photostat paper.

Whether original art or photostats are used, final illustrations are outlined, keyed, and cut out in the same manner as pencil sketches. However, rubber cement, invisible tape, or wax adhesive are used to construct the final paste-up.

The Mounting Surface

Most commercial paste-up is mounted on hard, smooth four-ply illustration board, and there are relatively few changes after the job has progressed to the paste-up stage. In our case, depending on the complexity of the teaching aid, there may be several drafts in "pencil paste-up" form before the artwork is inked in and transfer lettering is applied. Aside from being less expensive than board, paper originals can be changed more readily. Paper paste-ups are also more practical in making paper printing plates for offset printing. The original is passed through a plate-making machine that would not easily accommodate the thickness of four-ply illustration board.

AND NOW TO THE DRAWING BOARD

We began this discussion by confronting that old bugaboo—artistic talent. We hope that while reading this chapter the "monster" hasn't grown to unmanageable proportions. You may have decided—perhaps too prematurely—that the job of assembling pictures and print should be placed in the hands of an experienced expert. But before you set about recruiting a graphic artist or illustrator, why not try doing the work yourself? There's nothing like "hands-on" learning to build your understanding, skill, and self-confidence. You may surprise yourself with the amount of hidden talent you possess.

---

[1] Photostatic *enlargements* of illustrations have also proven very useful in developing teaching aids. An instructive diagram or illustration on $8\frac{1}{2}'' \times 11''$ paper is enlarged to poster size ($17'' \times 22''$) and printed on heavy photographic paper. The poster is then hand-colored with felt-tip markers or colored pencils. Covering the poster with clear self-adhesive plastic makes it more durable and easier to clean. Our health professionals use these posters with the Helping Hands for patient teaching. The posters also provide an invaluable tool for inservice education.

Start slowly and simply. Assemble some of the basic tools and graphic aids; you can always add to your inventory later as the need arises. Get to know your printer. Once he sees that you are sincerely interested in his trade, he may be an invaluable source of information and helpful, time-saving tips. Study the illustrations of printed materials that you particularly admire. Try to determine what graphic aids and techniques were used to produce these results. If your work is spontaneous, honest, meaningful, and memorable, it will certainly compensate for a lack of drawing skill. And if the pages are carefully planned to integrate elements of balance, space, and logical rhythm and flow, you can achieve results that compare favorably with the most professionally executed printed materials.

SELECTED READINGS

Arnold, Edmund C. *Ink on Paper: A Handbook of the Graphic Arts.* New York: Harper & Row, 1972.

Brown, James W.; Lewis, Richard B.; and Harcleroad, Fred F. *AV Instruction: Technology, Media and Methods.* New York: McGraw-Hill Book Co., 1973.

Croy, Peter. *Graphic Design and Reproduction Techniques.* New York: Hastings House Publishers, 1968.

Edel, D. Henry, Jr., ed. *Introduction to Creative Designs.* Englewood Cliffs, N.J.: Prentice-Hall, 1967.

Gill, Bob. *Illustration: Aspects and Direction.* New York: Reinhold Publishing Corp., 1964.

Maurello, S. Ralph. *How to Do Paste-ups and Mechanicals.* New York: Tudor Publishing Co., 1960.

Minor, Ed and Frye, Harvey R. *Techniques for Producing Visual Instructional Media.* New York: McGraw-Hill Book Co., 1970.

Nelms, Henning. *Thinking With a Pencil.* New York: Barnes & Noble, 1964.

Photodrawings. Rochester, N.Y.: Eastman Kodak Co., 1957.

Pocket Pal: A Graphic Arts Production Handbook. Rev. ed. New York: International Paper Co., 1974.

Stone, Bernard and Eckstein, Arthur. *Preparing Art for Printing.* New York: Reinhold Publishing Corp., 1965.

Taubes, Federic. *The Quickest Way to Draw Well.* New York: Viking Press, 1958.

chapter 6

Teaching the Health Professional to Teach

Jane Harman Hooker

"The great aim of education is not knowledge but action."

Herbert Spencer

"Do you feel confident that your patients and their families are well prepared to provide the necessary health care at home?" "Are you satisfied with the kind and amount of health teaching you are providing for your patients?" "Are you confident in your knowledge of *how* to teach?" If you answer "no" to any of these questions, it may indicate that you and the staff in your setting need to improve your skills in teaching patients.

As you develop patient teaching aids, such as the Helping Hands, you will also want to assess the teaching skills of the "teachers"—the health professionals. Educational opportunities should be provided for those who need to review patient education principles, improve teaching skills, or learn more about the teaching process. Education and training activities assist staff to acquire, to maintain, or to improve skills and knowledge which will produce desired outcomes for patient care (del Bueno, p. 44). This chapter discusses the process of teaching the health professional to teach and gives practical suggestions and direction to approach this endeavor.

THE STAFF DEVELOPMENT PROCESS

The recent emphasis in the health care field on quality assurance, continuing education, and peer review has increased the value placed on staff development by health care institutions and individual health professionals (Tobin, p. 40). With the rapid changes and advances in health care knowledge and practices, staff development and inservice education personnel have become increasingly involved in developing programs and strategies for implementing change. Education of the staff is one approach to implement change or improve performance of the health care provider. However, inservice training or education will produce improved performance and effect change only under two circumstances: (1) if the individual staff member has never acquired the specific knowledge or skill or (2) if the knowledge and skills are infrequently used and need reinforcement (del Bueno, p. 44).

Continuing education in nursing, as defined by the American Nurses Association, "consists of planned learning experiences beyond a basic nursing educational program. These experiences are designed to promote the development of knowledge, skills, and attitudes for the enhancement of nursing practice, thus improving health care to the public" (A.N.A., p. 69). Thus, inservice education for health professionals consists of planned learning experiences that are designed to increase the competence and skills within a specific area of knowledge.

In the literature we find numerous approaches for structuring and planning learning programs. The framework we use, the staff development process, is similar to the nursing care process. The first step in the process is *assessment:* identifying learner needs. The second step is the development of *goals and objectives* which are specific and stated in behavioral terms. Using the goals and objectives, a *plan* whereby the learner can achieve these goals is developed and implemented. The final step of the staff development process is *evaluation;* determining whether the learner achieved the objectives for which the learning opportunities were designed.

Using this process, we developed a patient/family teaching conference for our staff. Our experiences in planning and presenting the conference, as well as additional strategies and activities, are discussed in the following sections.

IDENTIFYING NEEDS

A need can be defined as a discrepancy or a difference between what is, and what is desired (Mager & Pipe, p. 7). There are several methods for assessing the need for staff development programs. *Direct observation* of the teaching practices of the staff provides the most reliable method for identifying needs. Staff development members and other leadership personnel make purposeful observations in the clinical areas. Attending patient care conferences, shift reports, rounds with the staff, and observation of interactions between health professionals and patients can provide information about the kind and amount of patient teaching performed. Learning needs are identified when the practices observed do not meet the standards for desired practice.

Another method is the review of *documentation on patients' charts.* Reviewing the reports of the nursing quality assurance program (nursing audit) can aid in retrieving information. Many of the educational needs of patients, individual health professionals, and various hospital departments can be identified by using these reports. For example, in our nursing audit of patients with fractured femurs, we identified a lack of documentation of patients' understanding of cast care (at the time of discharge). In this and other audits, the lack of documentation of patient understanding caused us to question the practice and

skills of our health professionals related to patient education. However, to validate whether audit findings are a result of deficiencies in documentation or practice requires further assessment.

Direct communication with the staff may also identify learning needs. Verbal communication with the staff in the work environment or informally during lunch or coffee breaks may elicit requests for specific learning opportunities. Written communication, in the form of a learning needs questionnaire or survey, can be used to gather information. The questionnaire may be general to allow for input on a wide variety of learning needs, or it may be specific in identifying learning needs related to a particular topic. An example of the latter is shown in Figure 6.1. We used this survey to compare patterns and attitudes toward patient teaching before and after the conference was offered. Thus, this survey was used as a learning needs assessment tool prior to the conference and as an evaluation tool after the program.

A fourth source for assessing learning needs is the identification of *internal and external changes* that influence the practice of the health professionals within the setting. For example, the proposed implementation of "primary nursing" within an institution would necessitate the re-education of the nursing staff, as well as all other health professionals who work with the nurses in providing patient care. External changes, such as the changes in health technologies and laws also generate a need for education.

No single method for identifying learning needs is complete and applicable in every situation. Direct observation is appropriate for assessing behavior, but pencil and paper tests may be more effective in assessing needs for knowledge. In identifying the needs of our health professionals we used several approaches; these included direct observation, review of nursing audit reports, written communications, and internal change. The introduction of the Helping Hands (an internal change) provided the primary stimulus for developing planned learning opportunities for the staff. Patient teaching skills as well as the intended use of the Helping Hands needed to be reviewed and learned.

DEVELOPING OBJECTIVES

After you have identified a learning need, the behavioral objectives can be written. A behavioral objective is a description of a pattern, behavior, or performance which we want the learner to demonstrate after successfully completing a learning experience (Mager, p. 3). Basic elements to include in the objectives are a description of the learner, statement of the kind of behavior the learner has to demonstrate to indicate learning, and statement of the content to which the behavior is related (Reilly, p. 31).

PATIENT/FAMILY TEACHING CONFERENCE

Teaching Practices Survey

Please answer each question as accurately as you can. This questionnaire will help us evaluate the long term effects of this conference on patient/family teaching.

* *

General Information

How long have you worked at Children's Hospital? _____

How long have you been a practicing health professional? _____

How often do you teach patients or families? _____

During the last week, how many patients/families did you instruct? _____

In which area do you instruct patients/families? (Check all that apply)

☐ Preoperative care
☐ Homegoing instructions
☐ Health guidance
☐ Other

* *

	Key:	Always 5	4	Sometimes 3	2	Never 1
1.	I enjoy teaching patients/families.	5	4	3	2	1
2.	I feel unsure of my teaching skills.	5	4	3	2	1
3.	I find myself making excuses to avoid teaching patient/families	5	4	3	2	1
4.	I feel confident that the families I have taught are well prepared to follow through at home with hospital initiated procedures.	5	4	3	2	1
5.	I feel that patient/family teaching is as essential to health maintenance as other responsibilities of health professionals.	5	4	3	2	1

(OVER)

-2-

	Key:	Always 5	4	Sometimes 3	2	Never 1
6.	I feel the responsibility for patient/family teaching should be shared equally among all health professionals.	5	4	3	2	1
7.	I assess individual learning needs before beginning an instructional program.	5	4	3	2	1
8.	I write down teaching goals and objectives before beginning instruction.	5	4	3	2	1
9.	I evaluate learning through observation, questions or other objective means.	5	4	3	2	1
10.	I ask the family to demonstrate what they have learned before they leave the hospital.	5	4	3	2	1
11.	I feel it is important to document in detail the teaching given on the patient progress notes.	5	4	3	2	1
12.	I feel that all patients/families with a similar diagnosis can receive the same instruction.	5	4	3	2	1
13.	Whenever possible, I try to use teaching aids such as dolls, charts or Helping Hands.	5	4	3	2	1

14. I am most likely to begin planning for patient/family teaching (Check one)
☐ At admission
☐ At discharge
☐ When the diagnosis is confirmed
☐ When patients/families ask questions
☐ Other _____

(OVER)

-3-

15. My greatest difficult in conducting patient/family teaching is: (Arrange in order of difficulty; 1 = most difficult)
☐ Arranging the time with the patient/family
☐ Arranging my own time
☐ Finding adequate teaching resources
☐ Stressing importance of patient education to others on the unit
☐ Knowing how to organize an instructional plan

16. I feel the amount of teaching I give is: (Check one)
☐ Enough
☐ Too much
☐ Too little

17. Within the last three months, I have read this many articles on patient education.
_____

18. Besides "more time", the following things would help me to teach more efficiently and effectively:
_____
_____
_____

FIGURE 6.1 A teaching practices survey is used to compare teaching attitudes and behaviors before and after the conference.

This formula, used for writing general objectives, communicates the intent of the program to others. Specific objectives which include the conditions under which the behavior is demonstrated and the standards of performance may also be written.

Learning behaviors are classified in three ways: *cognitive*—the knowledge and intellectual skills, *affective*—the states of feeling and valuing, and *psychomotor*—the manipulative or motor skills (Bloom, p. 7). For the purpose of our patient teaching workshop, we developed objectives with these three areas in mind. Our objectives for the learner were as follows:

The health professional will be able to:

1. Discuss trends in society and health care which influence the practice of health teaching

2. Identify the steps of the teaching-learning process

3. Plan a teaching session for a patient and family

4. Demonstrate use of Helping Hands in conducting a teaching session

5. Document on the patient record the learning demonstrated by patient and family

6. Evaluate a teaching-learning session

Developing behavioral objectives is an inexact process and requires practice. Use the references listed at the end of this chapter for assistance in developing objectives for your patient teaching program.

PLANNING AND PRESENTING THE LEARNING PROGRAM

Once you have identified the learning needs and developed the objectives, you are ready to plan your program. Many factors influence the approach you select for meeting the objectives, and the learning objectives may need to be revised as these factors are given consideration. These factors include scope of the program, faculty resources, audio-visual resources, time, place, and financial resources. The planning process can be considered a process of horizontal refinement; in other words, each of the factors become more specific as they interrelate to produce the final program. The factors influence and are influenced by the teaching strategy or learning activities designed to meet the objectives. Our planning committee considered these factors in designing our Patient/Family Teaching Conference.

THE PLANNING COMMITTEE

The purpose of the planning committee is to identify resources, to plan the program, to evaluate the feasibility and probable impact of the program design, and to generate support for the program. Some institutions have a permanent education or nursing inservice committee to identify educational needs and plan programs. We use an ad hoc committee for planning special programs or projects.

Who should be on the committee? Inclusion of representatives from various interest groups provides a broad base of knowledge and experience from which to draw information for decision making. Interest groups may mean members of the nursing department, education department, medical staff, and any other group that has interest or expertise in patient education. These members may serve in an advisory capacity or may have specific responsibilities such as faculty selection, program publicity, or facility scheduling.

In planning the program, use the expertise of each committee member. The member who has expertise in patient education can provide input relative to the content of the program; this person probably knows other resource people who could serve as faculty. The nurse-administrator member can provide input on administrative support and availability of staff to participate. The staff nurse can represent the interests of the staff nurses and their receptivity to various teaching approaches. The nurse-educator adds the dimension of adult teaching-learning theory, experience in program planning, and knowledge of resources. Representatives from other groups of health professionals can also share in the planning and implementation. Not all members of the committee need to be experts in patient education. It is helpful to have members who do not feel skilled in this area; they can provide valuable input about which approaches would be most helpful in learning the skill.

We use a program planning worksheet (Fig. 6.2) in developing a program. It serves as a reminder of the various factors that influence the program and reduces the chances of forgetting materials or equipment. Let's discuss some of the major factors which influence program planning.

DETERMINING SCOPE OF THE PROGRAM

How big shall we dream? How much time and effort should be spent on teaching how many people? Basically, the size of the potential learner group and the scope of the identified need determine the time and effort required to produce an adequate program. While determining the scope of your educational approach, give consideration to the following:

- Attitude and support of the organization toward continuing education
- Attitude and support of the organization toward the specific educational program, i.e., patient education
- Attitude of the learner and the learner's peer group toward continuing education and patient education
- Awareness of the learner that a learning need exists (a sense of uneasiness between what he can do and what he would like to do)
- Belief of the learner that the experience will assist him in meeting his learning needs.

In our setting, education of the staff is valued and supported. The nursing department has set patient education

program planning worksheet

Program:
Planning Committee Members: ______
Title: ______
Date: ______
Time: ______
Location: ______
Learner Group: ______
Objectives: ______

Program Faculty:
Names and Qualifications: ______
Honorarium: ______
Special Arrangements: ______

(OVER)

Publicity:
Announcements (In Newsletter, newspapers, journals, etc.): ______
Preregistration Form: ______
Send out on: ______
Send to: ______

Program Materials:
Name Tags: ______
Program (Complete): ______
"Hand Outs" (Titles, from whom): ______
Program Evaluation: ______
Program Certificates: ______
Audiovisual Equipment (What, for whom, time): ______

(OVER)

Facilities:
Room Arrangement (Tables, seating arrangements): ______
Refreshments ("Coffee breaks", etc.): ______
Registration Table: ______

After The Program:
Thank You to Speakers: ______
Summary Report (Including evaluation results) Send to: ______

FIGURE 6.2 A program planning worksheet is useful in organizing the details of the workshop.

as a priority for development and believes it deserves full consideration for effective implementation. Since we were introducing the Helping Hands (a change in available teaching resources), we identified a need to develop a program that would include the majority of nurses on our staff.

The challenge was to develop an approach that would reach the majority of our staff. Since we could not have all our staff personally participate in an extensive program, we decided to work toward developing the skills of representatives from each nursing unit. These nurses would serve as role models and consultants to others on the unit. To aid the "role model-consultant," we produced a 20-minute slide/tape program that reviews the teaching-learning process and illustrates the use of the Helping Hands. Following attendance at the Patient/Family Teaching Conference this audio-visual aid is available for the nurse to use during presentations in unit conferences.

SELECTING FACULTY

The selection of the teaching strategies and learning activities for the program depends in part on the availability of faculty: Who can best teach the health professional to teach? Do we invite an "outside expert" to present a program or do we use the "experts" on our own staff?

It is important to have some criteria in mind before selecting the program leader and individual instructors. Criteria we use are:

- The person has demonstrated expertise in the area of patient education.

- The person has gained the respect of the nursing staff.

- The person has established credibility.

- The person has demonstrated good teaching skills in a group situation; he/she is a dynamic speaker, one able to stimulate the interest of the group, to keep the program moving, and to be responsive to the needs of the learners.

Your first thought may be that the person must also be a nurse, but many health disciplines engage in patient teaching and you may find your dynamic educator to be a community physician, a physical therapist, or a dietitian. You may need to do some searching; perhaps *you* may be the one to fill this role.

External Educator

There are advantages to recruiting someone from outside your immediate setting to lead or to present the program. Such a person is generally viewed as having more expertise than an "inside expert." Having an external educator lends prestige to the program and sometimes produces better response for attendance. It is stimulating for the staff to hear about what is being done in other settings. It is also reassuring to know other places have many of the same problems you encounter. Yes, other health professionals *do* have difficulty planning their time to include the desired amount of patient teaching; and they *do* have difficulty finding a place, free of interruptions and distractions, in which to teach patients. It is also educational to hear how others approach and/or solve similar problems which frustrate the staff.

Assessing the qualifications of this educator may differ from assessing those of an in-house person. You may need to rely on second-hand information unless you have observed him in a similar teaching situation. Evaluate other aspects such as references from other professionals, publications of books or journal articles, prior experience as an educator or program speaker, work experience, and participation in professional organizations.

An educator from outside your setting also poses some different program planning considerations. The matching of time schedules may be a problem, especially if the person is frequently requested to present such programs. You may need to consider financing for an honorarium and travel expenses. You will want to share your program objectives with the educator to insure that they are consistent with the educator's ideas. If the educator already has a "packaged program" on patient/family education you need not develop the learning activities, but be sure to request his program objectives and outline for your review. Provide the educator with some information about your setting, the patient education needs you have identified, and the size and composition of the group who will attend the program. This information will help the educator to adapt his program for your setting. Ask if special equipment (such as chalkboard and overhead projectors) is needed or if specific room arrangements are desired.

Having an external educator can be a very positive approach. Beside the advantages already mentioned, you can also pick up some ideas on teaching styles and techniques. But you may decide to use teaching resources closer to home. Who do you have in your own setting that can do the job?

Internal Educator

There are several advantages to selecting an educator from within your setting. These are familiarity with your setting, recognition of the goals and needs of the personnel, knowledge of patient needs and of the current practice of patient education, and the ability to readily obtain needed information. Thus, the internal educator is in a better position to center the program around the specific needs of your setting.

If you have a "resident expert" on your staff, you have probably already involved him on your planning committee, at least in a consulting capacity if not in working out the details. Ask him to be the educator.

One person may not feel "resident expert" enough or

may be too involved with other commitments to lead the entire program. In that event, use several people, as we did. Perhaps you are thinking, "We don't have one expert, much less five." Think again. Look to the nursing leadership group. Look to the staff nurses. Look to other health care professionals. There are health professionals on your staff who do a lot of patient teaching. They are probably in a conference room right now, teaching a patient or family. Find out who does a good job with patient education and is enthusiastic about it. If they don't fit the criteria 100%, you can coach them and they can learn. Remember, one of the best ways to learn a subject is to teach it.

Prepare your group of educators by reviewing the program goals and objectives and the program flow as a group. They may have some additional ideas to improve your initial plan. Allow sufficient planning time with the group so each person has a clear picture of the overall program, as well as of his specific responsibilities. Determine the amount of time each participant will have to speak during the program. If the majority are not experienced in speaking before groups, you may want to discuss the management of time in relation to program flow. What will you do if someone uses less than the alloted time or if someone goes overtime? What do you do when discussion is planned but the group is nonparticipative? Plan for some flexibility in time. Provide your group of educators with some teaching tips. Build their self-confidence.

THE LEARNING CLIMATE

In planning and in conducting an educational program, give consideration to establishing an atmosphere that is conducive to learning. *Facilities,* including lighting, temperature, seating comfort, and seating arrangement, influence the participants' ability to concentrate on the task of learning. Some of these factors will be influenced by the availability and choice of classroom space. For example, our classroom allows for flexible seating arrangements; however, temperature control is a problem, and the student desk-chairs are uncomfortable to sit in for long periods of time.

The choice of the classroom and seating arrangement is considered in relation to the size of the group and the planned activities. Our conference consists of lecture, viewing of film strips, and small group work. Our seating arrangements changed throughout the program from the traditional classroom rows, to circles of ten, to triads. Separating the groups into different rooms for the small group workshops is ideal. But this is rarely possible in our immediate setting where available classroom space is in high demand.

Time, an important dimension of the learning climate, is also a factor in program planning. How much time is needed for the most effective learning of the objective? Consider a short-term course approach (such as 1- or 2-hour sessions once a week for several weeks) versus a compact, 1- or 2-day program. Compare the efficiency and feasibility of each approach in your setting. The advantages of the all-day approach are insuring continuity of learner participation, maintaining momentum of the learning experience throughout the program, and decreasing the amount of time needed to review or refocus the learners' attention from the work setting to the learning experience. The all-day program can also be a morale booster by affording more opportunity for interacting with other health professionals and for sharing common concerns. Sharing a meal together during a break in the day's program can be very refreshing and stimulating—usually quite a change from the hurried mealtime break during the work day.

There are also advantages in divided learning sessions. There is greater time to assimilate the material. Opportunities exist for testing some of the material in the work environment, then returning to the learning experience for discussion, confirmation, and clarification. Less time is lost in providing breaks although this may be balanced by the time spent on review and refocusing attention. Ability of the learners to arrange time for either the compact or divided approach will vary with the setting and the schedules for the individual learners.

We preferred the all-day conference to insure continuity. In our setting, it is difficult to find a time that is convenient for nurses from various areas to leave for an hour or two. We also find that situations arise in the work setting that prevent the nurse from leaving the unit to attend the program. Thus, we have no assurance that the nurse will be able to participate in all the sessions. The nurses also find it difficult to change pace from the work area to the classroom.

If your learner group is composed of people who do not know each other, plan a *get-acquainted activity* to start the program; this is also part of creating a learning climate. Divide the group into groups of about ten. Allow a few minutes for informal "getting to know each other." Then have each member introduce another member and give some information about him/her that is not work related. This is a change from "I am Sally Jones and I work on sixth floor Nursery" (name tags can include this identifying information). Activities such as this are part of climate setting and help to "break the ice," permitting learners to unwind and to begin group involvement.

Refreshments are a planned part of the all-day conference. They provide nourishment, as well as an opportunity for getting acquainted. The "coffee break" can be offered during the registration period or refreshments can be served at mid-morning break. As we mentioned previously, the lunch meal can provide a change from the usual break in the work day. We allow time for the learners to go out for lunch which is viewed by many as a special treat. This reduces the need for a catered luncheon and avoids a large influx of people in the hospital cafeteria.

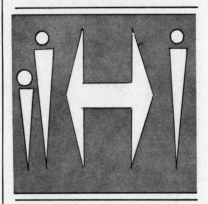

PATIENT/FAMILY

TEACHING CONFERENCE

March 17, 1978
8:00 - 4:30
Timken Hall

Sponsored by the
Department of
Staff Development
and Education
Children's Hospital
Columbus, Ohio

PATIENT/FAMILY TEACHING CONFERENCE

March 17, 1978
8:00 - 4:30
South Classroom
Timken Hall

8:00   Registration and Refreshments

8:15   Introductions & Objectives of
       the Conference

       Jane Hooker, RN, M.S.N.,
       Associate Director of Nursing,
       Staff Development

8:45   Patient/Family Teaching:
       Prescription for Better Health

       David Stein, Ph.D.
       Director, Education

       Jane Hooker, RN, M.S.N.

9:30   Intermission

9:45   Health Professional as Teacher

       Laurel Talabere, RN, M.S.N.,
       Clinical Specialist,
       Pulmonary Services

10:30 The Helping Hand

       Rose Marie McCormick, RN, B.S.N.
       Assistant Director of Nursing
       Continuity of Care

11:15 Lunch (on your own)

12:45 From Theory to Practice

       Jane Hooker, RN, M.S.N.

1:00   Workshop I

       Group A: Preparation for Surgery
       and Procedures

       Ruth Wheeler, RN
       Head Nurse, 4TN

       Raymond P. Davis, A.R.R.T.,
       Director, Respiratory Care

       Group B: Teaching for Home
       Therapy

       Syd Imes, RN
       Head Nurse, 5AE

       Lynn Holland, LPT
       Director, Physical Therapy

       Group C: Health Guidance

       Janet Smith, RN, P.N.A.
       Health Assessment Clinic

       Wynola Wayne, RN
       Coordinator of Diabetic Care

2:30   Workshop II - repeat of small
                      groups

4:00   Summary and Evaluation

       Jane Hooker, RN, M.S.N.

LEARNING OBJECTIVES

Following the conference the health
professional will be able to:

1. Discuss trends in society and
   health care which influence
   teaching patients and family.

2. Identify steps in teaching-
   learning process.

3. Plan a teaching session.

4. Demonstrate use of Helping
   Hands in conducting a teaching
   session.

5. Document teaching on the
   patient's chart.

6. Evaluate a teaching-learning
   session.

TO REGISTER, RETURN THIS FORM TO
STAFF DEVELOPMENT OFFICE BY
MARCH 10.

NAME: _____

UNIT: _____

FIGURE 6.3 The program announcement includes objectives and schedule of the activities.

These factors of time, place, and personal comfort influence the learners' receptivity to the program. Of course, your approach depends on the facilities available in your setting.

PROMOTING THE PROGRAM

Once you have planned the program, including the learning activities discussed in the next section, you will need to "sell" it. Two main groups need to "buy" it: the administrative personnel (the line managers who support and supervise patient care) and the personnel delivering that care. The administrative personnel must be convinced that the learning program is worthwhile, and that staff and patients will benefit from the time being spent away from direct patient care. The administrative representative on your planning committee can give you assistance in this area. Discuss the program at your management meeting to gain their support. Emphasize the intent of having at least one or more staff members from each unit attend if this is your identified learner group.

"Selling" to the second group, the desired participants or learner group, is less direct. For this group, you may want to distribute printed announcements, or "flyers," to publicize the program. The brochures should be attractive, neat, uncluttered, and easily read (Fig. 6.3). Art work, if used, should complement the information and not interfere with the written message. Colored paper and a combination of sizes of print attract attention and promote readability. Indicate date, time, place, and faculty. If the faculty is from outside your institution and is generally unknown in your setting, include a short summary of their credentials (at least each person's title and place of employment). If pre-registration is required, indicate the procedure and the deadline date. Sufficient information should be provided for personnel to decide whether the program will be of benefit to them. This may be done by including the objectives or questions that were used to identify learner needs. The program or schedule of events within the conference may also be part of the flyer. This is helpful when more than one person are presenting the program.

Various distribution systems for the announcements are probably used in your setting. Select a system that will insure high visibility to the health professional. We send the flyers to the head nurses and department heads to be shared with their staff and posted in the work area. We also place the brochures in strategic locations within the hospital such as the cafeteria, conference rooms, and the education bulletin board.

DEVELOPING LEARNING ACTIVITIES

Selection of the content and learning activities are based on the goals and objectives of your program. The objectives (page 140) relate to the attitude, knowledge, and skill you wish the learner to possess regarding patient education. In designing our learning activities, we gave consideration to the value of patient teaching and the knowledge of the teaching-learning process, as well as to the practice of the required skills. The learning activities and the supporting rationale presented in our conference and alternate approaches to meet the objectives are reviewed in this section.

An overview of the learning activities with the program flow is displayed as the learning activities design form (Fig. 6.4). We use this form during the planning process to map out the activities of the program. Let's concentrate now on the learning activities—the strategies developed to assist the learners in becoming more effective patient educators.

Promoting Positive Attitudes

Beginning the program with consideration of attitudes reaffirms and increases the health professional's positive feeling toward patient education and/or his sense of dissatisfaction with current practice. This captures his attention for the learning activities that follow.

Several learning activities related to attitudes toward patient education involve the learner actively in the learning process. For instance, have the participants list all their reasons for providing patient instruction. Or ask them to share a situation in which a child and family they cared for was significantly helped by the teaching. Or request them to identify a situation in which they, themselves, or their family were significantly affected by teaching related to their own health needs.

The approach used to develop a positive attitude toward patient teaching might be compared with an approach for selling a product: persuasive presentation of the values of the product—patient education. The selection of an approach to use in addressing the values or attitudes depends on the size of the group, time alloted, learners' needs to identify their own feelings, and the instructor or group leader's teaching style. In our program, we address issues of value and attitude related to patient education in a lecture format (most of this content is included in Chapters 1 and 2).

In addition to the value of patient education and patient rights, we emphasize the need to document the teaching performed. Documentation is the final step of the actual teaching session. Through documentation, the value, knowledge, and skills of the staff regarding patient education can be evaluated. In the discussion of documentation, we present standards such as those of Joint Commission on Accreditation of Hospitals and the nursing audit criteria. These standards form the base line against which teaching can be evaluated. Examples of documentation tools and documentation are presented and discussed; these include use of the teaching plans (Figs. 2.12, 2.13), the home-going

LEARNING ACTIVITIES DESIGN

CONFERENCE: Patient-Family Teaching
GROUP: Staff nurses and other health professionals
DATE: March 17, 1978
LOCATION: Timken Hall

Time	Activity	Instructional Strategy	Devices	Responsibility
8:00	Registration, coffee and donuts		Table in hall, name tags, program packets	Secretary
8:15	Climate setting	Chairs are arranged in four circles of ten seats each. When group is seated, moderator welcomes them to the program. Moderator asks the four seated groups to become acquainted and then introduce each other to the small group. Moderator describes the learning activities for the program and asks each participant to write down at least one personal learning objective for the day. These objectives will later serve as a basis of evaluation. A pre-test is administered, and collected. Moderator introduces first speaker.	3 X 5 cards Pre-tests	Jane Hooker
8:45	Patient/Family Teaching: Prescription for Better Health	Large group lecture defining the role of patient education in the hospital. Major points are: 1. Who is the learner in a pediatric hospital? 2. Patient education or family education? 3. The changing nature of the health care consumer. 4. What do we mean by learning - "change in behavior", effects of education. 5. Patient's bill of rights 6. Hospital's responsibility for patient education. 7. Delivery system for patient education 8. Documentation of patient learning.	Program packets: • Bill of rights • Charting forms	David Stein Jane Hooker

CONFERENCE: PATIENT/FAMILY TEACHING   Page 2

Time	Activity	Instructional Strategy	Devices	Responsibility
9:30	Intermission			
9:45	Health Professional as Teacher	A large group lecture: skills practice session on the instructional process. The following stages of the process are highlighted: 1. Assessing the need for learning 2. Assessing readiness 3. Objectives 4. Evaluation Learners are given a general teaching problem and must apply concepts presented to a real situation.	Program packet: • Lecture outline • Case study & teaching plan form Overhead projector & transparencies	Laurel Talabere
10:30	The Helping Hand - a slide/tape presentation	A brief introduction of the slide tape is given to the large group. Introduction stresses the following: 1. Teaching/learning occur all the time. 2. Materials are available This last point leads into a discussion of the Helping Hand materials concentrating on history of the project. After the conclusion of the introduction, the slide tape program is presented. Moderator concludes with a review of basic points presented and mentions availability of program for team conferences.	Slide/tape program 2 X 2 projector Cassette player	Rose-Marie McCormick
11:15	Luncheon	On their own		
12:45	Review	Moderator reviews afternoon activity. Divides participants into pre-selected groups for practice sessions.		Jane Hooker

CONFERENCE: PATIENT/FAMILY TEACHING   Page 3

Time	Activity	Instructional Strategy	Devices	Responsibility
1:00	APPLICATION OF TEACHING/LEARNING PRINCIPLES Workshop I	Group attends first choice session. Each small group meets with two resource persons. In an informal atmosphere, group leaders present their views of patient/family teaching as it occurs in a real setting. Group leaders touch on the following points: 1. Developing rapport with patients 2. Teaching techniques used 3. Resource materials available 4. Problems encountered in teaching Leaders encourage questions from the group. Presentation should not exceed 15-20 minutes. After the presentation, small group is divided into triads. Members of the triads take roles of health professional, patient/parent, and observer. A role play situation is devised. At the end of each role play the observes and group leader will critique the instructor.	Hand out - check list for teaching behaviors	Group A Pre-op and preparation for procedures - Ruth Wheeler, Ray Davis Group B Home Therapy a. Infants b. Children Lynn Holland Syd Imes Group C Prevention/ normal development Janet Smith Wynola Wayne
2:30	Workshop II	Same as Workshop I		
4:00	Conclusion/ Evaluation	Group reconvenes for summary of activities. Summary stresses importance of the teaching role, where and how to obtain resources, and wishes the group well in their future patient/family teaching efforts. Program evaluation is completed by participants.	Program evaluation	Jane Hooker

FIGURE 6.4 The learning activities design sheet indicates the time frame, activities, teaching tools, and person responsible.

```
NU-26
Rev. 10-77                    HOME—GOING INSTRUCTIONS
                                 CHILDREN'S HOSPITAL
                                  COLUMBUS, OHIO

To be completed by Physician and/or Nurse upon discharge.

Return to Clinic _____ Date _____ Time _____

       Office _____ Date _____ Time _____

Community Health Referral      No _____ Yes _____ To Whom _____

Date _____ Time _____ Signature _____

INSTRUCTIONS (Treatments, Medications, Diet & Activity) _____
_____
_____
_____
_____
_____
_____
_____
_____


NURSING DISCHARGE SUMMARY

Final Diagnosis _____ Vital Signs: T _____ P _____ R _____

General Appearance: _____
_____
_____

Appearance of incision or wounds: _____ ☐ N.A.

Supportive aids in use: _____ ☐ N.A.
SUMMARY OF PATIENT'S AND/OR FAMILY'S KNOWLEDGE AND UNDERSTANDING REGARDING MANAGEMENT OF HIS CARE FOLLOWING
DISCHARGE: _____
_____
_____
_____

Homegoing Instructions discussed with patient and/or family: Yes ☐

Helping Hand Instruction given (Title): _____

Discharged To:            Mode of Discharge:       Accompanied By:

Parent _____     Ambulatory   ☐          Family Member   ☐

Guardian _____     Wheelchair   ☐          Personnel       ☐

Agency _____     Cart         ☐

Representative _____  Carried      ☐          _____ RN Signature
```

FIGURE 6.5 The homegoing instruction and nursing discharge summary
form organizes patient record documentation.

instruction and nursing discharge summary (Fig. 6.5), and notations entered in the patient progress notes or nursing notes for ongoing teaching. These tools are also available for the participants to use during their practice teaching session.

The health professional's attitude toward patient education is implied by the amount of patient education that he performs and the documentation in the patient's chart. However, without knowledge of the teaching-learning process and the skill to implement the knowledge, the efforts in educating patients may be ineffective.

Providing A Knowledge Base

What knowledge must a person have to be effective in a teaching-learning situation with a patient and his family? In presenting a workshop for health professionals who care for children of various ages and with differing health problems, it is necessary to include information that is applicable in numerous situations. Thus, a theoretical base must be developed which the health professional can

apply to specific situations. This theoretical base of knowledge is presented in lecture format and is similar to the information in Chapter 2. Audio-visual aids such as overhead transparencies are used as much as possible. Providing the learner with copies of the speaker's outline during the lecture enables participants to jot notes without being distracted by continual writing. The learner can concentrate on the material being presented and still have information for later review.

Perhaps a lecture on the teaching-learning process is not your style or is not needed by the staff. Or maybe you do not want to spend time during the learning session for reviewing this information. Most recent graduates acquire a sound knowledge base for patient education while in school, and yet other health professionals in the group may need this material. Try giving assigned readings before your program. It's ironic that assigned readings are expected while in school but are infrequently used with inservice and staff development programs. A bibliography for patient/family teaching is included on page 35 and can be suggested readings before or after the workshop.

Developing Skills

The third major area of learning activity, and perhaps the most important, is the development and practice of teaching skills. It is now time to put the attitudes and knowledge into practice. Several activities in the workshop provide opportunity for skills development and practice.

Practice in planning As part of the session "Health Professional as Teacher," practice focuses on planning for patient teaching. We use this case study for one of the teaching situations:

Benjie Green, a 5-year-old, has recovered from his third episode of pneumonia; but he has a persistent infiltrate in the middle lobe of his right lung. Intravenous antibiotics were discontinued yesterday and oral antibiotics were begun. Benjie continues to receive postural drainage four times a day. He will probably be discharged in 2 days if his temperature remains normal.

While working with Benjie and his family since his admission to the hospital 2 weeks ago, you have obtained the following information: Benjie lives with his parents, his 3-year-old sister, and his grandmother in a house in a rural county. Mr. Green is a farmer and makes furniture during winter months. Mrs. Green is a homemaker. Grandmother Green has severe arthritis. The Green's have one car. They would like to visit Benjie more often but usually get to the hospital only one or two evenings a week and on weekends.

From this information, the learners are (1) to identify teaching needs, (2) to assess readiness, (3) to identify additional information the nurse would need, (4) to write behavioral objectives, and (5) to state criteria for evaluating that learning occurred. You may want the learners to do this individually followed by the full group discussion. Or you may have them divide into groups of three or four members for the exercise. We have found that the small group sessions followed by the sharing of results with the large group is more productive than the individual approach. Several minds working collectively usually generate more creative thoughts; these small groups also simulate team planning conferences which provide additional practice for future situations.

Demonstration A slide/tape program is also used to demonstrate a teaching situation. This presentation reviews the steps of the teaching-learning process and then demonstrates a teaching session of a nurse instructing a mother. The content of the teaching is the procedure of taking the baby's temperature. The Helping Hand *Taking a Temperature* and other aids are used in the teaching. The emphasis of this audio-visual aid is on the process of patient teaching and on the use of teaching aids, especially the Helping Hands.

Role play During the afternoon of the conference, we conduct a third activity for the development and practice of teaching skills. We identified three classifications, or types, of patient/family teaching opportunities and designed learning exercises for participants to practice skills. These teaching situations are: preparation for surgery and procedures, teaching for home care, and health guidance. Three teaching groups are designated and two facilitators assigned to lead each group. Two 90-minute practice workshops are scheduled into the conference, and each participant selects two of the three situations in which to practice teaching skills.

The group workshops begin with the group leaders sharing information about teaching in their area of expertise. They share "helpful hints" and teaching aids such as charts and pictures, teaching dolls, or Helping Hands that they frequently use. The participants then divide into groups of three to role-play a teaching situation. The content of the teaching episode is of their own choosing; this allows each participant to work with familiar content since the areas of expertise of the participants are usually varied. The Helping Hands and other teaching aids are available for their use.

After the triad decides upon a teaching situation, they develop a teaching plan for the patient and implement the plan in the role-playing session. During the role-playing, one participant acts as the nurse-teacher, one the patient-learner and one an observer.

The nurse-teacher in the role-playing situation sets the stage for her practice session. She selects content, characteristics of the patient, and introduces any other variables desired. This allows her to construct a teaching situation which would be most beneficial to her.

There may be skills which the nurse has identified for herself as needing improvement, and she may request the observer to note these specific teaching skills, such as establishing rapport with the patient or using open ended questions. A skills checklist (Fig. 6.6) is used by the observer to record the identified skills of the nurse-teacher.

Following the practice session, critique is done. This generally begins with the nurse-teacher sharing her thoughts and feelings about this teaching experience. Feedback is then given by the patient-learner concerning perceptions of the effectiveness of the teaching. The observer shares observations about the demonstrated skills and indicates those done well and those in need of improvement. The group decides if the objectives stated in the teaching plan were met. Several role-play situations may be done allowing

```
         PATIENT-FAMILY TEACHING SKILLS
             Observer Checklist
```

RAPPORT   Yes   No
• Did the instructor establish rapport with the family?   ☐   ☐

READINESS
• Did the instructor listen for possible learning
  needs identified through conversation with the   ☐   ☐
  family?
• Did the instructor have a prepared set of open   ☐   ☐
  focus questions?
• Did the instructor give the family adequate
  opportunity to express feelings and ask   ☐   ☐
  questions?
• Did the instructor assess the family's level   ☐   ☐
  of knowledge about illness?

INSTRUCTION
• Did the instructor place the family in an
  area in which they could adequately see and   ☐   ☐
  hear the demonstration?
• Did the instructor put the family at ease   ☐   ☐
  before beginning instruction?
• Did the instructor explain to the family what
  had to be learned in terms of behavioral   ☐   ☐
  objectives?
• Did the instructor state why learning was   ☐   ☐
  important?
• Did the instructor begin the lesson with   ☐   ☐
  something that was familiar to the family?
• Were terms used which were understandable to   ☐   ☐
  the family?
• Was the demonstration conducted step by step?   ☐   ☐
• Were steps organized in a way which would   ☐   ☐
  insure early success?
• Did the instructor remain alert for signs   ☐   ☐
  of confusion?

```
                      -2-
```
                                                               Yes   No
• Were questions asked and answered by the   ☐   ☐
  instructor?
• Were key points stressed?   ☐   ☐
• Was the instructor patient?   ☐   ☐

EVALUATION
• Was the family given an opportunity to   ☐   ☐
  demonstrate the task?
• Was the family instructed to explain each   ☐   ☐
  key step as it was performed?
• Were errors corrected in a constructive   ☐   ☐
  fashion?
• Was re-instruction given where necessary?   ☐   ☐

FOLLOW-UP AND DOCUMENTATION
• Did the instructor discuss with the family
  the need for instruction on other health   ☐   ☐
  concerns?
• Was the family given follow-up materials?   ☐   ☐
• Was the teaching session documented?   ☐   ☐

List general comments on the instructor's performance below.

_____

_____

_____

_____

_____

_____

_____

FIGURE 6.6 The skills checklist aids the "observer" during the role-play teaching situation.

each member of the triad to participate in the teacher role. Some participants may want to repeat a situation to incorporate feedback received in their critique.

Use of role-playing is an effective teaching strategy which permits the learner to experience and to practice a skill in a safe, nonthreatening environment. It enables the learner to experiment with new approaches and to receive feedback. However, some learners are hesitant to participate but do learn through observations of others in the group.

Several alternatives to role-playing also help to teach the skills needed for patient education. Demonstration of various teaching situations can be given. Small group problem solving and discussions of individual experiences is another approach which can be beneficial for some groups of learners.

If divided learning sessions are used, rather than the all-day program, the participants may be instructed to do some patient teaching between sessions. They can use the skills checklist for a self-assessment of the teaching experience. They may use an observer to provide feedback of their

skills demonstrated during a teaching session. These experiences can then be shared, and ways to improve can be discussed at the next learning sessions.

Conference Conclusion

Following the role-playing sessions, the large group is gathered for the conclusion of the program. The group facilitators share observations of the role-playing sessions with opportunity for open discussion by the participants. The program evaluation is completed. Finally the program leader summarizes the day's experiences and encourages the participants to take their learning into their work situation, to share with coworkers, and to implement more effective patient teaching.

EVALUATING THE CONFERENCE

Much time, thought, and effort go into planning and presenting a teaching program such as the Patient/Family

Teaching Conference. The process would be incomplete and, in fact, even discouraging if feedback were not obtained about its effectiveness. Evaluation is the process of ascertaining or appraising the value of something; for a staff development program, it is determining whether the objectives of the program have been achieved.

Even though we discuss evaluation at the completion of the program, the process begins at the program's inception. The behavioral objectives indicate *what* is to be evaluated and give clues as to *how*. The *who* of evaluation includes both the learners and the program itself.

It is difficult to evaluate the effectiveness of a staff development offering because of the number of variables that influence the staff before and after the program. For us, changes in the practice of patient teaching were also being influenced by the introduction of H.E.L.P. The participants varied in experience, unit, and shift assignment which made individual assessment of learning difficult. In this case, the evaluation method used can only provide a suggestion of the effectiveness of the program.

One approach to evaluation is using a survey to determine teaching attitudes and behavior of the participants (Fig. 6.1). The survey is administered at the beginning of the conference and then again 4 weeks after the program. To assess the appropriateness of the learning objectives we have the participants write their learning expectations on a card at the beginning of the conference. At the close of the program, they note whether or not their expectations

were met, and if not, *why not*. The third method for evaluation focuses on the learners' reaction to the program presentation; Figure 6.7 is the conference evaluation form we use.

THE SUMMARY REPORT

After the results of the various evaluation methods are tabulated, a summary report is written. Mean scores, or averages, are figured on items which are assigned number ratings. Specific comments may be included verbatim or generalized with only a few specific comments quoted for emphasis. An excerpt from our evaluation report follows:

The educational process consisted of a large group session followed by small group workshops (on applications of learning theory to specific hospital teaching situations). These clinic sessions were rated as highly valuable, since the learner was given the opportunity to interact with the "experts." Discussion centered on problems and techniques. Typical comments on the afternoon session were:

- *Afternoon workshop helpful for answering questions*

- *Small group sessions effective—demonstrated that we all need added training in teaching skills*

PATIENT/FAMILY TEACHING CONFERENCE EVALUATION
March 17, 1978

Please give us your candid evaluation of this staff development program. Your comments assist us in planning additional learning opportunities. Thank you.
* *

Morning Session

1. Express your reaction to each presentation by placing the appropriate number in each block. (Key: 1 = low; 2 = fair; 3 = good; 4 = excellent)

Lectures	Quality of Delivery	Content	Usefulness to my setting
Patient Education (Stein)			
Documentation (Hooker)			
Health Professional as Teacher (Talabere)			
The Helping Hand (McCormick)			
The Helping Hand (sound-slide program)			

2. How effective was the audio-visual presentation as a teaching device? (Circle one)

    Poor   Fair   Good   Excellent   Yes   No

a. Was the technical quality adequate? ☐ ☐

b. Was the length adequate? ☐ ☐

c. Were graphics legible? ☐ ☐

d. Was the narration clear? ☐ ☐

(OVER)

-2-

Afternoon Application Session

3. Did you have adequate opportunity to discuss your teaching problem? (Circle one)

    No opportunity   A fair amount   Yes - enough time and opportunity   Excellent opportunity for discussion

4. Did the small group discussion about teaching situations provide practical information? (Circle one)

    No   Some new information   Yes - practical points were discussed   Excellent session, this will help me tremendously

5. Did role playing improve your teaching skills? (Circle one)

    No, not al all   A little bit   Yes, gave me a chance to practice   Yes - helped a great deal.

COMMENTS:
_____
_____
_____
_____

OVERALL EVALUATION:
_____
_____
_____
_____

SUGGESTIONS FOR FUTURE STAFF DEVELOPMENT PROGRAMS:
_____
_____
_____
_____

FIGURE 6.7 The program evaluation is used to assess learner reaction to the program presented.

In general, discussion was rated more favorably than the role-playing. This may be due to the learner's lack of familiarity with the role-playing technique. Role-playing did bring out flaws and omissions that could possibly be present when dealing with real patients and families. Some individuals indicated that role-playing was effective for them.

The evaluation provides information to the planners about the effectiveness of the conference and thus aids in decisions concerning future programs. Should the program be repeated for additional staff members? Should it be shorter or longer? Comments may indicate a change in content or change in teaching strategy for a specific part of the program. Each program or workshop provides a learning opportunity for the planners and educators. Evaluations provide the feedback for improvements of future offerings.

RECORD KEEPING

Just as documentation of *patient teaching* is a requirement, so is the documentation of teaching of *health professionals.* Accrediting boards and professional organizations have set standards for staff development which include the need for appropriate documentation. The trend toward mandatory continuing education for health professionals carries with it the trend for increased documentation within the institution; records and reports are used to document the necessary information.

Two systems of records are maintained in our Staff Development Department: employee continuing education records and staff development program records. For the employee continuing education record, we document an individual's participation in the various structured educational programs: the date, title, sponsor and speaker(s) of the program as well as the number of continuing education units (C.E.U.'s). Attendance at both staff development programs conducted by the institution and continuing education programs offered elsewhere are recorded. Employees attending the Patient/Family Teaching Conference are also given a certificate of attendance for their own records (Fig. 6.8). We have a separate system for staff development program records. Folders are maintained for each program and include the following items: program planning worksheet, learning activities design sheet, attendance record, written communications related to the program, flyers, program evaluation forms, and summary report. Copies of all hand-outs and the individual instructor teaching outlines are also included.

Systematic, well-maintained records assist the staff development personnel in the planning of future programs and in the preparation of reports for the department. Reviewing the records of past programs can be helpful in

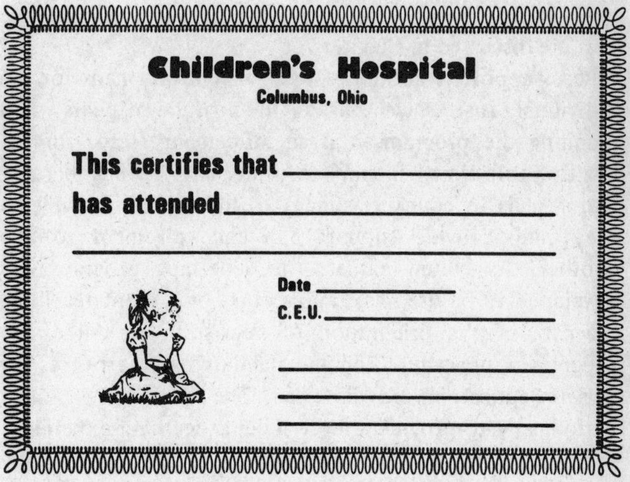

FIGURE 6.8 A certificate of attendance is presented to participants of the patient/family teaching conference.

planning future programs; programs can be repeated incorporating new knowledge, different teaching strategies, or other improvements suggested by former participants. Statistics can also be obtained from reports for use in annual reports and budgetary planning.

MAINTAINING NEW BEHAVIORS

Incorporating new or changed behavior into our usual or "old" work habits is not as easy as it seems. Attending a one-day conference on patient/family teaching is no guarantee that the health professional will be able to appreciably change work habits. How many times have you attended a conference, developed goals, then failed to accomplish these on return to the work setting? What may have been missing to assist you in maintaining your good intentions was *reinforcement.* "Behavior will occur if it is reinforced and will diminish and eventually stop altogether if it is not reinforced" (Berni, p. 114).

What can you do as an educator or manager to reinforce and encourage the health professional to maintain and even to expand new behavior? The best encouragement is a positive experience. After intensive teaching, Johnny learns to give his own insulin and proudly shows his mother. Following a discussion with the nurse, Susie explains to her father what will happen to her when she goes to the X-ray Department. These experiences give the health professional a sense of satisfaction, knowing that the teaching was effective. But the long-term results of much health teaching are not as readily apparent. So, information that is gathered about the effects of teaching should be shared with the staff. This information may be obtained through patient audits, statistics on return visits, reports returned by the community health nurse, or other evaluation methods that are discussed in Chapter 7.

Peer support is another source of reinforcement for the individual. Just as we consider the attitude of peers when planning the program, it is an influencing factor for the health professional in implementing what he has learned. Our goal is to educate as many of the staff as possible so they may provide support and encouragement to one another. As stated earlier, the slide/tape program was developed to be used as a mini-course on patient teaching. As part of the orientation of new staff, the slide/tape program is presented, and the standards and resources for patient education are discussed. The conference is held periodically to provide a more indepth learning experience for new staff. The slide/tape program is used additionally at unit conferences as a mini-refresher course for the staff.

Other types of unit conferences also serve to reinforce patient education. Patient care conferences include the discussion of identification of patient needs and the evaluation of patient learning. Discussion of teaching plans for specific patient populations may be the focus of a unit conference; articles and new ideas for patient education are shared.

The system for developing and maintaining of the H.E.L.P. program is itself a reinforcer; the staff are involved in writing and revising Helping Hands. The distribution of new Helping Hands and visits to the unit by the H.E.L.P. coordinator serve as reminders and reinforcers of patient teaching.

Second only to positive patient feedback as a reinforcer, is a word of encouragement. Telling the individual health professional when she has done a good job recognizes her efforts and steps toward improvement.

One other aspect should be considered in maintaining the behavior of the staff in patient teaching. If you have evaluated the educational approach used and the desired behaviors are still not evident, evaluate the environment and system within which the staff are working. Are there interfering barriers or obstacles which make it less desirable to provide patient teaching? We found that the writing of teaching plans were often neglected because they were time consuming and our patient charting system did not conveniently accommodate them. So we developed teaching plans and forms such as shown in Chapter 2 (Figs. 2.12, 2.13). We found the same to be true with documentation of homegoing instructions which led to development of the homegoing instructions and nursing discharge summary form (Fig. 6.5). Space and time factors may also be identified as barriers to patient teaching. Perhaps a system for reserving conference rooms can be devised. Or perhaps the health professional needs assistance in organizing work load and setting priorities.

Teaching the health professional to teach is our approach to influencing the quality and quantity of patient education. In this chapter we have discussed the staff development process and how it is used to present our Patient/Family Teaching Conference. We hope these ideas will generate enthusiasm and will assist you in designing your own program.

SELECTED READINGS

American Nurses Association. *Accreditation of Continuing Education in Nursing.* Kansas City, Mo.: American Nurses Association, 1975.

Berni, Rosemarian and Fordyce, Wilbert E. *Behavior Modification and the Nursing Process.* St. Louis: C.V. Mosby Co., 1973.

Bloom, Benjamin S., ed. *Taxonomy of Educational Objectives.* Handbook I: *Cognitive Domain.* New York: David McKay Co., 1956.

Del Bueno, Dorothy J. "What Can Nursing Service Expect From the Inservice Department?" *Journal of Nursing Administration* 6 (September 1976): 14-15.

Mager, Robert F. *Preparing Instructional Objectives.* Belmont, Cal.: Fearon Publishers, 1962.

Mager, Robert F. and Pipe, Peter. *Analyzing Performance Problems.* Belmont, Cal.: Fearon Publishers, 1973.

McKeachie, Wilbert J. *Teaching Tips: A Guideline for the Beginning College Teacher.* Lexington, Mass.: D.C. Heath and Co., 1969.

Mediaris, Naomi D. and Popiel, Elda S. "Guidelines for Organizing Inservice Education." *Journal of Nursing Administration* 3 (November–December 1973): 52-58.

National Task Force on the Continuing Education Unit. *The Continuing Education Unit: Criteria and Guidelines.* Washington, D.C.: National University Extension Association, 1974.

Reilly, Dorothy E. *Behavioral Objectives in Nursing: Evaluation of Learner Attainment.* New York: Appleton-Century-Crofts, 1975.

Rezler, Agnes G. and Stevens, Barbara J., eds. *The Nurse Evaluator in Education and Service.* New York: McGraw-Hill Book Co., 1978.

Tobin, Helen M.; Yoder, Pat S.; Hull, Peggy K.; and Scott, Barbara Clark. *The Process of Staff Development.* St. Louis: C.V. Mosby Co., 1974.

chapter 7
Evaluation: The Burden of Proof

David Stein and Barbara Turner Hord

"Basic to all processes of creativity is the ability to evaluate . . . to select, to reject, and to critically determine the value of what has been done."

George Conrad

Once upon a time, long, long ago and in a land far, far away, there was a hospital. Now this hospital was like any other; it had physicians, nurses, therapists, administrators, and all kinds of very expensive equipment. But, this hospital was a very special hospital—special because its patients were children, and we all know that children are very, very special people. At this hospital, the staff was genuinely concerned for the health of the children. The staff wanted to involve the parents in caring for their child's health. "Expand the patient and parent teaching program," the staff said. The children and their parents attended the classes offered. They read the printed health education literature. But something was missing! So the physicians examined the program with their stethoscopes and microscopes and endoscopes, but they could find nothing wrong. "The patient education program and materials are healthy," declared the physicians. The nurses and therapists continued to administer the literature in prescribed doses, and the parents and children

continued to attend the programs. But still something was missing! "Perhaps more money would buy more health education materials and more instructors," thought the physicians, nurses, and therapists. The hospital administrator studied the patient education budget, and said, "The program has adequate financial resources; it should be healthy! Request denied. In fact, how do you know that more money will improve the program?", continued the administrator, "What evidence exists to suggest that your educational efforts make any difference at all?" "Patient education is a necessary part of health care; patient education teaches patients to care for themselves; patient education is good, and it does make a difference!", replied the staff. "Yes", agreed the administrator, "the parents and children are interested in patient education, but how do you know the families understand and remember the information you seem so willing to impart? How do you know whether or not the families ever apply what you have taught? Can you demonstrate that patient education works? Come back with your request for funds when you have documented the answers to my questions."

The physicians, nurses, and therapists retreated to their units to collect the information that would convince the administrator to support an enlarged patient education program. Soon everyone was counting the number of programs offered, the number of hours spent in teaching and planning, the number of families attending the programs, the number of teaching aids distributed, and the number of hours spent in counting the numbers of everything else. But they still did not have the answers, and nobody knew why. Meanwhile, the administrator refused to spend more money on patient education. Confused and frustrated, the physicians, nurses, and therapists returned to their units to ponder their dilemma. The parents and patients were happy, the literature was good, and the program was good; still something was missing. "How can we possibly prove the effectiveness of the patient education program? We need H.E.L.P.!"

This fable has a moral. It simply is not enough to point to the magnitude and scope of our patient education efforts to justify the continued use of human and financial resources for patient education. A patient education program that can continue to attract support from administrators and from the patients must be able to produce results. You, as a patient educator, must be able to document and to demonstrate that families *do* acquire information and use skills that prevent further disability. Your programs must help families cope with the stress of hospitalization. As a patient educator, you must be able to identify and correct instructional experiences which do or do not contribute to the refinement of the patient's ability to maintain and improve health: this is the challenge which is before us.

Perhaps you too are confused and frustrated by the demand to clearly demonstrate the accomplishments of your patient education opportunities. Are you attempting to answer the questions posed to the patient education group in the fable? Is your patient education program building interest in "wellness"? Does the staff in your setting communicate effectively with patients and families? Is the teaching you provide, the teaching your patients *really* need? Do patients change their health behaviors because of participation in your programs? Do your educational materials assist you adequately in educating patients and families? You will not determine the answers to these questions without *evaluation*. This chapter will guide you through the evaluation maze.

WHAT IS EVALUATION?

Evaluation of patient education is an ongoing and systematic procedure for assessing the efficacy of your teaching skills and instructional materials to achieve intended outcomes. Evaluation should occur before you begin teaching, during your teaching session, and when you have completed the teaching. Evaluation procedures collect information that describe the instructor's goals, methods, content, and outcomes of patient education. In addition, evaluation involves making judgments concerning the quality and worth of programs and materials. Evaluation activities illustrate the achievements of your educational programs and materials, and the perceptions of the patients and staff toward reaching the objectives of your system. Evaluation highlights your successes and your failures, and above all, provides a blueprint for improving the quality of your teaching efforts and ultimately the quality of patient care.

QUANTITY AND QUALITY

The quantity and quality of patient education is addressed in evaluation reports. These statements lead to decisions concerning continued use, termination, or further refinement of program approaches and materials. Evaluation helps us to answer "how many?", "how much?", "how often?", and to visualize "how close" we come to achieving our instructional goals. Therefore, evaluation statements report *level of activity* and *results,* as well as *diagnose* instructional strategies necessary for refining your program.

Activity Level

Level of activity may be expressed in terms of numbers of patients and families participating, hours of instruction provided, and numbers of teaching aids used. This information is strictly descriptive; it does not comment on the effectiveness of efforts to bring about stated patient education goals and objectives. Activity levels may tell us that we have been working hard but do not tell us whether our efforts have made a difference in the lives of our patients and their families. Nevertheless, activity level is an important component of evaluation by providing necessary statistical data.

Results

The *results* of your patient education programs begin to demonstrate the *value* of patient education. Results may be reported in terms of reduced lengths of stay, compliance with instructions, increase in knowledge and skills, and reduction in repeated hospitalizations. However, the value of the results is a qualitative statement—a judgment made by you and your colleagues. These judgments are made in relation to statements of intended program outcomes. Knowing that 35% of your patients with diabetes can correctly perform a urine test is a statement of fact. Com-

Message (Content)	Resource (Tools)	Channel (Process)	Receiver (Learner)	Response (Outcome)
Diabetes: How to give insulin	• Staff • Audiotape • Videotape • Slides • Films • Booklets • Helping Hands	• Lecture to small group • Individual teaching • Demonstration in large group using TV	Diabetic children and adults	• Enjoyment of lecture • Score 90% on written exam • Can give insulin injection

FIGURE 7.1 Example of a patient teaching episode.

paring this figure with your goal of 100% of the patients receiving instruction allows you to make judgments about the quality of instruction provided. Thus, evaluation describes the activity level and results of your programs, and it also involves an interpretation of the results in terms of value.

Diagnostic Strategy

Undertaking an evaluation of patient education programs and materials is also a diagnostic function. As a diagnostic strategy, evaluation procedures will help you to continually refine the methods and techniques used to transmit information to patients and families. Through the evaluation process you can determine which educational methods (small group instruction, one-to-one teaching, printed literature, films) are appropriate and effective for your patient population. You can identify which staff members respond to the needs of the learning group and which staff members are in need of further inservice education. You can identify and revise the patient education materials that patients find cumbersome to read and hard to understand. Evaluation provides the feedback needed to improve the teaching-learning process within your institution.

Evaluation is collecting, describing, and interpreting evidence that the teaching-learning transaction works. The evaluation process helps us to demonstrate that patient teaching accomplishes our objectives. Through the evaluation process we can continue to improve our teaching-learning strategies. By conducting program evaluation, we demonstrate that we are accountable for effective and efficient health care. We can proudly and confidently document the results of our patient education programs and say that, as health professionals, we are *doing the right teaching and doing the teaching right.*

WHAT TO EVALUATE

The teaching-learning transaction is a form of communication designed to transfer information from you (the health educator) to the learner (the patient and the family).

Every teaching episode consists of a message, a resource, a channel for sending the message, a receiver, and a response (Fig. 7.1). The message is the information that the patient and family is to learn. The message is presented by the instructor who might use a resource such as a film, a book, or a Helping Hand. The channel for sending the message may be individual instruction, a small group session, or a discussion group. The receiver is the patient, family, or community. The response is an indication that the message has been interpreted by the receiver and has been acted upon; it provides evidence to you that the message has been effectively communicated.

The five elements of information transfer (source, message, channel, receiver, and response) are the focal points for our evaluation strategy.

RESOURCE AND MESSAGE

The patient is the key element in the evaluation process. You must evaluate all information in terms of its impact on the patient and family as learners. The patient interprets the program content and makes a response based on reactions to the instructors, the type and variety of learning activities provided, previous experiences with the health care system, and personal background, knowledge, and attitudes concerning health and illness. Your initial evaluation strategy should include a description of the patient. This description will help you choose the source and message style appropriate to the patient population. Questions to consider in evaluating resources of instruction and content are:

1. Do instructional materials or messages deal with events familiar to the patient?

2. Does the content contain references which may be offensive to the cultural backgrounds of the patients?

3. Are unfamiliar terms defined; is the literary level appropriate to the patient?

4. Does the patient possess background knowledge to profit from the content or other resources?

5. Is the information up-to-date?

6. Is the information accurate?

7. Has the content been endorsed by physicians, nurses, and other health professionals in your hospital?

8. Does the content hold the patient's interest?

9. Are materials and human resources available to achieve the goals—at a reasonable cost?

10. Are instructors trained in educational techniques?

When resources and content for instruction are evaluated, your frame of reference once again is the patient. The challenge is to select the appropriate methods which will result in effective teaching.

CHANNELING THE MESSAGE: EDUCATIONAL PROCESS

Evaluation is also concerned with the ability of the instructors to choose learning activities and to transmit the content of instruction to the patients. Thus, evaluation is concerned with the *educational process*.

Educational process describes the manner in which information is transmitted from the staff to the patient. This process is a mixture of *human and material* resources (instructors, teaching aids, films, slides), *techniques and methods* (lectures, discussions, and grouping of patients for teaching), and the *learning climate* established. Process evaluation gauges the flow of information from the instructor to the learner (receiver), indicating how effective the teaching process is in facilitating learning. The process evaluation is also conducted from the vantage point of the patient, and it examines patient satisfaction in relation to the design of the learning experience.

RESPONSE: THE OUTCOME

The "something missing" in our fable indicated that there is more to evaluation—more than just collecting data about the magnitude of the program, the content, source, and process. How can you judge if your patients have remembered any information or know more about their specific health education need?

Your evaluation activity should highlight the outcomes of your teaching program. At the conclusion of your instructional session you should be able to document a more favorable health status for the patient and family, an increase in knowledge about illness and prevention of disease, a more favorable attitude toward prevention, and/or an increased ability to perform health care procedures. These are the characteristics of patient learning. You are concerned with the ability of the patient and family to acquire and to apply information; your outcome evaluation will document changes in knowledge and behavior.

Again, the patient is the key in the teaching and evaluation process. The patient/family must be involved in determining outcomes if the teaching program is to be successful. When the evaluation points out deficiencies in the educational process, it may be due to deficiencies in the instructor, content, or materials used, or it may be that the patient does not want to learn. Activity involving the patient/family in planning the learning program can promote a successful outcome.

The components of the teaching-learning transaction (resource, message, channel, receiver, and response) will enable you to present a complete and thorough description of the activities occuring within your learning system. An examination of these components will provide feedback to the teaching staff, administrative staff, and community regarding the quantity and quality of health education delivered in your institution.

WHEN TO PLAN FOR EVALUATION

Evaluation is a process which compares intended standards of performance with actual standards of performance. This comparative process can only occur if you carefully establish an evaluation procedure when you establish your goals and objectives for the teaching plans. Thus, planning for evaluation occurs at the *beginning* of the instructional process. Evaluation will tell you if your standards are realistic, achievable, and relevant to the lives of your patients. Planning for evaluation before you conduct teaching programs will permit you to determine the data you will need to collect, the appropriate time to collect the data, the strategy for collecting the data, and to whom the data will be reported.

The patient education evaluation planning guide will help you to formulate the objectives of your evaluation and the tactics for collecting and analyzing the data (Fig. 7.2). The guide highlights decision points that you must consider when conducting an evaluation and lists the program components you may wish to evaluate. This will help you to clarify your thinking on the how, why, and when of evaluation.

In completing the patient education evaluation planning guide the questions you will ask are:

What do I want to know? List your objectives for conducting an evaluation. The statement you write should describe the elements of the program you want to evaluate. The phrase should be in question form.

Why do I need to know? This column helps you to decide the rationale behind your evaluation. It details how you will use the information collected. This column is primarily concerned with improvements in program design.

WHAT DO I WANT TO KNOW?
WHY DO I NEED TO KNOW?
WHO WILL BE MY DATA SOURCE?
WHAT WILL I LOOK FOR AS EVIDENCE?
HOW WILL I COLLECT THE DATA/EVIDENCE?
WHEN WILL I COLLECT THE DATA/EVIDENCE?
HOW WILL I ANALYZE THE DATA/EVIDENCE?
TO WHOM WILL I REPORT THE DATA/EVIDENCE?
HOW WILL THE INFORMATION BE USED?

COMPONENTS TO EVALUATE	WHAT DO I WANT TO KNOW?	WHY DO I NEED TO KNOW?	WHO WILL BE MY DATA SOURCE?	WHAT WILL I LOOK FOR AS EVIDENCE?	HOW WILL I COLLECT THE DATA/EVIDENCE?	WHEN WILL I COLLECT THE DATA/EVIDENCE?	HOW WILL I ANALYZE THE DATA/EVIDENCE?	TO WHOM WILL I REPORT THE DATA/EVIDENCE?	HOW WILL THE INFORMATION BE USED?
STAFF	Did the staff communicate	To develop an inservice	Parents in the program	Favorable comments	Satisfaction Tool	At end of program	Instructors should receive 3 on 4 scale	Instructors	To improve communication ability
CONTENT	Is the content accurate	Program revisions	Medical and Nursing	Opinions	Review of literature, interview staff	Prior to program	Content analysis	Medical, nursing consultants	Develop lesson plans, revise program
PATIENTS	Knowledge gain	Develop instructional strategy	Diabetic families seen in OPD	Three point gain in knowledge scores	Administer short multiple choice questionaire	Prior to program	Compare pre and post-test scores	Teaching staff	Determine effectiveness of teaching programs
PROGRAM/PROCESS	Were techniques appropriate	Choose tactics to facilitate learning	Patients in the program	Satisfaction with techniques	Administer Satisfaction Tool	At end of each session	# of individual responding positively to techniques	Teaching staff	Modify teaching approach
OUTCOME	Do parents perform urine testing accurately	Revise instruction conduct more classes	Parents, clinic staff	75% of parents with HH perform urine testing accurately	Interview staff observe parents	Upon next visit to clinic	Comparison of those receiving HH and those who do not	Director of Nursing, Helping Hand Staff	Allocate funds to continue educational programs

FIGURE 7.2 A completed patient education evaluation planning guide.

157

Data source. In this column, list the sources that will provide the information requested. Possible sources include physicians, nursing staff, patients, and families.

Evidence. List the criterion measured which indicates the successful accomplishment of your objectives. Criterion measures should be stated in percentages, change scores, length of stays, or return visits.

Collect and analyze the data. These columns describe appropriate times for collecting data. Before conducting an evaluation, decide on a method for analysis. Specify statistical tests that will be used or other methods for interpreting the evidence.

Report and use of data. Specify who will read the results of your evaluation report. This section is crucial since a report could be read and interpreted at various decision-making levels. Readers of your report (directors, administrators, instructors and others) may interpret your documentation from different points of view. During the planning stage it is helpful to anticipate the probable uses of the information you report. This may enhance the value of the report to those who have the authority to continue or to discontinue the teaching programs.

Now that you have formulated the objectives of your evaluation and the tactics for collecting and analyzing the data, you are ready to design your evaluation tools.

DESIGNING EVALUATION TOOLS

There are several steps in designing and using an evaluation tool. These are (1) determine the elements of the program that need to be measured, (2) design a simple form (tool) that can be easily tabulated, and (3) test the tool and (4) administer the tool. Your evaluation objectives indicated on the planning guide should be reviewed by those individuals who will make decisions concerning your program. Your group should represent medical, nursing, administrative, and other health professionals who will influence your program.

Design a simple evaluation tool that can be easily read, answered, and tabulated (such as a rating scale or a check box). Difficult forms, or ones which appear time consuming, discourage participants from completing the evaluation tool. Simple rating tools tend to increase response, permit standardization of response, and will save you time in summarizing the data. Remember that participants will opt for the path of least resistance.

EVALUATION

Evaluation is an important aspect of the program planning process. Please give us your candid reactions to the learning techniques and content presented in this program.

* *

Place in each block the appropriate number which expresses your reaction to each presentation. (1 = low; 2 = fair; 3 = good; 4 = excellent)

LECTURE	QUALITY OF DELIVERY	CONTENT	CLINICAL APPLICABILITY
Care of the Cardiac Patient			
Care of the Burn Patient			
Play Therapy			

Level of material presented was:
☐ too technical
☐ not clinical enough
☐ too basic
☐ satisfactory

Number of lectures presented was:
☐ too many
☐ too few
☐ just right

Length of presentation was:
☐ too long
☐ too short
☐ just right

Did the program promote an exchange of information:
☐ yes   ☐ no
☐ did not permit adequate discussion
☐ attempted to cover too much material
☐ other

FIGURE 7.3 Evaluating patient satisfaction with the instructor.

```
                              EVALUATION

    Directions:  Please indicate your candid reactions to the following questions.
    Please circle the number which represents your opinion.  Your responses will
    aid in planning future patient education programs.

    1.  How relevant was the workshop content to your life?

        | 1      | 2      | 3      | 4      | 5      |
        Use quite        Use              Not relevant
        frequently       occasionally     to life

    2.  How would you rate your instructor's estimate of your prior learning?

        | 1      | 2      | 3      | 4      | 5      |
        Assumed too      Taught at        Underestimated
        much prior       proper level     prior learning
        learning         of difficulty

    3.  Do you feel the workshop increased your knowledge or skills?

        | 1      | 2      | 3      | 4      | 5      |
        A great          Some-            Not at
        deal             what             all

    4.  Did you have adequate opportunity to discuss your problems?

        | 1      | 2      | 3      | 4      | 5      |
        Enough                            Would have liked
        time                              more time

    5.  How effective were audio-visual presentations as teaching devices?

        | 1      | 2      | 3      | 4      | 5      |
        Excellent        Fair             Poor

    6.  Technical quality of the audio-visual presentation    Comments: _____
                                            Yes      No
        Could you see clearly?              ☐        ☐       _____
                                                             _____
        Were you close enough               ☐        ☐       _____
        to the "action"?                                     _____
                                                             _____
        Was the choice of view             ☐        ☐       _____
        what you needed?                                     _____
                                                             _____
        Could you hear the                 ☐        ☐
        information clearly?
```

FIGURE 7.4 Evaluating the media.

Before actually using your evaluation tool, test it on several colleagues and patients—you may find a question that is confusing or that can be interpreted in several ways. Make sure that the information collected by the tool is what you want.

After a teaching session, most participants will want to return to their rooms or homes as soon as possible. It is, therefore, best to allow time within your teaching session for evaluation. Keep the form anonymous to insure honesty.

There are several types of tools you can use in evaluating patient teaching. Most effective are the "paper and pencil" variety, several of which are discussed in the following sections.

THE PATIENT SATISFACTION TOOL

A satisfaction tool is often used in conducting an overall evaluation of the learning episode and is usually administered at the immediate conclusion of the teaching session. To design a satisfaction tool it is necessary to determine which elements of the program are to be measured, then construct questions to which the learner can respond. Design your satisfaction tool to evaluate the instructor, visual media, learner interaction, environmental conditions, future planning suggestions, and objectives.

Instructor
This section of the tool examines the patient's satisfaction with the instructor (Fig. 7.3). The information obtained can be useful in improving the teaching skills of staff. You may also use this information to make decisions on future teaching assignments. Include questions such as: Does the instructor

- Speak clearly?

- Know the subject matter?

- Appear to be friendly?

- Illustrate and clarify important points?

Media
Many of our teaching materials are printed or audio-visual media. Feedback from patients can help us make decisions about the value of these materials in our program (Fig. 7.4). Feedback obtained may convince us of the usefulness of resource material, the appeal of the material, and the

technical quality. Some areas to consider are: readability, legibility, interest, audibility, and visability.

Content

Content questions are used to evaluate the perceived value of the information to the learner. When writing content questions, focus on the relevance of the information to the identified learning needs (Fig. 7.5). Content questions assess the degree to which learners report that they are able to understand and to apply new information. You may want to ask if the content is interesting, useful to the patient, relevant, applicable to the patient's life, and able to improve the patient's understanding.

Learner Interaction

Patients seem to learn more and to enjoy instruction when they are involved with the instructor and other members of the learning group. Therefore, it is important to obtain feedback to determine opportunity for interaction (Fig. 7.5). We have noticed that parents in our diabetic community class consider the opportunity to talk with other parents as the most effective component of our instructional design. When evaluating your patient teaching you may want to consider if there is opportunity for patients to discuss personal problems, and opportunity for patients to meet and talk with other patients and staff.

Learning Environment

A wise adage states that the brain cannot absorb more than the seat can endure. As designers of patient education programs, you need feedback on the environmental influences that can hinder or facilitate learning (Fig. 7.6). When designing your satisfaction tool, you may want to include questions such as:

- Were the seats comfortable?

- Did the seating arrangements encourage discussion and interaction?

- Was the room too hot? Too cold? Just right?

- Was the length of the session appropriate?

- Were adequate breaks provided?

Future Courses

Attending and participating in an educational session often stimulates the recognition of other needs for learning. It is useful to ask the group for suggestions concerning future topics for discussion; ask the group participants to list topics they would like to have presented (Fig. 7.7).

General Comments

While the other components of the satisfaction tool focus on particular aspects of the program, an open ended com-

---

EVALUATION

Directions

Please rate this workshop on each of the following items. Your candid reactions will help us to continue to plan quality education workshops. Circle the number that most closely approximates your rating of each statement.

1. Increased my understanding about diabetes.

   | 1 | 2 | 3 | 4 | 5 |
   | very low | | average | | very high |

2. Relevant to my home situation

   | 1 | 2 | 3 | 4 | 5 |
   | very low | | average | | very high |

3. Opportunity to discuss problems

   | 1 | 2 | 3 | 4 | 5 |
   | very low | | average | | very high |

4. Increased my child's understanding about diabetes

   | 1 | 2 | 3 | 4 | 5 |
   | very low | | average | | very high |

5. My overall impression of the program

   | 1 | 2 | 3 | 4 | 5 |
   | very low | | average | | very high |

6. My overall impression of the instructors was

   | 1 | 2 | 3 | 4 | 5 |
   | very low | | average | | very high |

FIGURE 7.5 Evaluating content and learner interaction.

-2-

7. In planning future workshops, please check your preference to the use of the following teaching techniques:

Technique	Increase	Decrease	As Is
Lectures			
Audio visuals			
Case studies			
Question-Answer			
Pre study materials			

8. What do you consider most effective about this workshop?

_____

_____

9. What do you consider least effective about this workshop?

_____

_____

10. Did the workshop session meet your needs?

    1   2   3   4   5
    A great deal   Somewhat   Not at all

11. Would you recommend this workshop to be given to other people? ___Yes ___ No

12. What recommendations do you have to improve today's workshop?

_____

_____

13. How well did the course accomplish its stated objectives?

    1   2   3   4   5
    Completely   Moderately   Not at all

14. Please rate the environment in which the course occurred:
    Hours per day   ☐ Too long   ☐ Too short   ☐ Just right
    Workshops: ☐ Too long   ☐ Too short   ☐ Just right
    Breaks ☐ Too few   ☐ Too many   ☐ Too long   ☐ Too short   ☐ Satisfactory

15. Please list suggestions for future topics and formats:

_____

_____

_____

_____

    PLEASE TURN IN AT THE END OF THE PROGRAM. THANK YOU!

FIGURE 7.6 Evaluating the learning environment.

ment section allows the patients to express their feelings about the course (Fig. 7.7). This information can be useful for course revisions, additions, or deletions in subject matter and design. You might want to ask the patients to indicate which aspects of the course were helpful to them, and which aspects of the course hindered their learning.

Objectives

A recent trend in the design of satisfaction tools is to list the course objectives and have participants indicate whether or not they think the course accomplished these stated objectives (Fig. 7.8). This information will provide an indication of the degree to which your instructional message was communicated to and received by your learner group.

A Word of Caution

When you are writing questions to be included on a patient satisfaction tool or any evaluation tool, avoid the use of questions that can be answered with a yes or no. Yes or no responses do not provide you with the information needed to correct deficiencies in your design. For example, the question "Was this Helping Hand useful", ☐ Yes ☐ No, could better be presented as:

How was this Helping Hand useful?

☐   Reviewed information for me

☐   Provided new information

☐   Not at all useful

You might indicate that the patient should check all responses that may apply. By following a question with explicit alternatives, you will be able to accurately revise your programs based on standardized responses. You will also be better able to describe why materials, staff, or program design facilitate or hinder learning.

```
Diabetes Education Program Questionnaire (Cont'd.)                    Page 2

What do you consider most effective about these workshops?

_____

_____

_____


What did you consider least effective about these workshops?

_____

_____

_____


Comments/Recommendations

_____

_____

_____

_____


Please list suggestions for future diabetes education programs

_____

_____

_____


Please return this evaluation to the Education Department at the end of the
session.
```

FIGURE 7.7 Open-ended questions allow patients to express feelings about the course.

THE TELEPHONE SURVEY

The telephone survey is a useful method for interviewing a random sample of parents receiving Helping Hands or other forms of patient teaching. Our experience with this tool indicates that it is not a time-consuming approach, with the average call lasting 6 minutes. We found that parents contacted in their homes were willing to talk about the instruction they received, as well as about their feelings about their experiences during hospitalization. Questions to ask when conducting a phone survey may include:

- Were written instructions used to supplement the verbal instruction received?

- When were written instructions received?

- Did the staff review the written instructions with the patient/family?

- Did the staff allow time for the patient/family to ask questions about the written instructions?

- What are the patient's/family's feelings about hospitalization and quality of care delivered?

Additional questions may be included if your objectives address a broader focus on patient education.

The telephone survey may be an expensive tool to use if part of your random sample necessitates long distance calls. However, careful scheduling may eliminate the need for calling the home more than once to receive the information necessary for your evaluation report.

DID THE PROGRAM MEET OUR OBJECTIVES?

DIRECTIONS: Place in each block the appropriate number which expresses your reaction to each point.	1 = Completely 2 = Moderately 3 = Slightly 4 = Not at all
A. To learn about and understand Diabetes	
B. To learn how to perform and interpret urine testing results	
C. To examine the emotional and social issues concerning Diabetes	
D. To learn how to live with Diabetes	

FIGURE 7.8 Evaluating the attainment of objectives.

Three advantages of the phone survey are (a) questions which are not clear to the patients/families can be explained, (b) you can increase the response rate by being persistent (we have been able to collect data from over 75% of the families receiving the Helping Hand *Having a T & A*), and (c) you can encourage patients/families to clarify and elaborate on their responses.

If you decide to use the phone survey as a method of evaluation, you will undoubtedly discover other advantages. Generally, families are very appreciative of your interest in their response, and they welcome the opportunity to discuss the hospitalization. In addition, it may provide a more objective evaluation, for the family to be able to respond from their familiar, less stressful surroundings.

THE STAFF SURVEY

The success of any patient teaching program depends on the cooperation of those staff members who actually conduct the teaching or use the teaching aids. The staff survey tool provides information on patient teaching as seen from the instructor's point of view. The staff survey tool (Fig. 7.9) is usually distributed to those individuals who conduct patient/family instruction on the units. Individuals who are not directly involved in teaching but are involved in the ordering or distribution of teaching aids should also be included. We also recommend sending the staff survey tool to physicians and administrators; this publicizes your program, generates interest among the medical and administrative staff, and identifies individuals who wish to become involved in your program. Areas to consider when designing a staff survey include: the frequency of use of instructional materials, satisfaction with content, family and patient reaction to the teaching approach, ease of the ordering and distribution system, and problems surrounding the teaching situation or use of materials.

To receive an adequate number of responses, the questionnaire should be clear, concise, and easy to complete; some thoughts to consider are:

- Will you be able to act on the information provided?
- Does the staff have the information necessary to answer the question?
- Are the questions concrete, specific, and related to the staff's experiences?

Unit ________
Level of Personnel ________
Primary shift ________

HELPING HAND
STAFF QUESTIONNAIRE

The Helping Hand Department would like to determine the impact and utilization of the Helping Hands. Your assistance in completing the following questions would help us to evaluate the program. Please return the questionnaire to ________ ________ by ________.

* *

1. How often do you utilize Helping Hands?

   ☐ 4 out of 4 patients
   ☐ 3 out of 4 patients
   ☐ 2 out of 4 patients
   ☐ 1 out of 4 patients
   ☐ Never

2. How have you used the Helping Hands? (Check all that apply)

   ☐ part of teaching plan
   ☐ as the only teaching resource
   ☐ just hand it to patients/parents
   ☐ have not used Helping Hands
   ☐ other (please specify) ________

3. How often do you use Helping Hands in preparing children for procedures and diagnostic tests?

   ☐ 4 out of 4 patients
   ☐ 3 out of 4 patients
   ☐ 2 out of 4 patients
   ☐ 1 out of 4 patients
   ☐ Never

4. When you have used the Helping Hands for preparation, (check all that apply)

   How did the children respond:

   ☐ asked more questions
   ☐ more complaint with instructions
   ☐ can describe what is happening to them
   ☐ cried less often
   ☐ less apprehensive
   ☐ no changes in behavior
   ☐ other (please specify)
   ____
   ____
   ____

   How did the parents respond?

   ☐ asked more questions
   ☐ less apprehensive
   ☐ no changes in behavior
   ☐ other (please specify)
   ____
   ____
   ____

(OVER)

-2-

5. How have the Helping Hands saved you time when teaching is indicated? (check all that apply).

   ☐ reviewed information for me
   ☐ helped me plan a teaching outline
   ☐ easy to use
   ☐ increased my confidence as a teacher
   ☐ made me want to provide instruction
   ☐ *did* not save time (please specify) ________

   ☐ other (please specify) ________

6. Have you found the Helping Hands helpful at the time of discharge as a supplement to written homegoing instructions? (check all that apply).

   ☐ yes - decrease time needed for discharge preparation
   ☐ yes - parents indicate Helping Hands are helpful
   ☐ yes (specify how) ________

   ☐ no (why) ________

7. Describe parent comments on Helping Hands (e.g. "wish I had this before").
   ____
   ____
   ____
   ____
   ____

8. Other comments and suggestions:
   ____
   ____
   ____
   ____
   ____
   ____
   ____
   ____
   ____
   ____
   ____

Thank you for your HELP in completing this survey.

FIGURE 7.9 The Helping Hand staff questionnaire.

Dear Parent,

The films your child saw today are part of our Health Education Program at Children's Hospital. It is helpful for us to know if our programs are meeting the needs of the children. Please answer the following questions and drop this card in the mail.

1. Did your child enjoy the films?   yes ☐   no ☐
2. Did you see any of the films yourself?   yes ☐   no ☐
3. Did the films teach your child any   yes ☐   no ☐
    useful information?
4. Did the films provide you with any   yes ☐   no ☐
    useful information?
5. Does the film program help your child   yes ☐   no ☐
    feel better about coming to the hospital?
6. Are the coloring books and pamphlets of   yes ☐   no ☐
    interest to the children after they
    leave?

Thank you for your assistance.   David Stein, Ph. D.
                                                       Director of Education

FIGURE 7.10 The post-card method of evaluation.

- Are any of the questions biased?

- Can the questions be misunderstood or misinterpreted?

- Is the response to one question likely to be influenced by the previous question?

- Is the form of response easy, definite, and adequate for your purpose?

In general, the survey method is an inexpensive tool to use, and is appropriate when the number of respondents is large and when the respondents are geographically dispersed throughout the hospital, health agency, or department.

THE CHECKLIST

A checklist is a useful technique for evaluating patient response. The checklist is used by the teacher or observer to evaluate the patient-learner and might include the following:

- How many questions/comments were offered by the group?

- Are patients paying attention?

- Are patients sharing experiences and trying to apply information to their own life experiences?

THE POST CARD

Often it may be impractical to administer an evaluation tool at the conclusion of the session. This may be the case in attempting to evaluate homegoing instructions, or programs presented in the outpatient clinic. In these situations, we use the postcard method. We have used this method to gather data from parents about their reaction to movies shown to the children in the outpatient waiting rooms. At the conclusion of the movie, each parent is given a card and requested to complete the card and then drop it in the mail (Fig. 7.10).

Data obtained from this method answer the question, "Do parents feel that time in the waiting room is being used productively?" Continuation of the program is based primarily on these responses. In our case, the response indicated that children did enjoy and learn from the health-related films, thus the program was continued.

TESTING

Many testing methods are available to evaluate learner retention of facts, principles, and concepts. Three common testing approaches include multiple choice, sentence completion, and true-false statements. In designing your evaluation tool, be sure that your questions are based on the knowledge or skills you expect your patients to possess at the end of the teaching session.

The multiple choice question consists of a stem question and several alternatives. The stem presents the situation to be solved, the conditions surrounding the decision to be made, or a statement that needs to be completed. The alternatives contain the correct answer as well as several distractors. Some general rules to follow in writing multiple choice questions include:

1. A multiple choice item has at least four or five distractors.

2. There is only one correct alternative; but, all others should be plausible.

3. Alternatives should be as short as possible.

4. The alternatives should be written in the same style.

The sentence completion question presents blanks which the patient must complete to demonstrate mastery of the content presented. General rules to follow in constructing a completion item include:

1. Provide enough information to cue the patient to what is required but do not provide too many hints.

2. Blanks should be of equal length to avoid clues to length of answer; do not put blanks at the beginning of a sentence.

3. Do not use articles before any blank (especially *a* and *an*).

4. Accept all reasonably correct responses.

An example of a correctly written completion question is: "Three tools you could use to assess patient learning include _____, _____, and _____."

The true-false question is the easiest question to write. However, it is the least satisfactory of all test items. By guessing alone, your patients could score at least 50% on your evaluation tool. Some guidelines for writing true-false items are:

1. Be sure the item is completely true or false.

2. Randomize the true-false responses to prevent pattern recognition.

3. Balance the number of true or false items on your tool.

4. Use correct grammar.

At this point we have established reasons for conducting an evaluation, and have presented a variety of evaluation tools available to collect information. The next section will describe how to collect and to analyze the evidence needed to support your evaluation objectives.

LEVELS OF EVALUATION

It may be your objective to demonstrate that patients and families enjoy the learning experiences provided by the staff. You may assume that attendance at a teaching session leads to learning. You may further hypothesize that your instructors are interesting, that the content is sound, and that the learning activities are well structured. Evaluations may be conducted at several levels. The patient *satisfaction* level of evaluation will provide evidence to support your hypothesis about course design.

The evaluation objective may be to demonstrate that patients have acquired increased knowledge about the disease process and increased skill in maintaining health or preventing further illness. Whatever the objective, the primary focus is on the patient and family. Evidence that the programs and materials are effective comes from the demonstrated or written performance of the patient. This is known as the *knowledge acquisition* level of evaluation. Evidence obtained at this level can support your assertion that patients who participate in your patient education program learn more than patients who are not provided with instruction.

Another evaluation objective may be to determine the effectiveness of your patient education program in reducing length of stay, preventing further illness, increasing compliance with homegoing instructions, or reducing return visits to the hospital. The primary unit of analysis is the manner in which patients and families apply their knowledge. This level of evaluation is termed *knowledge application*. Evidence obtained about behavior change will support your statements that patient education is effective in modifying the health habits of patients/families and leads to better health care at a lower cost.

PATIENT SATISFACTION LEVEL

Patient satisfaction evaluation is the easiest method of evaluation; it describes feelings of the participant, but it does not measure to any degree whether or not learning took place. Since evaluation conducted on satisfaction level is primarily concerned with patient reactions to the program, data obtained from evaluation instruments provide you with feedback only on the program's instructional design. Satisfaction evaluation does not tell you whether the patient has retained information, can apply information learned, or has changed his behavior in any significant way.

To develop and use a satisfaction evaluation, you should (1) decide which course components are to be judged (i.e., content, instructor, media, Helping Hands), (2) determine an appropriate form for collecting the data, (3) decide when and how to administer the form, (4) analyze the data, (5) prepare a report, and (6) distribute the report to appropriate individuals use the patient education evaluation planning guide (Fig. 7.2).

Satisfaction evaluation is a powerful diagnostic tool for providing you with information about what interests the patient. Evaluation conducted at the satisfaction level answers the question: "Does my patient education program generate interest in 'wellness'?"

If your goal is simply to attract learners to your patient education course, or to motivate them to use appropriate health measures, then indeed a satisfaction tool is appropriate. Satisfaction evaluations also provide you with data that can be used to improve the communication of health information between your staff and the patients. Your data should help you to demonstrate the instructional competence of your staff, the usefulness of your content materials as perceived by patients and staff, the interest in learning generated by your learning activities design, and the need for future teaching sessions.

Three tools have been useful in gathering evidence on learner satisfaction with our patient education programs; the "FAST" Evaluation, the Telephone Survey, and the Staff Survey.

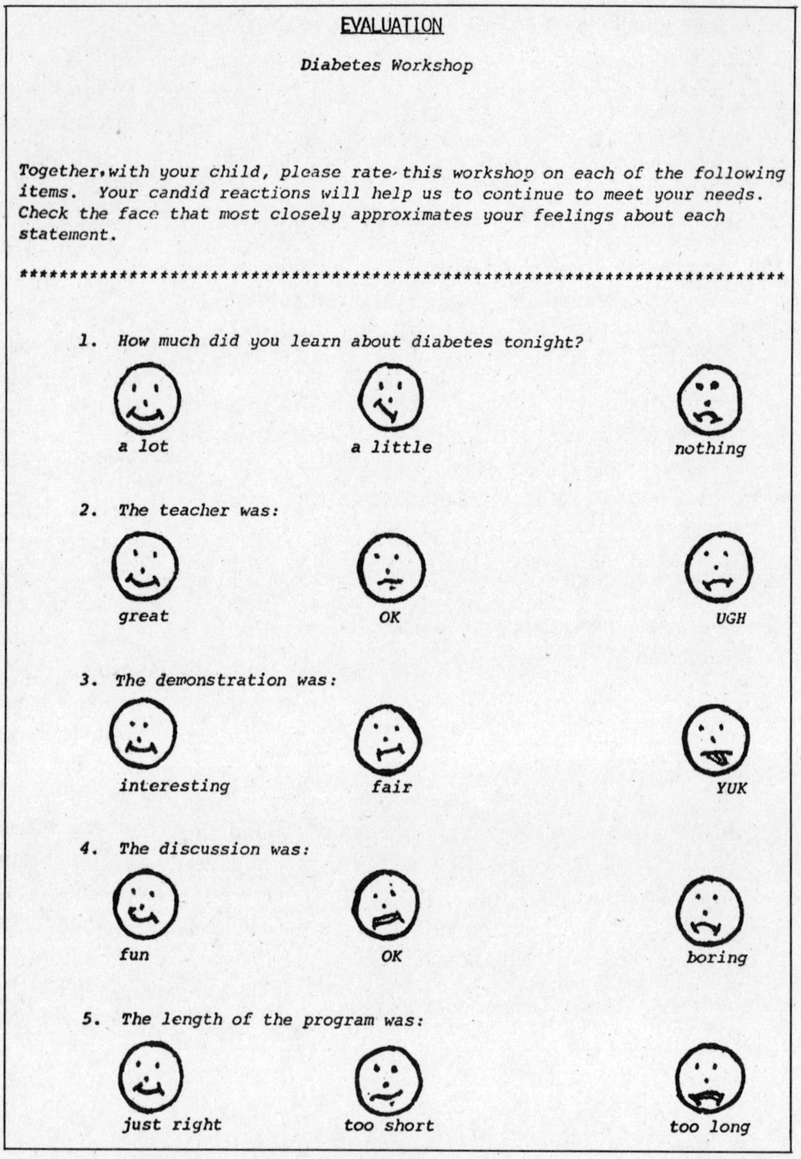

```
                            EVALUATION

                          Diabetes Workshop


    Together,with your child, please rate·this workshop on each of the following
    items.  Your candid reactions will help us to continue to meet your needs.
    Check the face that most closely approximates your feelings about each
    statement.

    ****************************************************************************
```

1. *How much did you learn about diabetes tonight?*

    a lot   a little   nothing

2. *The teacher was:*

    great   OK   UGH

3. *The demonstration was:*

    interesting   fair   YUK

4. *The discussion was:*

    fun   OK   boring

5. *The length of the program was:*

    just right   too short   too long

FIGURE 7.11 From a child's point of view.

"FAST" Evaluation

The Fun Assessment Satisfaction Tool (FAST), is administered at the conclusion of an instructional session. Administering the FAST tool is a quick and inexpensive method for obtaining feedback on your instructional design. The FAST tool will permit participants to communicate with you about topics that need more review or learning approaches that were effective or were not effective. Data obtained should alert you to needed revisions in your next teaching session. Of important consideration is the ability to elicit responses from the young patient on the various program elements. By developing a "fun" tool, improvements may be generated by the child who might otherwise not be able to relay this information.

The FAST tool has been applied to our community diabetic education classes. The tool is administered in two versions; a child version (Fig. 7.11) and a parent version (Fig. 7.5). Information obtained from the instrument has alerted us to techniques we could use to improve our program. We learned that in our session on urine testing more instructors were needed to effectively increase the child's learning. Therefore, rather than a group instructional approach, we modified our design and included an individualized one-on-one approach in the next group of classes. We learned that our introductory diabetes film, geared primarily for adults, was uninteresting to the children and did not stimulate conversation; so, we discontinued its use. Comments from the parents encouraged us to *listen more and talk less:* the parent group evaluation reflected a need for more discussion and problem solving with other parents rather than a lengthy lecture from the staff. These modifications of program design were also made. Information obtained from the FAST tool did provide us with valuable feedback on the strength of our instructional design. Through feedback we are able to continually correct those program features that hinder the flow of information to the children and parents.

Telephone Survey

We have used the telephone survey methodology to gauge parent satisfaction with instruction provided at the time of discharge and to identify the strengths and weaknesses of the Helping Hands and patient teaching. The telephone survey has been particularly useful in helping us to document that teaching was provided to the family, even though the teaching session may not have been entered on the patients's record.

Satisfaction evaluations conducted for *Having a Cystogram* and *Having a T & A* revealed that parents were appreciative of instructional efforts and did feel that the homegoing instructions were beneficial. The summary of the phone survey regarding *Having a T & A* indicated that 90% of the families received written instructions (70% received the instructions in the hospital and 20% before admission). The survey indicated that before leaving the hospital, all the families were asked if they had any questions on the care of the child at home. The survey further showed that all the families had received basic teaching with written instructions which were reviewed by the nursing staff; all the families were very pleased with the hospitalization experience. Sample comments in this telephone survey included: "Had instructions, very pleased"; "felt comfortable with what was expected at time of discharge"; "had lots of questions after discharge, more general written instructions from the hospital would have been helpful".

All this information was reported to the nursing group who provided the instruction and interesting results were noted thereafter. Previously, the nurses had not been charting patient teaching in the patient's record. An inspection of these records indicated that only a small percentage had the teaching sessions documented. The staff had recognized the need for patient teaching and had provided the instructions, but they did not consider documentation of their efforts a priority. After the survey was completed, and the report was discussed with the nursing staff, the percentage of records documenting patient teaching increased to 95%. The telephone survey had demonstrated to the staff that patients and parents did appreciate and did realize the value of their teaching efforts. In addition, it pointed out that the patients medical record had not accurately demonstrated the nursing care provided. The many hours of teaching had not been charted, and as the saying goes, "If it isn't documented, it isn't done." So not only from a legal standpoint, but more importantly for providing necessary information for patient

follow-up, the need for "appropriate documentation" was recognized and acted on.

The telephone survey will help you evaluate the reactions of your patients to: (a) the instruction presented, (b) the usefulness of the Helping Hands, and (c) the conditions surrounding the learning transaction. Data collected from the telephone survey will also aid in revising the content and format of your teaching aids and will provide feedback to your staff on the quality of their teaching efforts.

Staff Survey

The staff survey is a satisfaction level tool that evaluates the reactions of the health educators' content, format, and use of teaching materials; it aids in describing the teaching practices of the health professionals. In your setting the committee or staff responsible for the production of instructional materials would be the appropriate persons to develop this evaluation tool.

We have used the staff survey to generate data on the Helping Hands. The objectives of the evaluation were established by the Helping Hand staff, and the survey was reviewed by the nursing administration for comments, revisions, and support. The goals of the evaluation were also presented to the head nurses to elicit their support and assistance with explaining, distributing, and collecting the survey.

Two hundred questionnaires were distributed; 50% were returned by the requested deadline. The staff survey provided us with information on the use, distribution, and perceived value of the Helping Hands. Unlike other evaluation methods, this survey focused on the staff's needs and concerns. Instructors indicated that the Helping Hands (a) were used as part of the teaching plan, (b) decreased time needed for instruction and preparation of patients/families (c) provided continuity and uniformity in information provided to families, and (d) served as a reference or a refresher for the instructor.

The staff survey also served to validate responses obtained from parents about their level of satisfaction with the teaching program. Staff indicated that the Helping Hands did produce definite changes in patient behavior. Most replied that the use of the teaching aids and instruction help to reduce anxiety in patients and families and also seem to encourage questions.

All replies indicated that parents appreciated receiving the Helping Hands, they were easy to understand, and the Helping Hands aided the families in remembering the instruction. Representative examples of completed questionaires submitted by inpatient and outpatient personnel illustrate these points (Figs. 7.12, 7.13).

Limitations of Patient Satisfaction Evaluation

It must be remembered that evaluation activities conducted at the satisfaction level concentrate on the participants'

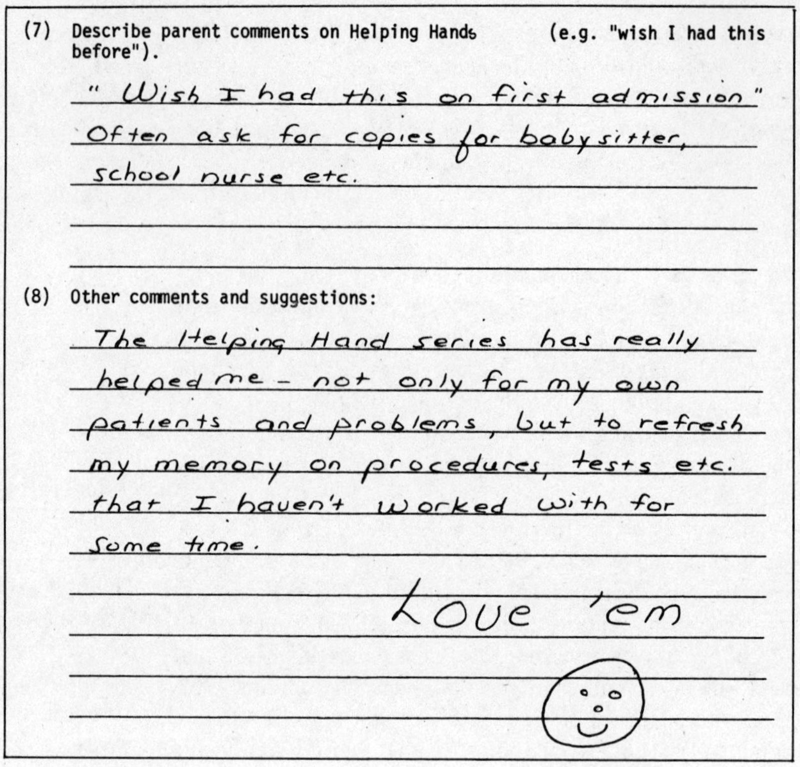

(7) Describe parent comments on Helping Hands (e.g. "wish I had this before").

"Wish I had this on first admission"
Often ask for copies for babysitter, school nurse etc.

(8) Other comments and suggestions:

The Helping Hand series has really helped me – not only for my own patients and problems, but to refresh my memory on procedures, tests etc. that I haven't worked with for some time.

Love 'em

FIGURE 7.12 Completed staff questionnaire from inpatient unit.

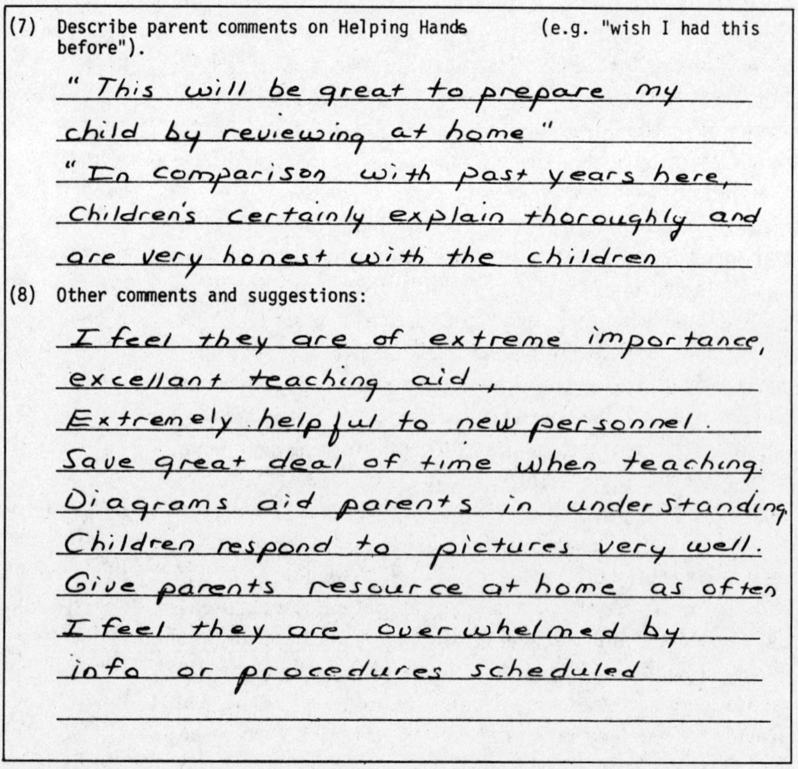

(7) Describe parent comments on Helping Hands (e.g. "wish I had this before").

"This will be great to prepare my child by reviewing at home"
"In comparison with past years here, Children's certainly explain thoroughly and are very honest with the children"

(8) Other comments and suggestions:

I feel they are of extreme importance, excellant teaching aid,
Extremely helpful to new personnel.
Save great deal of time when teaching.
Diagrams aid parents in understanding
Children respond to pictures very well.
Give parents resource at home as often
I feel they are overwhelmed by info or procedures scheduled

FIGURE 7.13 Completed staff questionnaire from outpatient clinic.

feelings. The information obtained is valuable from the diagnostic point of view of improving instructional design, *however, the ratings do not reflect information retained, information applied, or information that will result in behavioral change.* It is possible, and often happens, that the patients may not enjoy the program, but do learn. Conversely, they may enjoy an educational program (be entertained), but not learn enough to influence their ability to remain healthy. Thus, satisfaction evaluations do not reflect the learning that may have occurred.

A second limitation of satisfaction evaluation lies within the participants. Patients may have a tendency to over-rate the instructional session. This may occur for a number of reasons:

1. The patients may feel empathy with the instructor and do not wish to be overly critical.

2. The patients may not wish to critique a person in authority.

3. The patients may not wish to cause trouble for the instructor by giving a poor rating.

4. The patients may be appreciative of any educational efforts, even poor ones.

5. Learners may not want to take the time to provide adequate feedback and may consistently check one column.

KNOWLEDGE ACQUISITION LEVEL

Knowledge acquisition is a more complex level of evaluation. At this level we are interested in demonstrating the efficiency of our patient education programs in producing significant changes in the patients' and families' knowledge of illness, "wellness," and prevention. Our evaluation objective is to show evidence that patients who participate in education programs acquire more knowledge than patients who do not participate in any formal learning activity.

Knowledge acquisition consists of the retention of facts, principles, concepts, and procedural skills necessary to maintain health. Evaluation at the knowledge level will help you to answer the question: Are the materials I use or the courses I teach aiding the patient in retaining knowledge required to comply with health care routines and to prevent further illness?

We have found four approaches useful for gathering evidence to support the learning value of our programs and materials. These approaches include, pre-post testing, return demonstrations, self-assessment, and group reports.

The Pre-test/Post-test

To determine changes in knowledge, you must first have base line data on the patient's prior learning. The pre-test/post-test format is the method of choice for determining the entry level knowledge/skill of your group and measuring the effect of your program on knowledge acquisition and retention. The advantage of a pre-test/post-test approach, as compared with a post-test only, is that this method permits the health professional (1) to determine individual areas of weakness, (2) to provide a measure of success for the learner, (3) to attribute knowledge gain to the teaching presented, and (4) to judge the effectiveness and efficiency of different learning methods and techniques. As a diagnostic tool, the pre-test will cue the learner, as well as the instructor, to content areas that need greater or less emphasis than what was originally planned.

The pre-test challenges the background knowledge of the learner and provides measurable goals to be achieved during the teaching session. This method also helps the learner to complete a self-inventory of learning needs and may result in greater commitment and motivation toward completing the course. Try to incorporate a few questions that everyone will answer correctly since this technique will also increase motivation.

The pre-test/post-test should be based on the objectives of your program and should provide a measure of success for each learner. Each question or task required should refer to a particular objective, for example:

Objective:	*Question:*
The diabetic child will be able to choose five foods appropriate to his/her diet.	List five foods which you are permitted to eat.

It is possible that increases in knowledge scores obtained on a post-test given without a pre-test could be due to prior conversations with health professionals, reading journals, articles or books, or from previous life experiences. In the absence of a pre-test, you do not have a standard to compare post course performance. Unless base line data are available, it is unsound to make judgments comparing the effectiveness and efficiency of different instructional designs. More valid judgments can be made if control groups and statistical techniques are used to evaluate the education program.

We have used the pre-test/post-test tool to evaluate learning in two different situations. The testing format has been applied to the Helping Hands and also to the evaluation of knowledge acquisition and retention resulting from participation in dental and nutrition health education programs offered in the Outpatient Department waiting room.

The Helping Hand *When To Give Medication* (Fig. 7.14) was developed as a result of a nursing audit chart review of patients with appendicitis. The findings showed that appropriate documentation was necessary to indicate parent understanding of the use of medications. The Helping Hand was intended as reinforcement for discharge instructions, however, it was discovered that it could be used as a post-

HELPING HAND
Homegoing Education
and Literature Program

Let's talk about...

When to Give Medications

Child's Name: _____
Age: _____
Medication: _____
Dose (Amount): _____
Give this medicine _____ times a day at the times circled on the picture.

6 7 8 9 10 11 12 1 2 3 4 5 6 7 8 9 10 11 12 1 2 3 4 5
Noon   Midnight

HOW TO GIVE THE MEDICATION

☐ Take _____ (time) before meals
☐ Take with meals
☐ Take after meals

THIS DRUG IS USED FOR

_____
_____

CAUTION

• Store all medicine out of children's reach.
• Store in locked cupboard when possible.
• Give medicine only as ordered by your doctor.
• When medicine is no longer needed, flush it down the toilet.
• If a child accidentally takes too much of this medicine, it can make him very sick. Call your doctor (phone: _____), the Poison Control Center (_____), or the Emergency Room (_____) if this happens.

WHEN TO CALL THE DOCTOR

Call your doctor (phone: _____) if any of the following symptoms (signs) occur.

1. _____ 3. _____
2. _____

FIGURE 7.14 Post-test for medications.

test to evaluate knowledge acquisition. The staff member reviews the information with the family. After all questions are answered, the Helping Hand is given to the parent to complete. The information is then reviewed and any mistakes are corrected. Using this simple method, you can be reasonably sure that your families have achieved the necessary level of information acquisition required to comply with homegoing instructions.

More extensive assessment is conducted in our outpatient waiting room education programs. Before the dental or nutrition programs begin, parents and their children are requested to complete a self-assessment pre-test. The parents and children work in teams to arrive at the correct answers. Then the learners are instructed to listen for the correct responses during the teaching session and to tally their scores. At the conclusion of the program the post-test booklet is administered to parents and children (Fig. 7.15). The reverse side of the post-test reveals the correct responses. Our level of measurement is the change in scores from pre-test to post-test.

We can demonstrate the success of our program by comparing the scores of those individuals who have taken the test without attending the program. If all other elements in your design were identical except participation in your program, then it is highly likely that it was your program which resulted in patients and families acquiring and retaining information. By adopting this method you can truly demonstrate strength of your patient education program in producing results.

Return Demonstration

The objective of an instructional session may be to teach the patient how to perform a urine test, give an injection, or take a temperature. At the end of the session, if the instruction was adequate, the patient should be able to demonstrate the procedure correctly. At this level of learning, a precise description of the behavioral acts necessary to complete the task is needed.

The checklist is a useful tool for recording appropriate and inappropriate actions and provides immediate feedback to the patient-learner. The list also is a ready reference for the patient should the patient wish to review the steps in the procedure. In addition, the checklist serves as a tool to maximize learner involvement in evaluation. With a performance referenced checklist you can accurately record performance using the following steps:

1. The learner performs the task; the instructor records whether or not appropriate behaviors were exhibited.

2. At the conclusion of the task the instructor provides the learner with feedback.

3. The instructor reviews trouble spots.

4. The learner again performs the tasks.

A paper and pencil or oral evaluation may also be necessary. For example, before the child can perform a urine test, the child should be able (1) to identify necessary equipment, (2) to interpret the color chart, and (3) to list the steps for performing the task in correct sequence.

When designing the criteria to evaluate return demonstrations, a pass/no-pass standard should be adopted; the course has been successful when the learner can complete the task with complete accuracy. The return demonstration is the method of choice when evaluating the patient's learning of procedures. By observation of patient performance, the instructor is able to provide immediate feedback and to correct any mistakes that might have been made. In addition the patient will gain self-confidence when he is able to demonstrate the procedure correctly.

Self-evaluation

If you desire a less formal approach to evaluation, the self-evaluation technique is useful. For example, we use self-evaluation with parents in our diabetes program. Parents are requested to list three or more questions they

THE FANTASTIC FOUR FOODGROUPS QUIZ

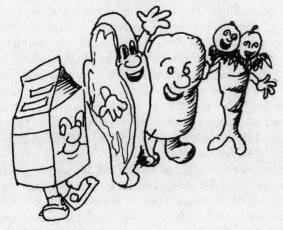

THE FANTASTIC FOUR FOOD GROUPS QUIZ

DEAR PARENT,

Please read each question to your child. Have your child select the correct response(s) and circle the letter. Answers to the questions are on the back.
****

(1) The four food groups are:

(a) 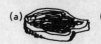 (b) (c)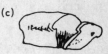

(d) 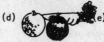 (e)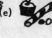

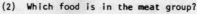

(2) Which food is in the meat group?

(a) (b) (c)

(d)

(3) Which food is in the milk group?

(a) (b)  (c)

(d)

(4) Which food is in the bread group?

(a) (b) (c)

(d)

---

(5) Which food is in the fruit/vegetable group?

(a) (b)  (c)

(d)

(6) The body builder protein...

(a) builds muscles
(b) builds strong bones & teeth
(c) builds red, healthy blood
(d) fights infections

(7) The body builder iron...

(a) builds muscles
(b) builds strong bones & teeth
(c) builds red, healthy blood
(d) fights infections

(8) Calcium builds strong bones and teeth.

TRUE   FALSE

(9) Vitamin C is found in fruits and vegetables.

TRUE   FALSE

(10) Carbohydrates supply energy to the body.

TRUE   FALSE

ANSWERS

(1) (a), (b), (c), & (d). The four food groups are bread, fruit/vegetable, meat and milk.

(2) (d) - beef is in the meat group. Other foods in the meat group are fish, eggs, peanut butter.

(3) (a) - ice cream is in the milk group. Other foods in the milk group are cheese and milk.

(4) (c) - bread is in the bread group. Other foods in the bread group are cereal, rice and spaghetti.

(5) (d) - tomatoe is in the fruit/vegetable group. Other foods in the fruit/vegetable group are carrots, green beans, apples, and strawberries.

(6) (a) - protein builds muscles. Protein is found in the meat group.

(7) (c) - iron builds red, healthy blood. Iron is found in the meat group.

(8) TRUE

(9) TRUE

(10) TRUE

FIGURE 7.15 A pre- and post-test used in our outpatient waiting room education program.

have concerning diets, urine testing, medications, and so forth. At the conclusion of the program, the questions are returned to the parent who submitted the list, and the parent is asked to answer the questions.

Group Interview

The group verbal interview is a useful technique when the learner group is composed of people with various educational backgrounds. This technique should be used when you think that patients or parents would feel threatened or insecure due to their lack of knowledge, experience, or educational level. We use the following guidelines to conduct a group interview:

1. Groups of no more than five members each are arranged in such a manner that each group has a variety of educational levels. You should be able to obtain this information from the medical history.

2. The instructor reads a question to the group.

3. Each group has 5 minutes to discuss a possible answer.

4. A member from each group reports answers to the larger group.

5. Variations in responses are discussed by the instructor.

6. The correct answer is agreed on.

This method provides immediate feedback to the group members about the success of their efforts at learning.

The goal of our instructional program is to provide patients with the knowledge, skills, and attitudes to cope with illness. Evaluation data will tell us whether or not our learning objectives were achieved. At this level we are primarily concerned with knowledge acquisition rather than knowledge application. Questions we are asking include:

Does the patient have the requisite knowledge to perform? (knowledge)

Can the patient perform? (skill)

Does the patient want to perform? (attitude)

To answer these questions, you must precisely:

1. State the objectives to be achieved.

2. Develop criterion referenced items to measure each objective.

3. Set standards which would indicate acceptable performance.

4. Administer an appropriate pre-test and record the scores.

5. Conduct the teaching program.

6. Administer the post-test and compare the scores.

7. Provide feedback to the learner.

KNOWLEDGE APPLICATION LEVEL OF EVALUATION: BEHAVIOR CHANGE

The measurement of knowledge application (behavior change) is the most difficult but most important level of evaluation. This level is difficult to measure since we cannot follow every patient home and observe the manner in which they implement new health care behaviors. Behavioral change is the level of evaluation in which we can observe the actual results of our teaching programs. At the behavioral level of evaluation information obtained answers the question, "Have our education efforts helped patients to achieve better health?" Our ultimate goal is the patient's/family's application of the knowledge gained to their everyday health patterns.

While behavioral change is difficult to measure, techniques are available for providing us with evidence that knowledge acquired has become knowledge applied. Techniques you may find useful in assessing the success of your program in helping patients acquire new health behaviors include the self-report diary, patient and family self-appraisal, and examination of medical records.

The Self-report Diary

The self-report diary is a technique used by the patient to record the practices that facilitate and maintain good health and the behaviors that lead to illness episodes. This technique relies heavily on patient and family involvement. The patient is simply asked to record events during a predetermined length of time that trigger the patient's illness. The patient also records the behaviors used to cope with the illness episode. It is hoped that the patient will recall and apply behaviors learned in the teaching program.

For example, in our diabetes class, children might be asked to record occasions in which they experience an insulin reaction. The diary entry would include a description of the precipitating causes, as well as the action taken to lessen the reaction; in the case of an insulin reaction, eating an appropriate food might be the correct action. The patient is asked to analyze reasons for the behavior exhibited. Through a process of self-introspection and practice with learned behaviors, the patient should exhibit a decrease in the frequency of diabetic reactions.

It is important to note that as health educators, it is our responsibility to provide the patient and family with a structure for recording in the diary. The structured diary could include: symptoms checklist, prescribed medications, restricted activity, health services utilization, and problems and experiences relating to health management. By providing a structure for analysis, the family and patient will have a clear indication of the requirements. Also, you will have a tool that will illustrate the patient's and family's use of correct procedures and their knowledge of the subject.

Patient and Family Self-appraisal

The self-appraisal is an interviewing technique. Through personal interviews or written instruments, the patient and family are asked questions on the use of behaviors learned in the teaching session. The patients appraise their behaviors in terms of successful applications, deficiencies in behavior, and further educational programs needed to maintain health adequately. Through informal discussion or analysis of written responses, you will be able to collect factual information that will provide insight into knowledge application.

Using a variation of the self-appraisal technique coupled with an observational strategy, we were able to evaluate the behavioral change occurring as a result of the Helping Hand *Cast Care*. The teaching aid was developed to provide parents with information about the care of the child and the integrity of the cast. In keeping with the philosophy of the Helping Hand Program, this information was reviewed with the parents and was reinforced by use of the Helping Hand. Our criterion measure was the number of casts that were found to have been kept in good condition on a follow-up visit to the orthopedic clinic. We interviewed the parents about their use of the Helping Hand; at the same time we observed the condition of the cast. We also interviewed the staff about conditions of casts. Our conclusion indicated that patients/families who received cast care instruction with use of the teaching aids kept their casts in better condition than those who had not previously received instruction. The data were further substantiated by the results of a nursing audit conducted before the teaching aid was available and a nursing audit conducted after distribution of the Helping Hand.

Inspection of Medical Records

The audit process can provide evidence to support the knowledge application benefits of your patient education program. Several Helping Hands have been developed from needs demonstrated in audit findings. A nursing audit on appendectomy indicated that there was a deficiency in information provided to parents whose children were taking the medication sulfadiazine upon discharge from the hospital. The teaching aid *When to Give Medication* was developed to help parents to understand and to avoid the side effects. The follow-up audit revealed that parents had received and retained the information. The primary evidence was obtained from examination of the patient chart.

Further evidence to support the value of patient teaching has been obtained from a nursing audit on charts of patients with head injuries. The Helping Hand *Head Injury*

was developed to prepare parents to recognize signs and symptoms indicating the need for immediate emergency treatment. Review of emergency room charts illustrated that parents had been able to recognize early signs and symptoms. The information was collected initially through a self-appraisal technique used by the emergency room staff. Documentation on the medical record provided the audit committee with the evidence needed to assess the value of the Helping Hand on head injury.

Just as nursing audits have demonstrated the need for improved documentation, in turn, Helping Hands have improved our documentation. It is a constant struggle to encourage staff to document inclusively, patient teaching and patient/family understanding. We have discovered that an effort must be made to facilitate this documentation, since patient education has become such a significant part of patient care. Therefore, through the development of Helping Hands for use in patient teaching, the staff may make reference to the Helping Hand in the patient record. With the Helping Hand available for reference, it is not necessary for the staff to record *all* the information covered in the teaching session. We have further facilitated this documentation by developing teaching plans and the nursing discharge summary, and revising the homegoing instructions form to include sections for recording Helping Hands used. The staff have appreciated these efforts to decrease the burden of charting and *have* improved their documentation. This has allowed us to place more emphasis on improving documentation on patient/family understanding which is the key to evaluating the success of your teaching efforts. It becomes very apparent that documentation is vital to evaluation. It is very difficult to evaluate what is not written, thus emphasis *must* be placed on developing skills and facilitating documentation.

The strategies suggested for evaluating knowledge application are indirect methods for assessing the value of patient education. In the hospital or clinic setting it is not always possible to use control groups for accurate verification of the results of teaching programs. The philosophy of your institution may state that it is unethical to deny patients the benefits of education regardless of the research value implicit in a control group. Yet in an era of cost containment, limited financial and human resources, and demands by the public for accountability, we cannot stand behind our rhetoric about the "goodness" or value of patient education. We must attempt to demonstrate the results and usefulness of patient education programs. We must illustrate through available tools: (1) that our programs do satisfy the educational needs of our patients, (2) that our patients do acquire information from attending our programs, and (3) that our patients do apply information gained, to reduce length of stay, to increase compliance with health regimes, and to maintain and to preserve good health.

PREPARING THE EVALUATION REPORT

The written evaluation report is a necessary component for documenting the individual patient's progress and the results of your teaching program. The key to accurate evaluation lies in recording each stage of the teaching-learning process. It is especially important when determining the outcomes of teaching activities from review of the medical records of patients who have been discharged from the hospital. These retrospective audits of care can only be accomplished from the information written on the individual patient record.

ELEMENTS OF THE REPORT

All information pertaining to content, process, knowledge acquisition, and behavior change must be recorded to determine if patient needs are being met and if we are meeting our responsibilities as health educators. Documentation provides the link of continuity from patient to patient and from program to program. We all need to reassess continually the quality of teaching provided, the needs of our patients, and new content areas. Our memories are often subject to failure; we remember only the best aspects of our programs—verbal wisdom passed down from staff member to staff member is not always reliable, consistent, or dependable. Written documentation provides a permanent reference and, in addition, provides a basis for revising our teaching programs.

We have found it helpful to record the results of our evaluations in a format that summarizes findings in a manner meaningful to the readers of our reports. A simple format which is useful as a diagnostic tool for future health teaching programs includes seven components; these components are:

- Description of the learner group
- Results of the program
- Analysis of content
- Analysis of process
- General comments from the participants
- Future courses
- Recommendations for program improvement

Description of the Learner Group

This component of the evaluation report describes the demographic, social, and other descriptive characteristics of the patients attending your program. Characteristics should be chosen that are relevant to the design and content of your teaching program; age, length of present illness, prior patient teaching received, educational level, and previous hospitalization experiences. This information

is useful when comparing the outcomes of similar programs with different patient groups. It will also help you to identify the appropriate teaching strategies and materials to use with various groups of patients.

Results of the Program

This section presents quantitative data that illustrate the accomplishments of your program. A simple format would include a description of each objective and the number of patients meeting the objective or reaching the recommended criterion level. The data can be summarized in percentages, average scores, or number of individuals. The information contained in this section will provide your reader with a clear illustration of your program's success.

The urine testing program results (Fig. 7.16) illustrate a format used to record patient satisfaction data for our diabetes education program. The mean score refers to the average of all participants rating each evaluation objective (labeled the variable). The standard deviation refers to the dispersion of scores around the mean. The standard deviation describes the degree to which scores departed from the mean. A small standard deviation means most scores were close to the average; a large deviation indicates that a significant percentage did not agree with the average. Practically speaking, a large deviation might indicate that some thought the program was excellent and some thought the program was poor. Without this information, the rating "good," which might be the average, would be misleading. The calculation of these statistical terms can be found in any standard textbook on research and statistics.

Figure 7.16 indicates that our diabetic session on urine testing needs to be reviewed and improved. Specifically, we need to correct the manner in which the information was transmitted, and to organize the program to facilitate patient learning.

Analysis of Content

The content component is a narrative which describes learner reaction to the information presented. This section is your opportunity to discuss and to analyze the factors influencing the ratings received. You should describe the objectives of your program and show how the content did or did not facilitate learning. You may wish to refer to the description of your learner group to help you analyze the results. When appropriate, present comments offered by the group to substantiate your claims; we have often found that including anecdotal data puts life into the report and makes reading more interesting as well as more vivid. For example, the content analysis of the urine testing program for patients and families included the following information.

The content components of this program were rated "fair." The information moderately in-

URINE TESTING

Variable	Mean	Standard Deviation
1. Quality of material	3.14	.36
2. Organization of material	2.86	.57
3. Improved my understanding	2.78	.70
4. Usefulness of material to you	3.86	.20
5. Speaker's delivery	2.78	.80
6. Quality of audio-visual aids	3.21	.43
7. Opportunity for discussion	2.50	.47

FIGURE 7.16 Urine testing program results summarize satisfaction (1 = poor, 4 = excellent).

creased the understanding of the learners. Some learning needs were not addressed—"would like to know more about different types of treatment," "would have been interesting to hear comments of parents and physicians." The participants also rated the information excellent on the "usefulness" variable. The content served mainly to provide the parents with a protocol for performing urine testing, for some parents the information served as a refresher."

Analysis of Process

The process section of your evaluation report describes the manner in which your educational design facilitated patient learning. This section should describe your rationale for choosing the educational methods and techniques used and the responses of the patient learners to your instructional strategy. As with the content section, you should include comments from the participants when feasible. Examination of comments received from patients in the diabetes education program revealed that the speaker did use visuals to reinforce learning, that discussion time was adequate, but that handouts reviewing the material would have been beneficial to the learning process. This last statement served as a cue for the development of the Helping Hand *Urine Testing*. The report stated:

The process components were rated "good." The speaker was commended for use of excellent visuals. Some suggested that handouts would have been a beneficial learning device. The participants rated discussion time as "fair." The instructional value of a film lesson can be enhanced by group discussion concerning the subject matter. This allows participants to comment and raise questions concerning the applicability of the material to individual settings.

Perhaps the rating on "usefulness" could have been improved if more time had been available for discussion.

General Comments

This section of the report presents comments from the participants on course content, and feelings and thoughts not elicited previously.

Future Courses

This section provides you with an indication of needs which could be met by additional education programs.

Recommendations

The recommendation section of your evaluation report completes the feedback function of an evaluation activity. This section provides you with an opportunity to consider improvements needed in your teaching program and to suggest educational approaches to improve the quality of your programs and materials. If an educational consultant is available in your hospital, you may want to share your findings and seek advice. The educational consultant will be able to suggest a variety of instructional strategies and tactics to remedy deficiencies that may arise in your programs or materials. The recommendations will serve as an instructional reference guide the next time the program is offered. The urine testing evaluation report indicated that:

During the planning phase, more thought should be given to the time allocation for information dissemination and for discussion. As a guideline, the planner should consider the projected number of learners and assign a time limit for comments from each person (two minutes per person). This will give a rough estimate of the time needed for discussion. The preparation of handouts detailing case histories and important lecture points is a recurring theme in these evaluation reports. These handouts could enhance the learning process.

DISTRIBUTING THE REPORT

Copies of the evaluation report should be kept on file as a reference for future planning. In addition copies of the report should be sent to the health professionals involved in the program to help them to improve their effectiveness as instructors and to complete the feedback system.

You may also want to include the patient in the feedback process. Perhaps patients who wish to receive evaluation reports could give you a self-addressed stamped envelope. Offering the opportunity to participate in the feedback process will demonstrate to the patient that you do value their input, and that you are continually assessing the quality of the educational programs.

THE MORAL OF THE STORY

Is "something missing" from your program? Just as we developed the Homegoing Education and Literature Program to answer our needs, we also identified evaluation as a vital part of making the systems work. Evaluation as an ongoing process, enabled us to examine and to make judgments about the H.E.L.P. program, as well as to provide feedback to the staff about their efforts.

We truly believed that our patients and families were happy, our program was good, the Helping Hands the best, and that our teaching made a difference. However, we also believe in the "value" of evaluation. Therefore, we have reviewed, revised, and rewritten to make the Helping Hands and the teaching methods even better.

In assessing the quality of care delivered to our patients, we must recognize documentation and evaluation as vital segments of the teaching process. In turn, patient education is a vital segment in quality care. Each of us has the desire to deliver health care at the optimum level of excellence. The primary objective is to benefit the patient and family, but in addition the health care team benefits as well. We benefit by realizing improvements in the skills of planning, recording, and delivering care. Evaluation strengthens our teaching programs, increases our body of knowledge, and leads to improved utilization of our resources. And in turn, who benefits? The patient and family!

SELECTED READINGS

Brethower, Karen S. and Rummler, Geary. "Evaluating Training." *Improving Human Performance Quarterly* 5 (Fall–Winter 1976): 103–120.

Esseff, Peter J. and Esseff, Mary S. *Criterion Test Items.* Langley Park, Md.: Educational System for the Future, 1974.

Froebe, Doris J. and Bain, R. Joyce. *Quality Assurance Programs and Controls in Nursing.* St. Louis: C.V. Mosby Co., 1976.

Green, Lawrence W. and Figa'-Talamanca, Irene. "Suggested Designs for Evaluation of Patient Education Programs." *Health Education Monographs* 2 (Spring 1974): 54–71.

Grobman, Hulda. *Evaluation Activities of Curriculum Projects.* Chicago: Rand-McNally & Co., 1970.

Hamblin, A. C. *Evaluation and Control of Training.* London: McGraw-Hill, 1974.

Mayers, Marlene G.; Norby, Ronald B.; and Watson, Anita B. *Quality Assurance for Patient Care: Nursing Perspectives.* New York: Appleton-Century-Crofts, 1977.

Nixon, George. *People, Evaluation and Achievement.* Houston: Gulf Publishing Co., 1973.

Phaneuf, Maria C. *The Nursing Audit: Self-Regulation in Nursing Practice.* 2d ed. New York: Appleton-Century-Crofts, 1976.

Tyler, Ralph; Gagne, Robert; and Scriven, Michael. *Perspectives on Curriculum Evaluation.* Chicago: Rand-McNally & Co., 1967.

Ulrich, Marian. "How Hospitals Evaluate Patient Education Programs." Paper presented at the National Conference on Hospital-Based Patient Education, Chicago, August 9–10, 1976.

Yura, Helen and Walsh, Mary B. *The Nursing Process: Assessing, Planning, Implementing, Evaluating.* 2d ed. New York: Appleton-Century-Crofts, 1973.

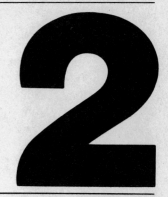

2

The
Helping
Hands

Whatever Your Gift

What is that you hold in your hand?
Nothing, you say? Look again.
Every hand holds some special gift—
A hammer, a broom, a pen,
A hoe, a scalpel, an artist's brush,
A needle, a microscope,
A violin's bow, a way with words
In the giving of faith and hope.
What is that you hold in your hand?
Whatever your gift may be,
It can open your door to abundant life—
You hold in your hand the key.

Helen Lowrie Marshall

Many of the Helping Hands developed at Children's Hospital are included in Part 2. We hope that the information contained, as well as the design and illustrations, are helpful to you in your patient education venture.

These teaching aids are presented as models. In order to reflect your particular setting and the specifics of care, some modifications will likely be needed. To assist you as far as possible, copyrights for the Helping Hands have been released. You may use the Helping Hands as is, or revise them as necessary; you may also use the illustrations included in the Helping Hands. We wish you much success and personal satisfaction as you meet the challenge of patient education.

—The Authors

Part 2 Contents

section 1
Diseases, Conditions, and Surgeries

HELPING HAND
Homegoing Education
and Literature Program

Let's talk about...

Dust Allergies

Dust particles float in the air. When breathed into the nose and lungs of the person who is sensitive to house dust, these particles cause allergic swelling of the mucous membrane. They may also cause a skin irritation called eczema. The main source of house dust is stuffed furniture, mattresses, box springs, pillows, rugs, rug pads, and stuffed toys. Kapok, feathers, "down," and animal hair can also be troublesome.

The best way to prevent symptoms from house dust allergy is to remove as much dust as possible from your home. It is important to pay special attention to the bedroom where your child spends much of his time. This list of ideas will help you make your child's environment more comfortable.

TO CLEAN AND "DUST-PROOF" YOUR CHILD'S BEDROOM

(If possible, do this cleaning while your child is away from the house.)

1. Remove all furniture from the room.
2. Wet mop and wet dust the room well from top to bottom, including lights, closets, window sills, shelves, and molding.
3. Clean all furniture well before it is put back into the room.
4. Wet mop and wet dust twice a week.

FURNISHINGS IN THE CHILD'S ROOM

- <u>Bed</u> - Beds in the child's room should have wooden or metal frames. Do not use a couch, sofa, or hide-a-bed.
- <u>Mattress</u> - Place the mattress in a vinyl (soft plastic) cover which has a zipper. If a box spring is used, it must have a plastic cover, too.
- <u>Pillows</u> - Pillows should be made of Dacron or other synthetic fiber. Do <u>not</u> use kapok, foam, feather, or "down" pillows.
- <u>Blankets</u> - Do not use comforters, quilts, or a bedspread on the bed. Use only cotton, rayon, or synthetic fiber blankets. These should be washed often.
- <u>Rugs</u> - Small, washable cotton rugs may be used if washed often. If you use a rug pad, be sure it is made of rubber.
- <u>Furnishings</u> - Remove all upholstered ("stuffed") furniture, rugs, rug pads, pillows, stuffed toys, window drapes, and dust-catching ornaments from the bedroom.
- <u>Closet</u> - Remove all stored toys, packages, and other articles from the closet. The closet should contain only your child's clothing and should be as dust-free as the room.
- <u>Furnace outlets</u> - Cover all furnace pipe outlets in the room with ten thicknesses of cheesecloth. This will catch dust in the furnace air. Change the cheesecloth when it gets dusty underneath.
- <u>Doors</u> - Bedroom closet door and bedroom door must remain closed as much as possible.

(continued)

THE FAMILY CAR

The family car is also a source of dust. Following these suggestions will make it a healthier place for your child.

- Before winter, turn on the car's heater (with the car doors open) to clean out the heating system. Vacuum the heating outlets.
- Wash and vacuum the inside of the car often.
- Wash the car floor mats with Lysol to kill molds. Dry well.
- Use only Dacron pillows in the car.
- Do not allow smoking in the car. Tobacco smoke is especially irritating in an enclosed area.

OTHER IMPORTANT TIPS

- <u>Sleeping and napping</u> - Your child should nap or sleep only in his own bed, which has been prepared as directed. If your child is confined to bed because of illness, do not give him extra feather or kapok pillows. When your child visits or travels, he should take his nonallergic pillow with him.
- <u>Other rooms</u> - If child plays in a room other than his bedroom, it also must be as dust-free as possible.
- <u>Playing</u> - Do not allow child to jump on furniture or beds nor to wrestle on carpeted floors.
- <u>Pets</u> - Dogs and cats often cause allergy troubles. The child should not have pets nor visit a home where pets are kept.
- <u>Cleaning</u> - Avoid cleaning fireplaces and furnaces when child is around.
- <u>Chalk dust</u> - Child should avoid chalk dust.
- <u>Dusty objects</u> - Child should not handle objects that are covered with dust; such as books, boxes, or clothing if they have been stored in shelves or cupboards for long periods of time.
- <u>Attics or closets</u> - Child should stay away from attics and closets.
- <u>Odorous products</u> - Child should avoid things that smell strong; such as perfumes, moth balls, tar, wet paint, gasoline, insect sprays, and room deodorizers.
- <u>Smoking</u> - Discourage family and friends from smoking inside the house.

If you have any questions, please call _____.

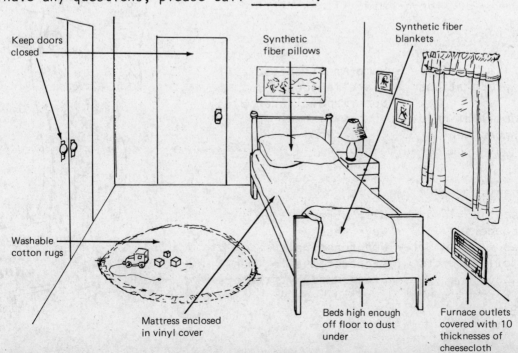

Keep doors closed

Synthetic fiber pillows

Synthetic fiber blankets

Washable cotton rugs

Mattress enclosed in vinyl cover

Beds high enough off floor to dust under

Furnace outlets covered with 10 thicknesses of cheesecloth

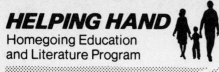

HELPING HAND
Homegoing Education
and Literature Program

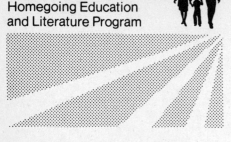

Let's talk about...

Karaya or India Gum Allergies

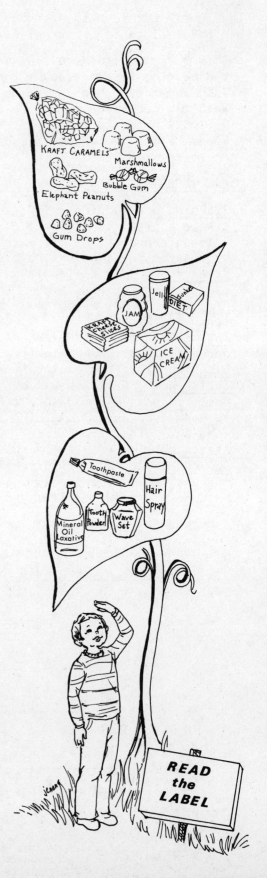

Karaya (ka-RYE-ya) gum comes from trees or shrubs that grow in tropical (warm) climates. This gum is found in many products children eat, breathe in, or touch.

Some of the products that have Karaya gum in them are listed below. <u>The allergic child should stay away from these products.</u>

KARAYA GUM IS FOUND IN

Candy and Gum

- Gum drops
- Jelly beans
- Marshmallows
- Elephant peanuts

- Kraft caramels
- Most chewey candies
- Bubble gum (not regular gum)
- Mint slices

Some Foods

- Some jellies or jams
- Gelatin preparations
- Junkets
- Ice creams that hold their shape when melted

- Some Kraft cheeses
- Dietetic foods
- Some manufactured pies

Other Products

- Toothpastes
- Dental powders
- Laxatives
- Mineral oil products

- Hair sprays
- Wave sets
- Nongrease hair preparations for men
- Drier used by printers

(continued)

LOOK FOR THESE WORDS ON THE LABEL

If any of these words are on the label, <u>do not</u>
<u>use the products</u>.

- Belleypentali
- Gulu
- Kadaya
- Koln
- Karaia

- Katila
- Katira
- Kawila
- Kuteera

- Loli
- Panduk
- Penari
- Sterculia

FOODS YOU MAY EAT

The manufacturers state that the following foods
do not contain Karaya gum unless stated:

- Jello
- Jello Puddings
- Knox Gelatin

- Kremel desserts
- Royal Pudding
- Royal desserts

OTHER INFORMATION

If you cannot find out if Karaya gum is added by
reading the label, call your local Poison Control
Center (phone:_____). They will help you get
the information.

If you have any questions, please call _____.

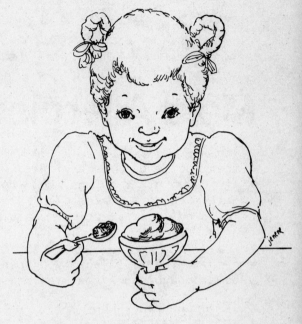

There are still special treats
you can eat.

Let's talk about...

Mold Allergies

A mold (or fungus) is a simple form of plant life. It cannot make its own food, so it feeds on other things. Mold does not need sun as most other plants do, so it can live in dark places. The seeds (or spores) are blown around by winds or are carried by insects, animals, and man. This means that molds can be found almost everywhere. But most molds live in damp, dark, cool places where moisture collects.

The following lists tell you some of the places and things that have molds. These should be avoided as much as possible by your child.

WHERE MOLDS ARE FOUND

Around the House

- Attics
- Basements - Especially if musty
- Bathrooms - Especially shower curtains and tiles, behind the toilet, under the sink
- Garages
- Cement - One third of cement dust is mold, so do not sweep cement when your child is around.
- Dust - Old dust (like that found in attics) has a lot of mold.
- Fireplace logs - Do not allow your child to stack logs or to play with them.
- Mildewed articles - Mildewed articles should not be used or worn.
- Sawdust

Plants and Outdoor Areas

- Potted plants - If you have potted plants, keep them in a room where your child does not play. The child should not keep plants in his bedroom.
- Trees - Avoid climbing trees.
- Leaves - Avoid raking, burning, or jumping in dry leaves.
- Shrubbery - Avoid playing under bushes, hedges, and shrubs.
- Christmas trees - Use an artificial tree if possible. If you use a live tree, put it up late in December, and take it down soon after Christmas. Keep it well watered.
- Weedy areas - Avoid vacant lots, fields, wooded areas, and tall grass.
- Water areas - Avoid creeks, river beds, or swampy areas.

Around Farming Areas

- Barns and silos
- Compost
- Grains - Avoid combining and shoveling.
- Hay and straw
- Peatmoss

(continued)

Other Places

- <u>Buildings that are unheated</u>
- <u>Caves</u>
- <u>Cottages</u> - If the cottage has been unheated, avoid using pillows, mattresses, and upholstered furniture in it.
- <u>Greenhouses</u>

In Some Foods

- Blue cheese and some other cheeses
- Cottage cheese (eat only when very fresh)
- Moldy bread
- Mushrooms (including mushroom soup)

OTHER INSTRUCTIONS

- DO NOT USE A VAPORIZER. Molds grow in moist containers.
- Do not allow fallen leaves to collect in downspouts, gutters, and screens. Leaves grow mold.

THE USE OF CAPTAN OR PHALTON (ORTHO)

Captan is a product used to reduce the growth of mold, which is nontoxic to humans and animals. It is used by gardeners and dairy farmers. It is available in a 50% wettable powder and can be purchased at most plant nurseries.

To use this product, mix 4 ounces of Captan or 2 ounces of Phalton in one gallon of water. Spray this on the walls, floor, ceiling, bedframe, and furniture of the area to be treated. Spray the bedroom closet, bathroom, and family room if they are damp. The solution should be sprayed with a portable spraying device. These rooms should be sprayed with <u>Captan</u> every 6 months.

Two ounces of <u>dry Captan or one ounce of Phalton</u> may be stirred into a gallon of paint if the room is to be painted.

If you have any questions,
please call _____.

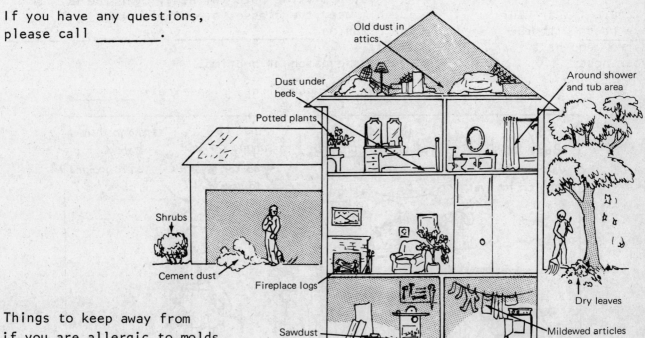

Things to keep away from
if you are allergic to molds.

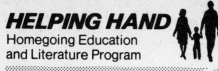
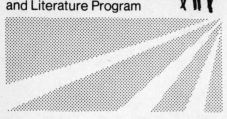

Let's talk about...

Amblyopia

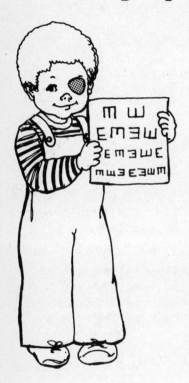

Picture 1 Wear your
eye patch with the
narrow end next to
your nose.

Amblyopia (am-blee-O-pee-a) or "lazy eye" happens when
a child uses only one eye. The "good" eye takes over
the work of seeing for both eyes. Your child's eyes may
look normal. The only way "lazy eye" can be found is
with an eye examination.

TREATMENT

Amblyopia is treated by covering the good eye with a
patch. This will make the lazy eye start working. If
the lazy eye is not treated early, the child may never
be able to see with that eye.

It is hard to tell how long your child will need to
wear his eye patch. Usually the number of wearing hours
is slowly decreased by the doctor until the patch is
not needed.

HOW TO PUT ON AN EYE PATCH

1. Remove the gauze backing. (The side that goes next
   to the skin will be sticky.)
2. Have child close his eye.
3. Gently place the narrow end of the patch toward the
   child's nose (Picture 1). (If the child wears
   glasses, apply the patch directly over the eye, and
   let him wear the glasses over the patch.)
4. Put patch on _____ eye _____
   day.
5. Remove the patch at bedtime.

If you have any questions, please call _____.

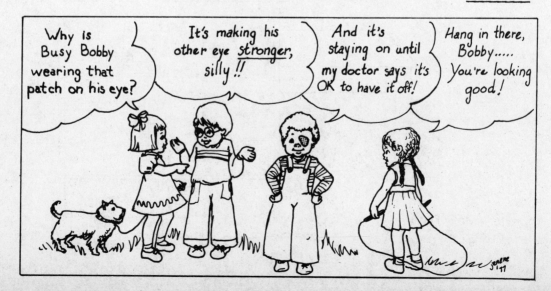

HELPING HAND
Homegoing Education
and Literature Program

Let's talk about...

Iron Deficiency Anemia

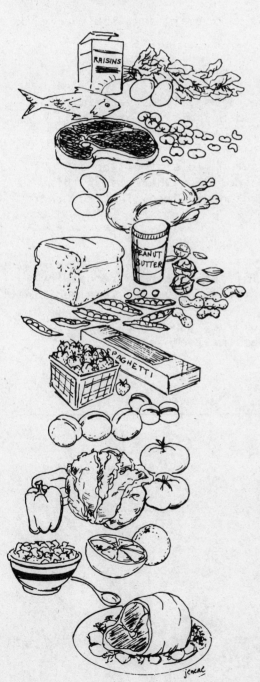

Iron deficiency anemia (I-urn dee-FISH-un-see ah-NEE-me-ah) means there is not enough iron in your child's blood. Iron is important because it carries oxygen in the blood. An anemic child tires easily, looks pale, and has a poor appetite. Certain foods rich in iron must be eaten to overcome the anemia.

Here is a list of foods rich in iron. Suggestions will be given to you on what foods your child should have. The foods chosen will depend on your child's age and on his likes and dislikes.

FOODS RICH IN IRON

Meat

- All meats
- Liver
- Giblets
- Kidney
- Turkey
- Fish
- Chicken

Vegetables

- Greens
- Broccoli
- All leafy green vegetables
- Dried peas and beans

Dried Fruit

- Dried apricots
- Dried peaches
- Prunes
- Raisins

Other Foods

- Egg yolks
- Molasses
- Enriched cereals
- Foods high in vitamin C
- Peanut butter
- Enriched macaroni
- Enriched noodles
- Iron enriched baby cereal
- Iron enriched formula

(continued)

2 Iron Deficiency Anemia

FOODS HIGH IN VITAMIN C

Foods high in vitamin C may help your child's body use iron. Some of these foods
are:

- Grapefruit
- Oranges
- Strawberries
- Tomatoes
- Cantaloupe
- Bell peppers
- Broccoli
- Raw cabbage

MILK

Your child should have no more than _____ ounces of milk every day. Too much milk
can prevent iron from being used in the body.

IF IRON MEDICINE IS NEEDED

The doctor may want your child to take iron medicine. If so, it is very important
that the child takes it every day. Give _____ drops of iron at (time):
_____ each day.

After the medicine has been given for a few days, your child's stool (bowel
movement) will look black. This is expected. It does not mean there is anything
wrong. What it means is your child's blood is getting enough iron. The iron that
is not needed is going out in the bowel movement.

Care of the Teeth

Iron medicine will stain your child's teeth brown. This stain can be removed by
brushing the teeth with baking soda or toothpaste after you give the iron medicine.

If the teeth are not as white as you think they should be, you may call your
dentist or the Dental Clinic (phone: _____) to get the teeth cleaned.

FOLLOW-UP APPOINTMENT

Your follow-up clinic appointment is on (date): _____
at (time): _____.

If you have any questions, please call _____.

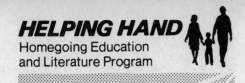

HELPING HAND
Homegoing Education
and Literature Program

Let's talk about...

Aspirin Ingestion

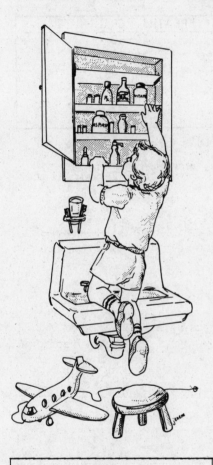

Your child has recently been seen in the Children's Hospital Emergency Room for the ingestion of aspirin or an aspirin-like product. Although we do not feel admission to the hospital is necessary at this time, there are several things we request that you do at home.

CHECK YOUR CHILD'S BREATHING

Check your child's breathing rate every hour for 8 hours. To check, count the number of times he breathes per minute. Count one breath each time he breathes in. Write down the number of breaths per minute. Count the breaths when your child is sleeping or quiet. Do not count the breaths if he has been running or playing.

To check how deep the breaths are, place your hand in front of your child's mouth and measure how far away you can feel his breath. Write down the distance (number of inches) from his mouth where you can feel his breath.

GIVE THE CHILD PLENTY OF LIQUIDS

Encourage your child to drink as much water, 7-Up, ginger ale, fruit juice, or other liquid as he will take. Keep offering liquids for _____ hours.

WARNING

A child who eats or drinks medicine is likely to do so again. Lock up anything he might swallow. Remember: your child may take dangerous medicines again unless you stop him.

KEEP ALL MEDICATIONS AND OTHER DANGEROUS MATERIALS LOCKED UP AND OUT OF THE REACH OF CHILDREN!

(continued)

WHEN TO CALL THE DOCTOR

Call your doctor (phone: _____) or the Emergency Room (phone: _____):

- If your child begins to breathe faster than the normal rate for his age. Find the normal rate on the chart below.

CHILD'S AGE	BREATHS PER MINUTE
Newborn	30-50
2 years	24-32
6 years	22-28
10 years	20-26
12 years	18-24
Adult	16-22

- If you can feel the child's breath 5 inches or more from his mouth
- If your child vomits for more than 2 hours after he returns home

If you have any questions, please call _____.

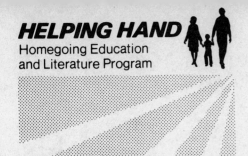

HELPING HAND
Homegoing Education
and Literature Program

Let's talk about...

Circumcision

A circumcision (sir-cum-SI-zhun) is the surgical removal of extra skin from the end of the penis.

WHAT TO EXPECT AFTER SURGERY

- Your child will "wake up" in the Recovery Room near surgery. He will be returned to his room when he recovers from the anesthetic. Parents may wait in the surgery lounge.
- There is usually no bandage over the surgical area. If there are stitches, these will dissolve and will not need to be removed.
- There will be some swelling of the penis after surgery. This will gradually go away during the next week.
- There is usually only a small amount of soreness after surgery. Pain medication is rarely needed, however, if your child has pain, your doctor will want to know.

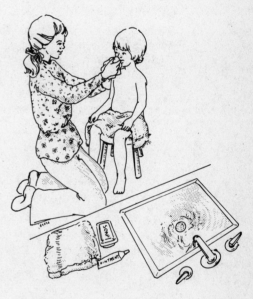

Picture 1 Take sponge baths for the first week.

HOME CARE AFTER SURGERY

- Loose clothing should be worn by older children.
- Child may sleep on stomach if comfortable.
- Do not place any medication on the penis unless instructed to do so by your doctor.
- The skin of the penis should stay pulled back. If it slips up over the incision, gently push it back with your fingers. Check with your doctor or nurse about this if you have any questions.

BATHING

☐ Your child should have a daily sponge bath (not a tub bath) for 7 days (Picture 1). After the penis has healed, bathe as before. Keep the penis dry at all times for at least 7 days.
☐ Your child may be bathed in the tub after surgery.
☐ Other instructions:

(continued)

2 Circumcision

PLAY

Your child should walk and play quietly for the
first 7 days after surgery (Picture 2). (No
riding toys or unsupervised play with other
children is allowed.)

FOLLOW-UP APPOINTMENT AFTER SURGERY

Please call the Surgery Clinic (phone: _____)
a day or so after surgery to make an appointment.
The doctor will want to see your child 2-3 weeks
after surgery.

If you have any questions, please call _____.

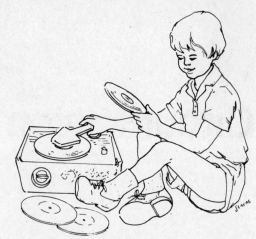

Picture 2 Play quietly for
the first 7 days.

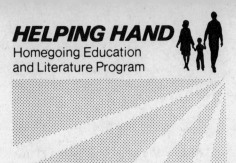
Let's talk about...

Croup

Croup is a spasm (tightening of the muscles) around the larynx (voice box). This spasm causes frightening sounds. Your child will have a cough that sounds like a seal barking. When your child breathes in you will hear a high-pitched rasping sound. The voice may be hoarse.

Croup may come on suddenly in the night and is usually caused by a virus. Usually croup causes breathing problems in children 2-6 years old. A child that has it once probably will have it again. The best thing parents can do is to be prepared.

WHAT YOU WILL SEE

- The hollow in the child's neck may "pull in."
- His chest may "pull in" when he breathes in.
- His face will be pale.
- He will look "frightened."

This happens because your child cannot move air in and out of his lungs easily.

STAY CALM

Croup is frightening to the child <u>and</u> parents. A crying, upset child tends to make the croup worse. Parents can help to relieve croup by being calm themselves, which helps to quiet the child. This relieves the tightness of the voice box and allows the child to breathe easier.

WHAT YOU SHOULD DO

1. Stay calm.
2. Take your child into the bathroom and shut the door. Turn on the shower and hot water faucets to <u>make steam</u>. Be careful to keep away from the hot water (Picture 1).
3. Sit with the child and let him breathe in the steam.
4. Do not leave the child alone.
5. Have someone start a vaporizer in the child's room.
6. When breathing is easier for the child (10-15 minutes), give him a popsicle. Later give the child more clear fluids to drink. This will help to keep the throat moist.

Picture 1 Stay with your child and let him breathe in the steam.

(continued)

2 Croup

AFTER A VISIT TO THE EMERGENCY ROOM

Your child has had a breathing treatment with a medicine that reduces the swelling in his throat. After you get him home he may have the same breathing problem he had when you brought him in. If this happens, take him into a steamy bathroom as explained on page 1.

You can treat his fever (if temperature is above 102° rectally) with Tylenol/Tempra: _____ teaspoons or _____ droppers, or with baby aspirin: _____ tablets.

WHEN TO CALL THE DOCTOR

CALL THE EMERGENCY ROOM (phone: _____) OR BRING YOUR CHILD BACK:

• If child does not improve after being in a steamy bathroom for 10-15 minutes
• If child's breathing becomes more difficult (chest continues to "pull in")
• If child begins to drool
• If child has difficulty swallowing

If you have any questions, please call the Emergency Room (phone: _____) or _____.

HELPING HAND
Homegoing Education
and Literature Program

Let's talk about...

Rotating Insulin Injections

Rotating injection sites means giving your injection into a different place each day. If you give your injection in the same place each day, this area of your skin will become sunken (atrophy) or hard and lumpy (hypertrophy). When insulin is given into these hard or sunken areas, the insulin may not be absorbed well.

You should rotate your injection sites every day to keep your skin in good condition.

INJECTION AREAS AND INJECTION SITES

Injection areas are the places on your body where you can give your insulin.

Injection sites are the spots where you actually put the insulin in. There are several "sites" in each "area" (see Picture 2).

You will be giving most of the injections into your upper, outer leg (thigh) or into your upper arm. Other areas where injections may be given are in the lower abdomen and upper hip (see Pictures 1 and 4).

To Begin Your Rotation Plan

Choose one of your legs to start your rotation plan. When all injection sites are used on this leg, move on to the next area in a clockwise pattern. For example, go from your left leg to your right leg. Then to your right arm to your left arm then back to your left leg. By doing this, you will be giving each area a few weeks of "rest." Read the following pages for more information.

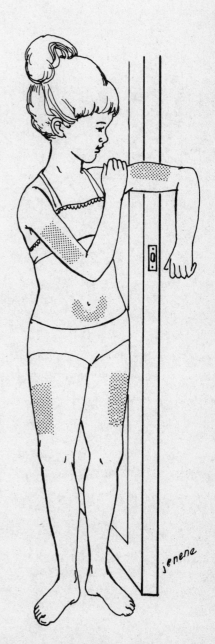

Picture 1 Shaded places show injection areas.

(continued)

INJECTION AREAS FOR UPPER ARMS

1. Fold your lower arm across your waist (see Picture 2).
2. Draw an imaginary line down the center front of your arm from the shoulder area to elbow.
3. Draw an imaginary line down the outer side of your arm from shoulder to elbow.
4. Put your hand over your upper arm at elbow level. Measure one hand's width and connect the imaginary line <u>above</u> your hand.
5. Put your hand over your upper arm at shoulder level. Connect the imaginary line <u>below</u> your hand.
6. The area inside these imaginary lines is where injections may be given into your arms (see Picture 2).

ROTATING INJECTION SITES ON UPPER ARMS

1. Draw three imaginary lines 1 inch apart from shoulder to elbow (see Picture 2).
2. Call the first line (large dots in Picture 2) on the center front of your arm "week 1."
3. Divide this line into seven sites, one for each day in week 1. (These dots should be about 1/2 inch to 1 inch apart.)
4. One injection should be given at each site down the first line (the line nearest your body) until week 1 is completed.
5. The next week ("week 2") is the next line moving toward the outer side of the arm. This line is 1 inch away from the first line.
6. If you are unable to complete seven injections in each line, the remaining two or three injections should be given in the buttocks inside the area shown in Picture 4.

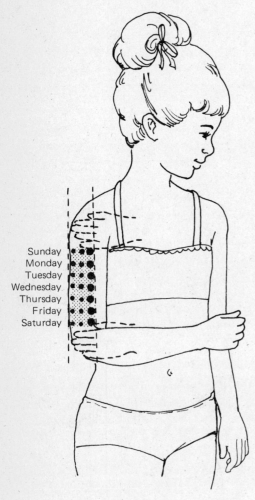

Sunday
Monday
Tuesday
Wednesday
Thursday
Friday
Saturday

Picture 2 Shaded area on arm shows injection area and sites.

(continued)

INJECTION AREAS FOR UPPER LEGS (IN SITTING POSITION)

1. Draw an imaginary line down the middle and top of your leg (from your hip area to your knee).
2. Draw an imaginary line down the outer side of your leg from hip to knee.
3. Put your hand on top of your knee and measure one hand's width. Connect the imaginary line <u>above</u> your hand.
4. Put your hand on your upper thigh next to your hip area. Connect the imaginary line <u>below</u> your hand.
5. The area inside these imaginary lines is where injections may be given on your legs (see Picture 3).

ROTATING INJECTION SITES ON UPPER LEGS

1. Draw three imaginary lines 1 inch apart from hip area to knee.
2. Call the first line (large dots in Picture 3) "week 1."
3. Divide this line into seven sites, one for each day in week 1. (These dots should be about 1/2 inch to 1 inch apart.)
4. One injection should be given at each site down the first line until week 1 is completed.
5. The next week ("week 2") move to the next imaginary line going toward the outer side of the leg (Picture 3). This line should be 1 inch away from the first line.

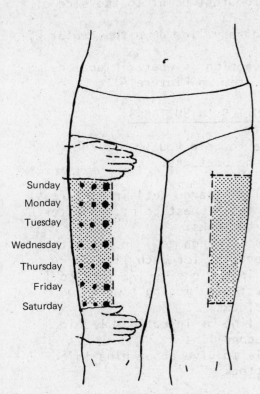

Sunday
Monday
Tuesday
Wednesday
Thursday
Friday
Saturday

Picture 3 Shaded area on legs show injection areas and sites.

(continued)

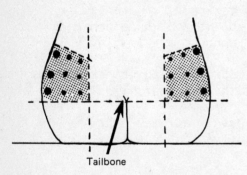

Picture 4 Shaded area on
buttocks shows injection areas
and sites.

INJECTION AREAS FOR BUTTOCKS

1. Find your tail bone (see Picture 4) and draw an imaginary line from that point to the side of your buttocks.
2. Draw another imaginary line down the center of the buttock.
3. The upper outer section is where injections may be given (shaded area in Picture 4).

ROTATING INJECTION SITES IN BUTTOCKS

You may need someone to help you to use the injection sites on the buttocks.

1. Start the first line (large dots in Picture 4) of injections at the highest point and outer most area of the buttocks.
2. Each injection is 1/2 inch to 1 inch apart (about three injections for each line).
3. The next line of injections is 1/2 inch to 1 inch from the first line moving toward the center of the buttocks.
4. Continue a third line of injections 1/2 inch to 1 inch from second line.
5. You should be able to give about nine injections in each buttock.

POINTS TO REMEMBER

- Injection sites must be changed every day.
- Change the injection area after all injection sites are used.
- Start each line in the injection area at the highest point of the area and continue down toward the point farthest away from the body. For example, upper arm down toward elbow; upper part of thigh down toward knee.

If you have any questions, please call _____.

Pictures adapted from illustrations by Millie Rinehart.

Let's talk about...

Giving an Insulin Injection

Picture 1

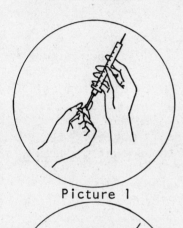

Picture 2

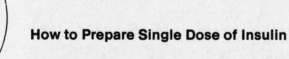

Picture 3

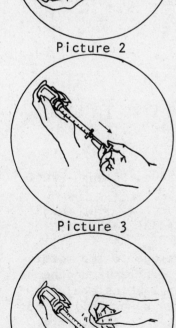

Picture 4

Name of Child: _____

Diabetes mellitus is caused by too little insulin being produced by the pancreas. Your body needs insulin every day to stay healthy. So, you must give the insulin every day to meet your body's needs. The following guide will help you do this.

YOU WILL NEED

Insulin
100 U disposable syringe and 26- or 27-gauge needles
Bottle of 70% alcohol
Cotton balls
Heavy cardboard container for disposal

How to Prepare Single Dose of Insulin

1. Wash your hands.
2. Read label on the insulin bottle.
3. Gently roll bottle between your hands, mixing well (if "cloudy" insulin is used).
4. Clean top of insulin bottle well with a cotton ball dipped in alcohol.
5. Remove needle cover from disposable syringe. Push plunger back and forth to make sure it moves freely.
6. Pull air up into syringe equal to the amount of insulin to be given (Picture 1).
7. Push needle through rubber top of insulin bottle (Picture 2). Push air into bottle.
8. Turn bottle upside down. Be sure the tip of the needle is in the insulin.
9. Pull insulin into syringe. Pull plunger several units past the number of units to be given (Picture 3).
10. With needle still in bottle, tap syringe gently to make air bubbles rise (Picture 4).
11. Push insulin back into the bottle to the number of units to be given.
12. Check syringe for dosage and air bubbles. (If bubbles are present, repeat steps 9, 10, and 11.)
13. Keeping bottle upside down, remove syringe from bottle.
14. Put the needle cover back on the needle.

(continued)

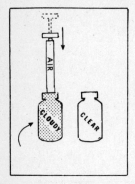

Picture 5

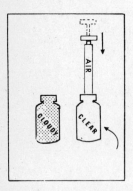

Picture 6

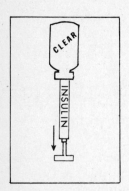

Picture 7

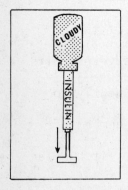

Picture 8

How to Prepare a Mixed Insulin Dose

A "mixed dose" of insulin means mixing clear (short-acting) insulin with cloudy (intermediate-acting or long-acting) insulin in the same syringe.

To give a mixed insulin dose, make sure the <u>clear insulin (short-acting) is drawn up first</u>. This keeps the cloudy insulin from getting into the clear insulin bottle.

1. Wash your hands.
2. Read label on insulin bottle.
3. Gently roll cloudy insulin bottle between your hands, mixing well.
4. Clean tops of insulin bottles well with a cotton ball dipped in alcohol.
5. Remove needle cover from disposable syringe. Push plunger back and forth to make sure it moves freely.
6. Pull air up into syringe equal to the amount of <u>cloudy</u> insulin to be given (Picture 1).
7. Push needle through rubber top of cloudy insulin bottle. Push the air into bottle (Picture 5). Pull needle out of bottle.
8. Pull air up into syringe equal to the amount of <u>clear</u> insulin to be given.
9. Put needle through rubber top of clear insulin. Push air into bottle (Picture 6).
10. Turn clear insulin bottle upside down. Be sure tip of needle is in the insulin.
11. Pull clear insulin into the syringe. Pull plunger several units past the number of units to be given (Picture 7).
12. With needle still in bottle, tap syringe gently to make air bubbles rise (Picture 4).
13. Push insulin and air bubbles back into the bottle to the number of units to be given.
14. Check syringe for dosage and air bubbles. (If bubbles are present, repeat steps 11, 12, and 13.)
15. Keeping bottle upside down, remove syringe from bottle.
16. Figure out total number of units needed. <u>Clear insulin + cloudy insulin = Total units.</u>
17. Turn bottle of <u>cloudy</u> insulin upside down. Put needle through rubber top. Be sure that tip of needle is in the insulin.
18. Slowly pull cloudy insulin into syringe to the total number of units needed (Picture 8). There should be no air bubbles in the syringe. (If air bubbles are present, both insulins must be drawn up again.) <u>Do not push any of this mixed insulin back into the bottle.</u>
19. Check syringe for dosage. Keeping bottle upside down, remove syringe from bottle.
20. Replace needle cover.

(<u>Note</u>: Semilente is a cloudy short-acting insulin. It should be drawn up the same as clear insulin.)

(continued)

How to Give the Injection

1. Choose correct injection site. (Refer to instructions: Rotating Insulin Injections.)
2. Clean the skin with alcohol.
3. Hold syringe like a pencil. Remove needle cover.
4. If site area is chubby, push down and spread skin out with first finger and thumb. If site area is thin, grasp skin between thumb and index finger. Do not pinch skin too tightly (Picture 9).
5. Quickly thrust the needle into the skin to the hub at a 45-90° angle (Picture 9). (The faster the needle goes in, the less it will hurt.)
6. Pull back on plunger to see if blood appears (Picture 10). (If blood appears in syringe, do not inject insulin. Withdraw needle and start all over with a new syringe and insulin. Choose another injection site.)
7. Inject insulin at a steady rate within 5 seconds.
8. Place cotton ball dipped in alcohol next to needle (Picture 11).
9. Withdraw needle quickly.
10. Hold alcohol cotton ball on injection site for 2 or 3 seconds. Do not rub skin.
11. Break off needle of disposable syringe and put it into the special container (Picture 12).

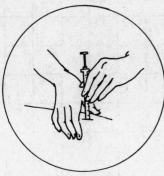

Picture 9

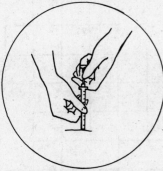

Picture 10

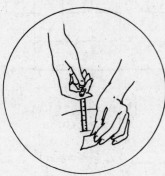

Picture 11

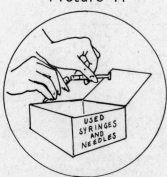

Picture 12

> CAUTION: Be sure to keep syringes and supplies out of the reach of children and others who might misuse them.

CAUTION: The law states that the syringe must be "rendered inoperable." This means the needle must be broken off, and the plunger must be taken out. This will keep anyone from reusing a disposable syringe.

If you have any questions, please call _____.

(continued)

Insulin Crossword Puzzle

ACROSS

1. One treatment for _____ is insulin.
5. Another word for Mom
7. Be sure to _____ injection sites.
9. _____, two, three!
10. If blood appears in syringe, start _____.
11. Opposite of Jr.
12. NPH and Lente are _____ insulins.
15. Use a new _____ and syringe for each injection.
16. A preposition
19. There should be _____ air bubbles in the syringe.
20. Short way of saying advertisement.
22. Many years _____, insulin was discovered.
23. _____ up the area before giving injection.
26. Cloudy and clear insulin in the syringe is a _____ dose.
28. _____ of injections means changing injection sites daily.
30. Amounts of medicines are called _____.
32. "_____ unto others. . . ."
33. For a _____ dose, you use one type of insulin.
35. "_____ frog" (game).
36. _____ the syringe to get rid of air bubbles.
37. Wash your _____ before preparing insulin.

DOWN

1. _____ of all used syringes.
2. There are injection sites on the _____.
3. The place for an injection is called a _____.
4. _____ insulin can be mixed with cloudy.
6. _____ must be put in the bottle before insulin can come out.
7. _____ the bottle of cloudy insulin between the hands.
8. Opposite of Off.
11. A _____ is used to inject insulin.
12. _____ the injection site with an alcohol swab.
13. Dispose of all _____ syringes and needles.
14. Giving medicine with a syringe and needle is called an _____.
17. Eating proper _____ is important.
18. The syringe _____ protects the needle.
21. Mud; soil.
22. A chopping tool.
24. Opposite of Yes.
25. Laughing sound.
26. Sound a cow makes.
27. Your medicine is called _____.
29. Short for "I would."
31. _____ is another name for cotton balls.
32. A well-balanced _____ is important for health.
34. A space between things.

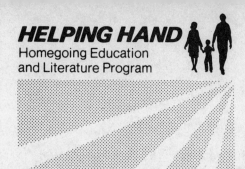

HELPING HAND
Homegoing Education
and Literature Program

Let's talk about...

Urine Testing

Daily urine testing is done to measure the amount of sugar (glucose) and acetone (ketones) in the urine. The results of the test aid in adjusting the amount of food or insulin needed to help control diabetes.

WHEN TO TEST THE URINE

Testing urine for sugar and acetone should be done before each meal and before the bedtime snack. Be sure to follow your doctor's instructions.

STORAGE AND CARE OF EQUIPMENT

The testing materials may be damaged if they are exposed to heat, light, or moisture. To keep materials in good condition, you should:

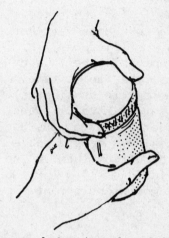

Picture 1 Cap bottle tightly.

- Store them in a cool, unlighted cupboard or drawer.
- Store at room temperature not over 86° F (30°C). Do not refrigerate tablets or Ketostix. Do not store in the bathroom.
- Keep bottle tightly capped (Picture 1).

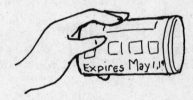

Picture 2 Check expiration date on label.

- Do not remove desiccant capsule from Ketostix bottle. (This keeps moisture from damaging the strips.)
- Do not transfer testing tablets or strips from the original bottle to another container.
- Rinse test tube and dropper after each use. Store with open end down so water can drain out.
- Store tablets and other testing materials out of the reach of other children.

CHECKING THE TESTING MATERIALS

- Check the expiration date on all testing materials (Picture 2). Do not buy testing materials that do not have an expiration date.
- Do not use any testing materials after the expiration date. Replace with new materials.
- Clinitest tablets will turn from white with blue specks to dark blue if they are too old for use. Replace old tablets with new ones, and flush old ones down the toilet.
- Acetest tablets will change from white to tan, beige, or brown if too old for use. Replace with new tablets.

(continued)

CHECKING THE TESTING MATERIALS (continued)

- If the Acetest tablet does not absorb the urine in 30 seconds, it has absorbed moisture and should not be used. Replace with new tablets.
- When the rubber bulb of the Clinitest dropper becomes weak or sticks together when squeezed, replace it with a new special Clinitest dropper. You can buy a new dropper at the drug store. Throw away the old dropper.

SAFETY TIPS

- Do not touch the bottom of the test tube. The bubbling of the testing materials causes the tube to become very hot, and it will burn the fingers (Picture 3).
- Do not hold the tube of solution close to the eyes. The tablets and solution can cause chemical injury (burns).
- Do not pick up Clinitest tablets with bare fingers. The tablets can burn the skin.
- Flush any damaged tablets down the toilet rather than putting them in the garbage. If pets or children swallow the tablets, they will burn the mouth and throat.

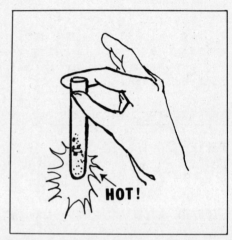

Picture 3 Hold test tube at top.

FIRST AID

- If someone swallows the tablets, do not make the person vomit. Call the Poison Control Center (phone: _____) or your doctor for advice.
- If any of the solution or tablets gets into the eyes, wash the eyes with cool tap water for 15 minutes, then call your doctor for advice.

Collecting Urine for Testing

SECOND-VOIDED SPECIMEN

Urine that has been in the urinary bladder for a time does not give an accurate measurement of sugar and acetone. A fresh urine specimen will give results which are closest to the actual blood sugar level. To collect a fresh specimen ("double-void" or "second-void") follow these directions:

1. Urinate (void). Do not save this specimen.
2. Drink some water (it will help you to void).
3. Wait 15 to 30 minutes.
4. Urinate into a clean container.
5. Use this second-voided urine specimen for the testing.

SPECIAL INSTRUCTIONS

_____

_____

_____

(continued)

Urine Testing for Sugar — Clinitest 2-Drop Method

YOU WILL NEED

Clean container for fresh urine specimen
Clean glass test tube
Clinitest tablets
Clean Clinitest dropper
Small container for clean water

Small container for rinse water
Clock or watch with second hand
Color chart - "2-Drop Method"
Clinilog or record book
Pen or pencil

CLINITEST 2-DROP METHOD

1. See Directions on page 2 on how to collect a urine specimen.
2. See Directions on page 4 for how to do the urine test.

OTHER INFORMATION

· The amount of sugar in the urine is found by comparing the color of the test tube solution with the color chart. Do this at the end of the 15-second waiting period. Pay no attention to any color changes after this 15-second waiting period.
· The more sugar there is in the urine, the more the colors will change. The colors will also change very quickly, if there is much sugar in the urine.
· If the sugar is very high, you may see "pass-through."

Pass – Through

When the sugar is over 5% the colors change quickly from green to tan to orange, and back to a dark greenish-brown. This color change may happen before the 15-second wait is over. So, you must watch the complete reaction the whole time the solution is bubbling. If this quick pass-through of orange to dark greenish-brown happens, record it on your record book as over (↑5%) (do not compare it with the color chart).

SPECIAL INSTRUCTIONS

_____

_____

_____

_____

_____

_____

_____

_____

(continued)

Clinitest 2-Drop Method

1. Place the test tube in Clinitest kit holder.

2. Place 2 drops of urine in the tube. Hold the dropper straight up and down.

URINE

3. Rinse dropper with water.

RINSE WATER

4. Place 10 drops of water in the tube.

CLEAN WATER

5. Shake 1 Clinitest tablet into bottle cap and drop it into test tube.

6. Recap bottle tightly.

7. Hold test tube at the top (bottom gets very hot). Allow to bubble. Watch for "Pass-Through!"

HOT

8. When the bubbling stops, wait 15 seconds. (Time with second hand of clock or watch.)

9. Shake tube gently.

10. Compare color of test solution with color chart.

11. Record result, date, and time in record book.

12. Rinse test tube and dropper well and store in upside-down position.

PLACE COLOR CHART HERE

(continued)

Testing for Acetone

Testing for acetone is done to see if acetone bodies are present in the urine. Acetone in the urine means that the body is using fat as a major source of energy instead of sugar (glucose).

The test should be negative (no color change). If the test is positive, it means the body is not working right. <u>This is a danger signal</u>. This can mean the beginning of a serious illness.

<u>THINGS THAT CAN CAUSE THE URINE ACETONE TO BE POSITIVE</u>

- Too much food
- Too little insulin
- Injury or illness
- Infection (mild or severe)

<u>TESTING URINE USING ACETEST TABLETS</u>

<u>YOU WILL NEED</u>

Clean white paper
Bottle of Acetest tablets
Fresh urine specimen (second-voided)
Special dropper

Clock or watch with second hand
Color chart
Clinilog or record book
Pen or pencil

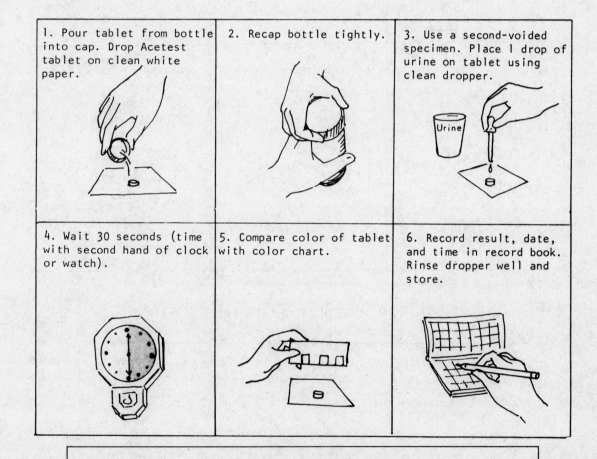

1. Pour tablet from bottle into cap. Drop Acetest tablet on clean white paper.

2. Recap bottle tightly.

3. Use a second-voided specimen. Place 1 drop of urine on tablet using clean dropper.

4. Wait 30 seconds (time with second hand of clock or watch).

5. Compare color of tablet with color chart.

6. Record result, date, and time in record book. Rinse dropper well and store.

PLACE COLOR CHART HERE

(continued)

TESTING URINE FOR ACETONE USING KETOSTIX

Ketostix is another method to test urine for acetone. Remember: <u>Urine that is positive for acetone is a danger signal.</u>

<u>YOU WILL NEED</u>

Bottle of Ketostix   Color chart
Fresh urine specimen   Clinilog or record book
Clock or watch with second hand   Pen or pencil

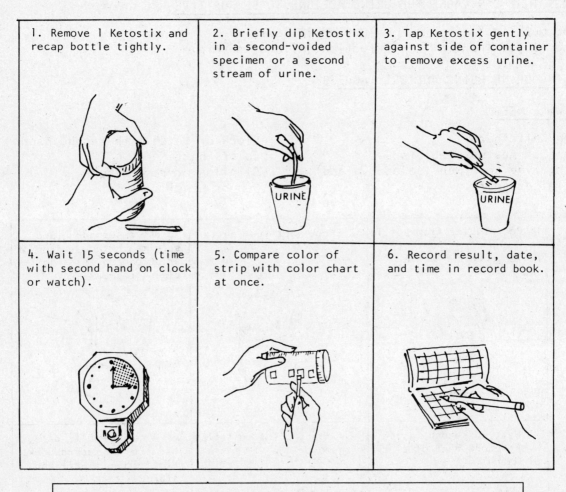

1. Remove 1 Ketostix and recap bottle tightly.	2. Briefly dip Ketostix in a second-voided specimen or a second stream of urine.	3. Tap Ketostix gently against side of container to remove excess urine.
4. Wait 15 seconds (time with second hand on clock or watch).	5. Compare color of strip with color chart at once.	6. Record result, date, and time in record book.

PLACE COLOR CHART HERE

HELPING HAND
Homegoing Education
and Literature Program

Let's talk about...

Diaper Rash

Diaper rash is caused by irritation of the skin from urine and bowel movements. Baby's skin becomes sore and hurts when the diaper is wet or soiled. There are several things you can do to heal the diaper rash.

WHAT YOU SHOULD DO

Do the following things several times a day:

1. Remove the baby's diaper.
2. Clean baby's bottom and all skin folds well with mild soap and water. Rinse skin well and pat dry (Picture 1).
3. Turn baby on his stomach with a folded diaper under him.
4. Let baby play on his stomach with his diaper off. The air helps dry and heal the rash (Picture 2).
5. You may apply a soothing ointment to baby's bottom as ordered by your doctor.
6. If the rash does not improve, call your doctor.

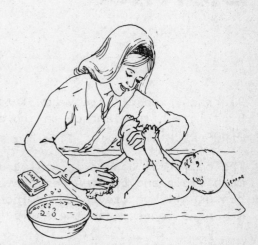

Picture 1 Wash baby well with soap and water.

SPECIAL HINTS

- Change the diaper as soon as baby wets or has a bowel movement.
- Gently wash and dry baby's bottom every time you change his diaper.
- Keep diaper off as much as possible.
- Plastic pants or throw away diapers may make diaper rash worse. Try not to use these while baby has a rash.
- If the diaper has a strong ammonia odor, give the baby more water to drink between feedings.
- If the bowel movements are loose or runny, cut down on the fruit you give.

TO WASH DIAPERS

Soak diapers in cold water. Then wash diapers in hot water using mild soap. Rinse well and dry. If rash continues, add 1/2 cup of white vinegar to the last rinse, then dry the diapers well.

OR you may put one crushed tablet of Diaperine into 2 quarts of water. Soak clean diapers in Diaperine solution, then dry the diapers well.

If you have any questions, please call _____.

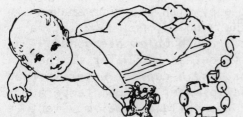
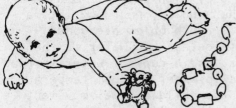

Picture 2 Let baby play on his tummy, with diaper off.

Let's talk about...

Diarrhea

Name of Child: _____
Date: _____
Doctor: _____

Diarrhea (loose, watery bowel movements) is a common problem of growing children. Once in awhile diarrhea may be due to a serious illness, but usually it is only a minor problem.

The only real danger in having diarrhea is dehydration. If your child loses too much fluid and becomes dehydrated (dried out) he can become very sick. Dehydration can usually be prevented by increasing the amount of liquid the child drinks. You may need to decrease the solid foods so he will drink more.

We think this diarrhea can be treated at home. The following suggestions may be helpful to you.

HOW TO GIVE LIQUIDS AND SOLID FOODS

- Give liquids in small amounts quite often. For example, give 1 or 2 ounces every half hour. If the child takes this well, increase the amount a little every half hour. If your child is forced to drink more than he wants he may vomit. Some vomiting is common during diarrhea, but we don't want it to get worse by giving more liquids than he wants to take (Picture 1).

- Solid foods should be given in small amounts. Milk is one food that sometimes makes diarrhea worse. It is best not to give milk for a day or two.
- Do not give the child salty soups or broths.

LIQUIDS YOU CAN GIVE THE CHILD

- Soda pop (<u>not</u> diet pop) with the fizz shaken out. To take out the bubbles, pour pop into a glass and stir until the bubbles are gone.
- Jello water - add twice as much water as the directions call for (use 4 cups of water instead of 2). Leave the Jello water at room temperature. The color of the child's bowel movement will be the color of the Jello.
- Apple juice   • Tea
- Kool-Aid   • Solid Jello
- Ice popsicles   • Gatorade
- Oral electrolyte fluids (such as Pedialyte, Lytren) - available at local drugstores without a prescription.

Picture 1 Give liquids in small amounts quite often.

(continued)

SOFT FOODS YOU CAN GIVE (IN SMALL AMOUNTS)

• Apple sauce
• Raw apples (remove the peel and chop or
  scrape very fine)
• Bananas
• Simple unsalted crackers and cookies
• Any meats
• Carrot juice

WHEN TO CALL THE DOCTOR

You should call the doctor (phone:
_____).

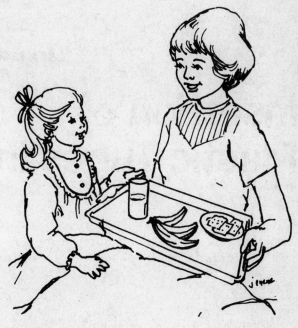

• If the child suddenly develops a very
  high fever
• If stomach pain becomes severe or is more
  than occasional cramps
• If the diarrhea becomes bloody (more than
  a streak of blood)
• If the diarrhea becomes more frequent or
  is more severe
• If the child becomes dehydrated (dried
  out)

Picture 2 At first, give soft foods
in small amounts.

SIGNS OF DEHYDRATION

• Child has not urinated (passed water) for 6 or _____ hours.
• There are no tears when child cries.
• Child's mouth becomes dry or sticky to touch.
• Child's eyes are sunken.
• Child is less active than usual.

WARNING

Do not use stool "binders" or antidiarrhea medicines for children under 6 years of
age, unless you are specifically directed to do so by your doctor. These medicines
can be very dangerous if they are used improperly.

If you have any questions, please call your physician (phone: _____), the
Emergency Room (phone: _____), or the Pediatric Clinic (phone: _____).

HELPING HAND
Homegoing Education
and Literature Program

Let's talk about...

Insertion of Plastic Tubes in Ears

Plastic tubes have been put in your child's ears to prevent fluid build-up behind the ear drums. Here is some information you will need to know.

AFTER SURGERY

- There may be some drainage from the child's ear for 2-3 days after surgery.
- The plastic tubes usually stay in the ears for 3-6 months. The tubes will not have to be removed, they will come out by themselves.
- Your child can have a normal diet after surgery.
- Do not allow your child to chew gum for 2 weeks after surgery.

PERSONAL CARE

- Hair may be washed 1 week after the tubes have been put in.
- The child may take showers after returning home.

ACTIVITY

- School - Your child may return to school the day after surgery.
- Swimming - Swimming is not allowed for 3 weeks after surgery. Regular swimming is allowed after that EXCEPT FOR:
    No jumping into the water
    No diving
    No swimming under water
  All swimming skills will be allowed after the tubes fall out (in 3-6 months).
- Play - Other types of play activities are allowed.

FOLLOW-UP APPOINTMENTS

Please return to the clinic for a check-up in 3 weeks. Call the Ear, Nose, and Throat Clinic (E.N.T.) for an appointment (phone: _____).

If you have any questions, please call the (E.N.T.) Ear, Nose, and Throat Clinic or _____.

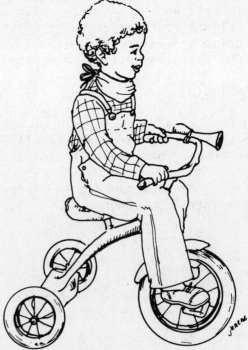

Your child may play normally, except for swimming.

HELPING HAND
Homegoing Education
and Literature Program

Let's talk about...

Care After Ear Surgery

Your child has had an ear operation. There are a few things you should do after the child goes home.

WHAT TO DO

- Give your child the medication as directed.
- The child may have slight pain in the ear. You can give aspirin or Tylenol _____ if the child has pain.
- If the child's bandage falls off at home, go to the hospital Emergency Room and have the bandage replaced.
- When you wash the child's face, keep the bandage dry.
- Keep the child from blowing his nose until 4 weeks after surgery. The pressure from blowing can cause the incision to come apart and ruin the operation.
- Do not let the child chew gum or blow bubbles with bubble gum for 2 weeks. Blowing bubble gum can make pressure in the ears and cause the incision to open.

ACTIVITY

- The child may play outside.
- The child should avoid contact sports such as football and swimming for several weeks.

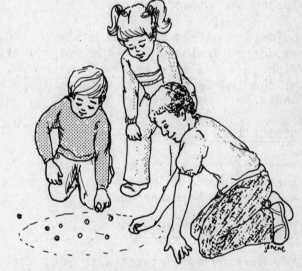

Your child is free to play, but no contact sports.

WHEN TO CALL THE DOCTOR

Call the Ear, Nose, and Throat (E.N.T.) Clinic (phone: _____):
- If child complains of a lot of pain.
- If you see a lot of drainage coming out of the child's ear.

FOLLOW-UP APPOINTMENT

You will be given an appointment to visit the Ear, Nose, and Throat Clinic every week for several weeks.

If you have any questions, please call _____.

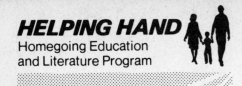

HELPING HAND
Homegoing Education
and Literature Program

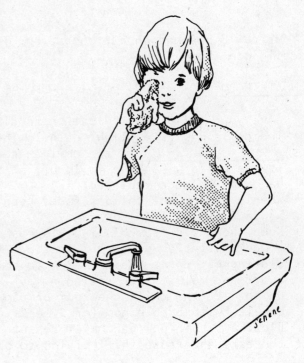

Let's talk about...

Care of an Artificial Eye

A "conformer" has been placed in your child's eye socket. This conformer is left in the eye socket after surgery and keeps the eye socket ready for the artificial eye. The conformer will be removed <u>by the doctor</u>.

TO KEEP THE EYE SOCKET CLEAN

Gently wash around the eye with a soft clean wash cloth and warm water. Make sure the lashes are clean. Pat dry.

Colds and allergies cause an increased amount of drainage from the eye socket. Wipe this drainage away with a tissue. Start at the inside of the eye (next to the nose) and wipe toward the ear.

MEDICATIONS

Your doctor may have given you a prescription for drugs or ointment. Use these medications as directed.

FOLLOW-UP APPOINTMENTS

You have an appointment with your doctor or at the clinic on (date): _____ at (time): _____. It is important to keep this appointment.

WHAT TO EXPECT AT YOUR APPOINTMENT

Your eye doctor will remove the conformer and examine the eye socket. He will then direct you to a prosthesis (pros-THEE-sis) technician who will make the prosthesis (artificial eye). The technician will teach you how to put in the artificial eye and how to keep it clean. The conformer will be used until the permanent artificial eye is made.

(continued)

WHEN TO CALL YOUR DOCTOR

Call the eye clinic or your doctor:
• If pain develops
• If eye tissue becomes red and swollen
• If the drainage from the eye socket increases or changes color (for example, clear to yellow)
• If any problems develop in the other eye

If you have any questions, please call the Eye Clinic (phone: _____).

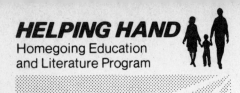

HELPING HAND
Homegoing Education and Literature Program

Let's talk about...

G6-PD Deficiency

Your blood test shows that you have a shortage in the glucose-6-phosphate dehydrogenase enzyme (G-6-PD) (GLUE-kose six de-HY-droe-gin-ace EN-zime). G-6-PD is a hereditary hemolytic condition which means it can cause problems with your blood. Several things can cause these problems, such as drugs, infections and fava beans. Therefore you cannot take certain drugs and products because they will make you ill and anemic (have "low blood"). NO DRUGS OR PRODUCTS SHOULD BE GIVEN TO THE CHILD WITHOUT FIRST CHECKING WITH THE DOCTOR OR PHARMACIST. The drugs you should not take are listed on Page 2.

COMMON DRUGS AND PRODUCTS

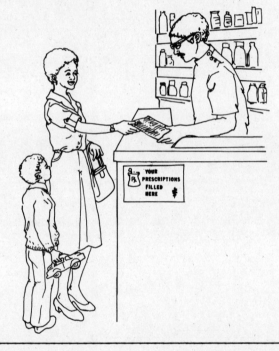

Many drugs and products you buy in a drug store or grocery store contain "hidden ingredients" such as aspirin, acetaminophen, or others which may be harmful to your child. When you buy these products, it is important to read the labels or have your pharmacist help you. Some of these products are for:

- reducing fevers (such as aspirin, Tylenol, Tempra, Liquiprin)
- colds (such as Coricidin, Dristan)
- itching (such as Caladryl)
- constipation
- diarrhea
- upset stomach (such as Alka-Selzer)
- Naphthalene (moth balls) (clothing protection)
- Fava bean products (foods)

SPECIAL INSTRUCTIONS

- Never give medicine of any kind to your child without a doctor's advice.
- Be sure to read labels on prescriptions and household products before giving them to the child.
- Take this list of drugs with you whenever you take your child to the doctor, pharmacy, or to an emergency room. Show this paper to the doctor, nurse or pharmacist.
- Give a copy of this Helping Hand to your child's school teacher and nurse.

WHEN TO CALL THE DOCTOR

Call your doctor if any of the following signs of anemia occur. These usually are noticed 1-3 days after the drug is taken.

- abdominal pain
- back pain
- paleness
- dark urine (it may even look black)
- yellow skin or eyes

(continued)

NOTE TO PATIENT AND/OR PARENT:
- DO NOT TAKE ANY OF THE FOLLOWING DRUGS OR PRODUCTS
- Carry this list with you at all times.
- Show this list to your doctor or pharmacist before medications are prescribed or filled.

NOTE TO THE PHYSICIAN AND PHARMACIST
This patient has a Glucose-6-Phosphate Dehydrogenase deficiency. The following list of most common offenders is available for your information.[1]

A PERSON WITH G-6-PD DEFICIENCY SHOULD NOT USE ANY OF THESE DRUGS OR PRODUCTS

(NOTE: The drugs marked with an asterisk (*) are those that cause clinically significant hemolysis. The other drugs listed usually do not cause hemolysis unless abnormal conditions are present, i.e., infections.)

ANTIPYRETICS AND ANALGESICS - These drugs are used to reduce fever, or relieve pain and discomfort. These are usually given when children have colds, flu, headaches or pain.

Aspirin (Acetylsalicylic acid) and aspirin containing products	Acetophenetidin (Phenacetin)
Acetaminophen (Tylenol, Tempra, Liquiprin)	Antipyrine (Felsol tablets and powder)
* Acetanilide	P-Animosalicylic acid (PAS)

ANTIHISTAMINES - These drugs are used for colds and "stuffy nose" and also for itching of the skin.

Antazoline (Antistine)	Tripelennanine (Pyribenzamine)
Diphenhydramine (Benadryl)	

ANTIBACTERIALS - Antibacterials are used for children who have bacteria-caused diseases such as sore throats, infected ears, or urinary tract infections.

* Salicylazosulfapyridine (Azulfidine, Sulcolon)	* Sulfamethoxypyridazine (Kynex, Midicel)
Sulfacetamide (Sulamyd)	* Sulfapyridine
Sulfadiazine	Sulfisoxazole (Gantrisin)
Sulfamerazine	Sulfamethoxazole with trimethoprim (Bactrim, Septra)

NITROFURANS - This is a group of drugs used to treat infections in the urinary tract, on the skin, or in the bowels.

	* Nalidixic Acid (Negram)
Furaltadone (Altafur)	* Nitrofuratoin (Furadantin, Macrodantin)
Furazolidone (Furoxone)	Nitrofurazone (Furacin)

ANTIMALARIALS - These drugs are given to prevent or to treat malaria. Malaria is a disease carried by a mosquito which lives in warm climates. Malaria is given to people by the bite of this mosquito.

Chloroquine (Aralen)	Pentaquine	Pyrimethamine (Daraprim)
* Dapsone (Avlosulfon)	Plasmoquine	Quinacrine (Atabrine)
Pamaquine	* Primaquine	Quinine
		Quinocide

OTHER HARMFUL PRODUCTS TO AVOID

Acetylphenylhydrazine	Orinase
Ascorbic Acid (vitamin C)	Phenylhydrazine
Chloramphenicol (Chloromycetin)	Polycillin PRB
Dimercaprol (BAL)	Probenecid (Benemid, Col Benemid)
Fava Bean	Principen with PRB
Isoniazid	Procainamide (Pronestyl)
Methylene Blue (M-B, Trac Tabs, Urised, Uristat, Urolene Blue)	Quinidine
	Sulfoxone
Napthalene (moth balls)	Vitamin K (water-soluble analogues)

---

[1] Information sources:
Carlstedt, Bruce C. "The Clinical Lab: Hematology: G-6-PD". U.S. Pharmacist, (Nov.-Dec. 78): 10-16.
Oski, Frank and Naiman, J., Lawrence, M.D. Hematologic Problems in the Newborn. 2nd ed. Philadelphia: W. B. Saunders Co., 1972.
Shirkey, Harry C. Pediatric Therapy. 5th ed. St. Louis: C. V. Mosby Co., 1975.

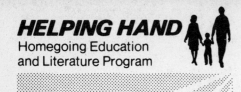

HELPING HAND
Homegoing Education
and Literature Program

Let's talk about...

Head Injury

Your child has had a head injury and is now ready to go home. For your child's safety, there are several things you will need to do at home.

WHAT TO DO

1. Watch your child for signs of head injury (signs are listed below).
2. Call your child's doctor (phone: _____) if you see any of the signs of head injury. If you cannot reach the doctor, call the Emergency Room (phone: _____) or bring your child to the Emergency Room.

SIGNS OF HEAD INJURY TO WATCH FOR

- Change in your child's behavior such as extreme irritability (cross)
- Nausea (upset stomach)
- Vomiting (throwing up)
- Complaints of headache or stiff neck
- Bleeding from nose or ears
- Increased sleepiness (does not respond when you offer a favorite toy)
- Temperature of more than 101°
- Convulsions (seizures)
- Staggering or swaying while walking
- Weakness of one side of body
- Eye changes (crossed eyes, droopy eye lids, trouble using eyes)
- Blurred or double vision
- Loss of consciousness (does not waken when you touch and talk to him)
- If child does not "look right" to you

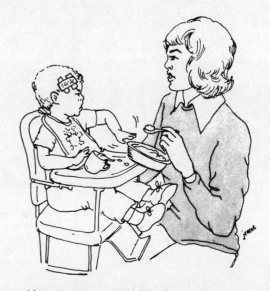

Watch your child for change in behavior.

ACTIVITY

Your child may return to school. The child should avoid rough activities until after his follow-up visit with the doctor. The types of activities to avoid are:

- Bike riding
- Swimming
- Skateboard riding
- Tree climbing
- Contact sports
- Gym class

FOLLOW-UP APPOINTMENT

Your child should see the doctor 2 or 3 weeks after leaving the hospital. Call the doctor for an appointment if the appointment has not already been made.

If you have any questions, please call your doctor (phone: _____) or _____.

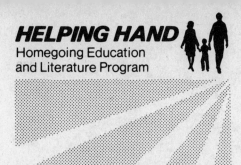

Let's talk about...

Hepatitis

Hepatitis (hep-a-TIE-tis) is often called "yellow jaundice." It is an infection of the liver. It may be caused by a virus. It is spread by contact with urine, feces (bowel movements), water, or milk that has the virus in it.

TO HELP STOP THE SPREAD OF DISEASE

There are several things you can do to help stop the spread of this disease. Please follow these instructions until your doctor tells you that the child with hepatitis is completely well.

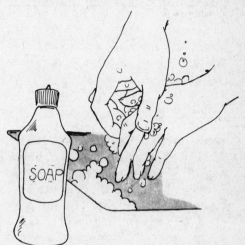

Picture 1 Good handwashing is very important!

HAND WASHING

The hands of all family members must be washed well with liquid soap or detergent and rinsed. Good hand washing by all members of the family MUST BE DONE:
· Before meals
· After using the bathroom
· Before preparing or serving food

GOOD HOUSEKEEPING

To prevent the spread of infection, the following steps must be taken in the home:
· The home must be free of rodents (rats and mice) and insects (flies and roaches).
· Clean the bathroom every day. Carefully wash the sink and toilet bowl with full strength Lysol or other disinfectant. Wear rubber gloves to protect your hands (Picture 2).
· Place tissues that have been used to clean the nose and mouth in a separate bag and throw it into the garbage.
· Wash utensils used in eating (glasses, dishes, forks, spoons, and knives) in soapy water and rinse in hot water.
· Flush urine, feces, and toilet paper down the toilet. (Urine, feces, or toilet paper that cannot be flushed down the toilet must be soaked with full strength Lysol or Chlorox every day for at least 12 hours before it is discarded.)

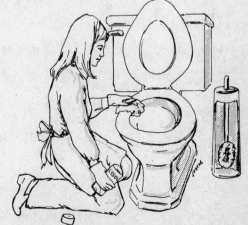

Picture 2 Clean toilet daily with disinfectant.

(continued)

222

2   Hepatitis

GOOD DIET AND REST

- The family should eat a well-balanced diet using the basic four food groups as a guide (Picture 3).
- Food left on the plate of an ill person should not be eaten by other family members.
- All family members should get at least 8 hours of sleep each night (Picture 4).
- Young children should have naps when possible.

MEDICAL CARE

- Your doctor may give medication to all family members who have been exposed to hepatitis.
- The Public Health Department will be asked to visit your home to help you to control this disease. They will ask several questions and will answer any questions you may have.

WHEN TO CALL THE DOCTOR

Call your doctor or the Medical Clinic (phone: _____) if any of the following signs occur:

- If the child does not feel hungry or does not want to eat
- If the child's temperature is more than 99.6° for more than 2 days
- If child has abdominal discomfort (stomach ache)
- If child is vomiting (throwing up) more than two times in an hour
- If child's skin or the white part of the eyes turns yellow

If you have any questions, please call _____.

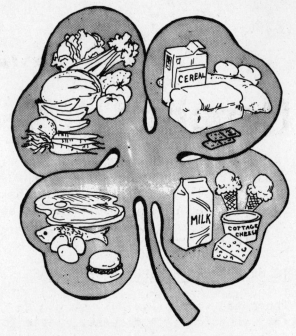

Picture 3 The Basic Four Food Groups:
1. Fruit and Vegetable Group
2. Bread and Cereal Group
3. Meat and Egg Group
4. Milk and Cheese Group

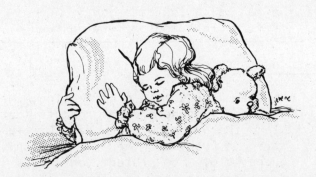

Picture 4 Get at least 8 hours of sleep each night.

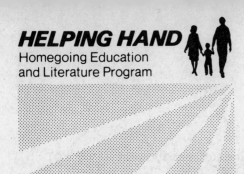

HELPING HAND
Homegoing Education
and Literature Program

Let's talk about...

Umbilical Hernia Repair

Your child is having his umbilical hernia (um-BIL-e-kal HER-nee-a) repaired.
During the surgery, parents can wait in the surgery lounge on the second floor.

WHAT TO EXPECT AFTER SURGERY

- Your child will "wake up" in the Recovery Room near the surgery area.
- The child will be returned to the unit as soon as he recovers from the
  anesthetic.
- The child will have a gauze dressing (bandage) over his incision (wound).
- Usually the child will have only a small amount of discomfort after surgery.
  Pain medication is rarely needed.

DIET

- The child can have clear liquids when he first wakes up after surgery. Clear
  liquids are: water, Kool-Aid, Jello, and popsicles.
- If the child has no trouble drinking the liquids, he may then have a regular
  diet.
- DO NOT give carbonated beverages (soda pop) or gas-producing foods for a few
  days.

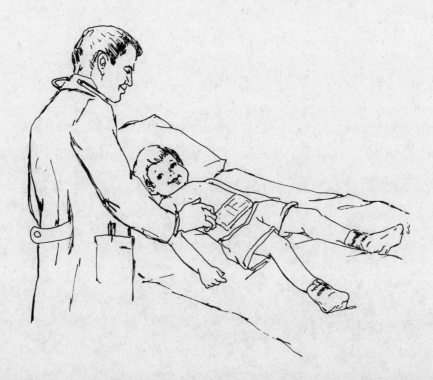

(continued)

2 Umbilical Hernia Repair

CARE OF THE WOUND

· Keep the bandage clean, dry and in place until the doctor removes it. <u>DO NOT</u> <u>TAKE OFF THE BANDAGE</u>.
· You may put more tape over the bandage to keep it on.
· If the bandage comes off or gets wet, call the doctor or clinic for advice.
· Give the child a "sponge bath", not a tub bath, as long as the dressing is on.
· The child may sleep on his tummy if he wants to.

ACTIVITY

· Your child should play quietly for the first 7 days after surgery or until he sees the doctor at the follow-up appointment. (No running, jumping, wrestling, or rough play.)
· The child should not climb steps for 7 days after surgery unless he has to.
· An older child should not take gym class or play sports until the doctor says he can.
· The child may return to school _____.

FOLLOW-UP CARE

· Call the clinic (phone: _____) a day or so after surgery to make a follow-up appointment. This appointment will be 5-7 days after surgery.
· At this appointment, the doctor will remove the bandage. The doctor will also tell you when the child can play normally.

If you have any questions, please call _____.

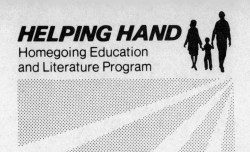

HELPING HAND
Homegoing Education
and Literature Program

Let's talk about...

Hydrocarbon Ingestion

Your child has been seen in the Emergency Room because he drank a hydrocarbon-type product. A hydrocarbon is a liquid like turpentine, gasoline, kerosene. Hydrocarbons are also found in certain types of cleaning fluids. Although we do not feel admission to the hospital is necessary at this time, there are several things we request that you do at home.

WATCH FOR THESE SIGNS

Watch your child closely for the next 3 days and nights. Wake your child several times during the night. Ask him to name familiar persons or toys.

It is very important to watch for the following signs:

- Fever, temperature over _____ °
- Trouble with breathing
- Frequent coughing
- Pain in stomach, vomiting, or diarrhea
- Excitement
- Increasing sleepiness (does not respond normally when you call his name)
- Difficulty in waking up
- Does not waken when you touch or talk to him.

WHEN TO CALL THE DOCTOR

Call your doctor (phone: _____) or the Emergency Room (phone:_____) if you see any of these signs.

WARNING: Keep all harmful liquids out of children's reach.

GIVE THE CHILD LIQUID FOODS

Give your child liquid foods for the next 12 hours. Some liquid foods are:

- Fruit and vegetable juice
- Milk
- Strained soup
- Plain ice cream
- Cereal gruel (like Cream of Wheat)
- Sherbet
- Gelatin (like Jello)
- Custard
- Plain pudding
- Popsicles

> WARNING: Children who drink harmful products once, are likely to do it again. Children are naturally curious. KEEP ALL HARMFUL SUBSTANCES OUT OF THE REACH OF CHILDREN.

If you have any questions, please call _____ .

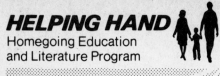

HELPING HAND
Homegoing Education
and Literature Program

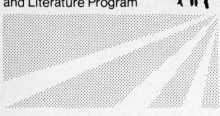

Let's talk about...

Impetigo

Impetigo (im-pe-TIE-go) is a skin infection which can be spread to other parts of the body and to other people. It first appears as a discolored pimple. Then small blisters form and quickly break. This spreads germs to the skin. The "weeping" sores form yellow crusts and the skin around them is red.

To keep impetigo from spreading, follow these instructions carefully three times a day.

YOU WILL NEED

Water
Mild soap
Ointment (as ordered by your doctor)
Clean wash cloth and towel
Nail clippers

WHAT TO DO

1. Wash your hands.
2. Read label on the ointment.
3. Have a person help hold your child if necessary.
4. Soak crusty areas on the skin with warm soapy water to loosen crusts.
5. Remove all crusts by using wash cloth (see Picture 1). IT IS VERY IMPORTANT TO REMOVE THE CRUSTS.
6. Apply ointment to the sore and to the area around it. Rub it in well.
7. Wash your hands well when finished.
8. Continue to apply ointment for 3 days after the sores have healed.

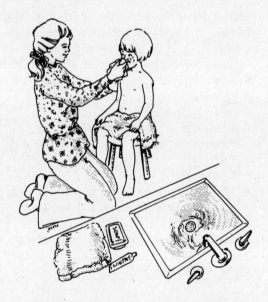

Picture 1 Wash sores three times a day.

(continued)

OTHER INSTRUCTIONS

- Wash bath tub, bathroom sink, or pan well after each use. DO NOT USE KITCHEN SINK FOR WASHING.
- Wash the towel, wash cloth, and bed linen after each use.
- Explain to your child that he should use only his wash cloth, towel, or bed linen - not anyone else's, and no one should use his linens either.
- Keep your child's fingernails cut short. Teach him not to touch the sores.
- Your doctor will tell you when your child may return to school.

WHEN TO CALL THE DOCTOR

Contact your doctor (phone: _____) if sores have not improved in 2 or 3 days, or if sores spread rapidly.

If you have any questions, please call _____.

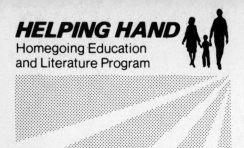
Let's talk about...

Head Lice-
Treatment and Prevention

Lice are small, sucking insects. They lay their eggs (nits) and attach them to the hair shafts. The nits look like bits of dandruff in the hair.

Lice can be passed from one person to another by direct contact or by the clothing the lice are living in. The lice cause itching. If the skin is scratched open, sores can develop. The lice and sores must be treated by your doctor.

To destroy the lice and nits you must follow these directions carefully.

YOU WILL NEED

Shampoo (as ordered by your doctor)
Fine-toothed comb
Soap
Towels

HOW TO SHAMPOO

1. Have child take a hot soapy bath. Rinse. Towel dry.
2. Pour 2 tablespoonfuls of shampoo on child's hair and on the skin around the hair.
3. Wet the hair with a small amount of warm water.
4. Rub briskly for 4 minutes to make a good lather. (Picture 1) (Try not to get shampoo in child's eyes. If this happens, rinse eyes with clear warm water.)

Picture 1 Make a good lather.

5. Rinse hair and skin around the hair well, and rub with dry towel.
6. Comb hair with fine-toothed comb to remove nits.
7. Look at the hair and scalp in 24 hours to be sure all lice and nits are gone. Repeat shampoo if necessary; do not give more than two shampoo treatments.
8. Call your doctor for advice if more than 2 treatments are needed.

(continued)

OTHER INSTRUCTIONS

• Wash all washable clothes, towels, wash cloths, and bed linens. Dry clean all nonwashable clothes that the child has used (Picture 2).
• Wash combs and brushes in soapy water after each shampoo. Use a little of the shampoo in the water.
• Look at the hair and scalp of all family members. Treat their hair if lice and nits are found.
• Ask the doctor when the child should return to school.

FOLLOW-UP CARE

Please report this condition to the nurse at the child's school. The nurse can check other children for nits and see that they are treated too.

If you have any questions, please call _____ or your local Health Department.

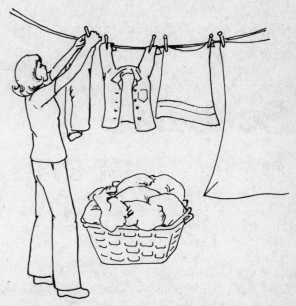

Picture 2 Wash clothes and bed linens.

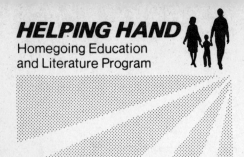
HELPING HAND
Homegoing Education
and Literature Program

Let's talk about...

Scabies

Scabies, "the itch," is a skin condition caused by a mite. A mite is a spider-like insect so small that it can only be seen under a microscope. The female mite burrows under the skin and lays eggs. The path where the mite burrows looks like a tiny scratch mark. This burrowing causes severe itching. If the skin is scratched open, it can become infected.

Scabies is "caught" by having body contact with a person that has it or by wearing clothes that have scabies mites living in them.

TO TREAT SCABIES

1. Buy the lotion prescribed by your doctor.
2. Give your child a warm soapy bath or shower.
3. Shampoo the child's hair with the lotion.
4. Rinse the soap off and dry.
5. Apply a thin coat of the prescribed lotion to the child's entire body, from the neck down. The mites like to live in warm moist areas (between fingers and toes, in the armpits, and in the skin around the waist and genital area). Make very sure the lotion is applied to these areas.
6. Have your child dress in freshly washed clean clothes (Picture 1).
7. Leave the lotion on for 24 hours; then have your child take a bath or shower.
8. Repeat the treatment in 4 days if the itching continues.
9. If itching does not stop after two treatments, call your doctor.

CARE OF CLOTHING AND LINENS

- The mite that causes scabies can live in clothing and bed linens for a week.
- Using hot water, wash all clothing, bed linens, towels, and wash clothes that have been used or worn within the week before your child was treated (Picture 2).
- Freshly washed clean clothes should be worn and clean bed linens used after each application of lotion.

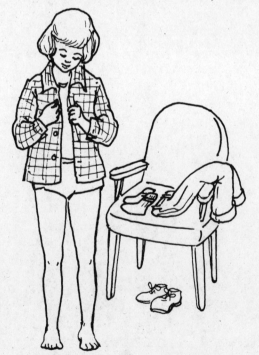

Picture 1 Dress in clean clothes after putting on lotion.

(continued)

TO PREVENT SCABIES FROM SPREADING

- Family members should be examined and should be treated if they have signs of scabies on their skin.
- If you know where your child got the scabies, have the child avoid contact with that person until the person is treated and well.
- Damp dust the child's bed daily.
- Wash toilet seat once a day until all family members are well.

SAFETY TIPS

Store the lotion out of children's reach. If any of the lotion happens to get into the eyes, wash the eyes with cool water.

If you have any questions, please call _____.

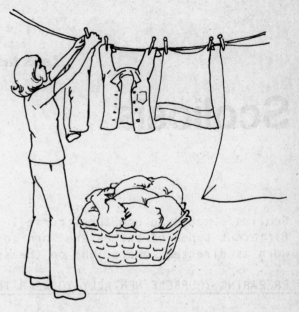

Picture 2 Wash all clothing and linens well.

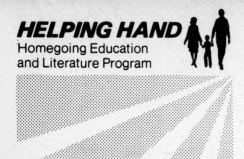

HELPING HAND
Homegoing Education
and Literature Program

Let's talk about...

Scoliosis

Scoliosis means an unnatural curve in the spine. The cause is usually not known. Different types of braces are worn to prevent more curving. If the braces are worn as directed, operations on the spine can sometimes be avoided.

PREPARING YOURSELF MENTALLY TO WEAR THE BRACE

Sometimes it is hard to stick with wearing the brace. The first 2 weeks are the hardest time. After that, the brace becomes more familiar, and it won't bother you as much to wear it.

When the brace is first put on, you will have feelings that you "can't stand it." But keep it on as long as you can. If you feel you can't go through with it, take it off for a while. When you can get yourself together, put it on and try again. You may cry at times because you feel trapped, but stick with it. In a short time you will feel better and will be doing most of the things you did before.

The feeling that the brace is "too long" will decrease with time. It is important to keep the brace snug.

CARE OF THE BRACE

Wash the brace daily with a wash cloth and mild soap. Rinse with wash cloth and clear water and wipe dry. Do not put any part of the brace into water.

SKIN CARE

Wash and rinse your body thoroughly every day. Apply rubbing alcohol to toughen the skin. After it dries, dust lightly with corn starch to help prevent friction spots from forming where the brace might rub.

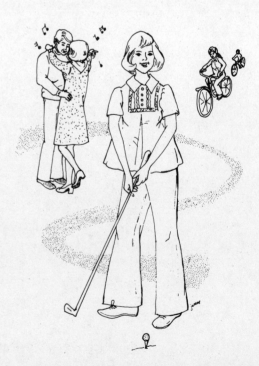

Check your skin for red spots. If necessary, use a mirror to see all areas.

The skin will itch a lot when the brace is first removed. Apply rubbing alcohol to the skin. It will help stop the itching.

(continued)

SPORTS AND OTHER ACTIVITIES

It is important to get plenty of exercise. You can continue most sports and activities such as swimming, volleyball, biking, and golf. You should wear your brace for all these sports, except swimming. Do not go horseback riding because the jarring is uncomfortable. Do not play football or other contact sports.

Your doctor will advise you when you can return to school and continue activities.

DIET

A well-balanced diet will help to keep you healthy. It will also help the treatment to be a success. If nausea (feeling "sick to your stomach") occurs, eat smaller amounts of food and liquids more often.

DENTAL CARE

Consult your dentist about how often you should have a dental check-up.

CLOTHING

Wear a cotton sleeveless undershirt under the brace. Buy one size larger than normally worn. Make sure it is 2 or 3 inches below the end of the brace. Smock-like tops are easy to get into. Shift-type dresses make the brace less noticeable. Buy jeans or slacks a size larger than you usually wear.

SPECIAL TIPS

- When you have to be some place at a certain time, allow yourself more time to get ready. Don't hurry getting into a car. You might tilt back and cause the brace to hurt you.
- Raise the height of the table or desk for eating and studying. A portable tilt table may help. Microscopes can be slanted or can be put on a higher level. Prism glasses can be worn for reading. Wedge-shaped pillows can help to maintain the desired position.
- A special toilet seat can be purchased at a hospital supply company. This will raise the height of the toilet and will make it easier to use.
- Try to sleep on the side that is curved out, as often as possible.
- Try to resume your normal activities as soon as possible. Don't lie around and feel sorry for yourself. Let your close friends know you are wearing a brace. They can help you be less self-conscious about "being different."

WHEN TO CALL YOUR BRACE SPECIALIST (Phone: _____)

- If there are any breaks in the brace
- If the brace feels too tight
- If there are any pressure areas on your skin

You will have appointments to see the brace specialist about every 6 weeks.

(continued)

3 Scoliosis

<u>WHEN TO CALL YOUR DOCTOR</u> (Phone: _____)

_____

_____

_____

_____

_____

_____

_____

<u>WHEN TO CALL YOUR ORTHOPEDIC NURSE</u> (Phone: _____)

_____

_____

_____

_____

_____

_____

_____

<u>FOLLOW-UP APPOINTMENTS</u>

Be sure to keep the appointment with your doctor and brace specialist as
scheduled.

If you have any questions, please call _____.

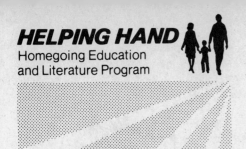

HELPING HAND
Homegoing Education
and Literature Program

Let's talk about...

Having a T&A

"T & A" means having tonsils and adenoids taken out.

Your child is scheduled for surgery on (date): _____. You will be told the time of surgery when you come to the hospital.

PREPARING FOR SURGERY

- If your child develops a cough or fever before coming to the hospital, call the Ear, Nose, and Throat Clinic (E.N.T.) (phone: _____), or call your doctor (phone: _____).
- Explain to your child what will happen at the hospital. You may tell your child that he is going to have two little lumps taken out of the back of his mouth. He will be taken to a big room. Then he will be given some sweet smelling air to make him sleep for a while. When he is asleep, the doctor will take out his tonsils. After his tonsils are out, he will go back to his room and will be awake.
- Your child can bring his favorite toy from home.

Picture 1 How to get to Children's Hospital

THE EVENING BEFORE SURGERY

Please <u>do not</u> give your child any food to eat or liquids to drink after midnight the evening before surgery. <u>This is very important</u>.

The child should have nothing to eat or to drink the night before surgery, so he won't choke while under anesthesia.

ON THE DAY OF SURGERY

- Bring your child to the Patient Services office in the main lobby at 8:00 A.M. The main lobby is at the entrance to the new building that faces Parsons Avenue (Picture 1). At this office you will be interviewed. Then you will be taken to the nursing unit by a volunteer.
- If you have hospital insurance, please bring the forms with you.
- Please do not bring any other children who are not having surgery.

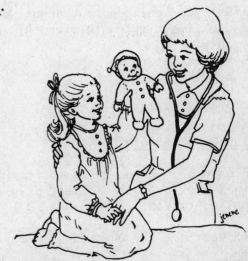

Picture 2 Your child may bring a favorite toy from home.

(continued)

2 Having a T&A

ON THE NURSING UNIT

- Your child will have a medical examination.
  Parents - <u>please remain on the unit until you
  have talked with the doctor.</u>
- A parent may stay overnight with the child.
  Most children go home the next morning.
- A supervised playroom is available for older
  children to enjoy.

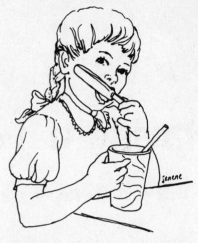

WHAT TO EXPECT AFTER SURGERY

- Your child may have a temperature of 100-102°
  for 1-7 days. If it is higher than that, call
  the E.N.T. Clinic (phone: _____).

Picture 3 Give plenty of
liquids.

- Pain in the ears may last as long as 2 weeks.
  These pains are usually worse in
  the morning but decrease during the day. Swallowing is painful. Have the child
  take the prescribed medication as directed to ease the pain.
- Raw white areas will appear where tonsils were removed. These will disappear in
  about 2 weeks.
- Occasionally, children will bleed from the nose or mouth, even 1 week after the
  operation. This bleeding is rarely serious, but we want to see your child if it
  happens. Call the E.N.T. Clinic (phone:_____), your private physician (phone:
  _____), or the Emergency Room (phone:_____), and take your child to the
  Emergency Room.

DIET AFTER SURGERY

Your child may eat or drink whatever he wishes. Food will not injure his throat.
If he does not want food, be sure he drinks plenty of liquids (Picture 3). This
will keep his fever down and keep his nose and throat from feeling dry.

ACTIVITY AFTER SURGERY

- Get your child up and about, do not keep
  him from playing (Picture 4). He may play
  outside.
- He may return to school 7 days after the
  operation.
- No swimming is allowed for 2 weeks after
  the operation.

FOLLOW-UP APPOINTMENT

Please bring your child to the E.N.T. Clinic
in 3 weeks. An appointment slip will be
mailed to you.

If you have any questions, please call
_____ .

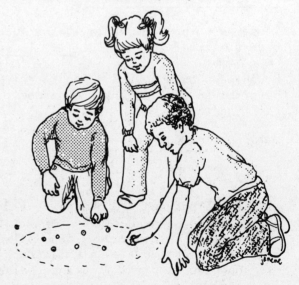

Picture 4 Your child may play outside.

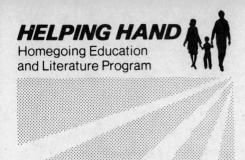

HELPING HAND
Homegoing Education
and Literature Program

Let's talk about...

Vomiting

Child's Name: _____
Date: _____

Your child has been seen by Doctor _____ at Children's Hospital
for vomiting (throwing up). The following information and suggestions will be
helpful to you as you care for your child at home.

Vomiting is usually caused by a minor infection. Vomiting will usually stop in a
couple of days and can be treated at home. There are a number of serious illnesses
that may cause vomiting, but we do not think your child has any of these illnesses.

WARNING: Some medicines used for vomiting in older children or adults are very
dangerous for young children. DO NOT use any medicines unless your doctor has told
you to use it for this child.

The main danger from vomiting is dehydration (dee-hi-DRAY-shun), being "dried
out." To keep your child from getting dehydrated, you should give liquids in a way
that will allow him to "hold them down."

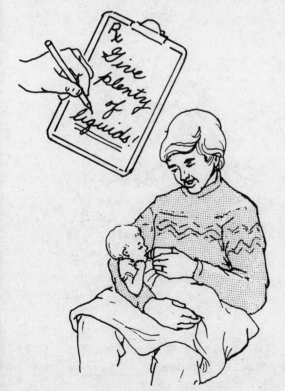

GIVE YOUR CHILD CLEAR LIQUIDS TO DRINK

Some clear liquids you can give are:

- Soda pop with the fizz shaken out (not diet
  pop). Pour pop into a glass and stir until
  bubbles are gone.
- Jello water - Add twice as much water as the
  directions call for (use 4 cups instead of 2).
  Allow Jello water to reach room temperature.
- Apple juice
- Kool-Aid
- Ice popsicles
- Oral electrolyte fluids (such as Pedialtyte,
  Lytren) - available at local drug stores
  without a prescription
- Gatorade
- Tea
- Solid Jello

(continued)

2 Vomiting

HOW TO GIVE LIQUIDS

You should give small amounts of these clear liquids often. For example: give 1/2 ounce (1 tablespoonful) every 20 minutes for a few hours. If your child takes this without vomiting, increase to 1 ounce (2 tablespoonfuls) every 20 minutes for a couple of hours. If your child takes this well, allow him to increase the amount he drinks. If the child vomits, wait for 1 hour before offering more liquids.

SOLID FOOD TO NIBBLE ON

If your child wants solid foods to nibble on and you think he can hold them down, try small amounts of:

- Soda crackers
- Graham crackers
- Vanilla wafers
- Toasted bread

DO NOT GIVE THESE FOODS FOR A DAY OR TWO

- Solid foods (other than soda crackers, graham crackers, vanilla wafers, or toasted bread)
- Milk
- Orange juice
- Salty soup or broth

WHEN TO CALL THE DOCTOR

You should call the doctor if you think your child is getting worse, or:

- If your child vomits blood or material that looks like "coffee grounds"
- If vomiting becomes more severe, or more frequent
- If your child is lethargic or difficult to waken
- If your child acts confused ("out of his head") or does not know what he is doing
- If the child has constant abdominal pain (tummy ache)
- If the child seems to be getting dehydrated (dried out)

SIGNS OF DEHYDRATION ARE

- Child has not urinated (passed water) for 6 or _____ hours
- There are no tears when child cries
- Child's mouth feels dry or sticky
- Child's breathing is hard or fast

If any of these things happens, please contact your doctor (phone: _____), the Emergency Room (phone:_____), or the Pediatric Clinic (phone:_____).

section 2
Procedures

Let's talk about...

Changing a Gauze Bandage

Dry sterile gauze dressings (bandages) are used to protect wounds and to absorb drainage from infected wounds. To prevent other infections, all items needed to care for your child's wound must be kept as clean as possible. Good handwashing is also required.

THE DOCTOR'S ORDER

☐ Change bandage and clean wound with _____ solution _____ times per day.

☐ Change soiled bandage. <u>Do not</u> clean the wound.

☐ Do not remove bandage. If bandage is soiled, apply sterile gauze bandage on top of the bandage that is on the wound.

You Will Need:

FROM THE PHARMACY	FROM HOME
☐ Gauze squares, size _____	☐ 1 tray for all supplies
☐ Cotton balls	☐ 1 small tray for bandage change
☐ Cleansing solution (as ordered by the doctor)	☐ Large pan with lid
☐ Roller gauze bandage size _____	☐ 2 8-oz. jars with lids
☐ Nonallergic adhesive tape _____	☐ 1 jar (holder for tongs)
☐ Rubbing alcohol	☐ 1 small drinking glass
☐ Q-tips	☐ Tongs
	☐ Scissors
	☐ Paper towels
	☐ Plastic bags
	☐ Rubber bands

(continued)

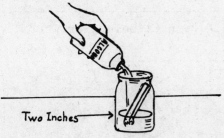

Picture 1 Sterilizing the equipment.

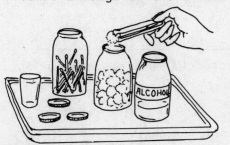

Two Inches →

Picture 2 Tongs in the alcohol.

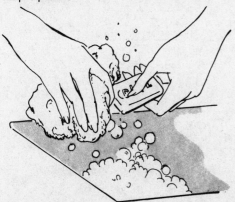

Picture 3 Preparing the equipment.

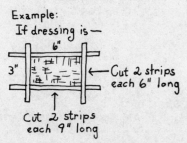

Picture 4 Wash hands well.

Example:
If dressing is —
6"
3"
← Cut 2 strips each 6" long
Cut 2 strips each 9" long

Picture 5 To cut adhesive strips.

TO PREPARE EQUIPMENT

1. Place the three glass jars, lids, tongs and small drinking glass in the pan (Picture 1).
2. Cover items with water.
3. Bring to a boil.
4. Put lid on pan.
5. Boil 10 minutes. (Start timing after the boiling starts.)
6. Let cool.
7. Remove tongs, touching the handles only. Pour the water out of the jars, glass and lids. Using the tongs, place them on the tray.
8. Pour 2 inches of alcohol into a jar. Then, place the tongs into this jar (Picture 2).
9. Allow the other jars to air dry.
10. Using the tongs, fill one jar with cotton balls and one jar with Q-tips (Picture 3).
11. Put the other items on the supply tray (gauze squares, roller gauze bandage, adhesive tape, scissors, rubber bands, paper towels, and plastic bags).

TO PREPARE TRAY FOR ONE BANDAGE CHANGE

1. Wash your hands well. Rinse and dry.
2. Pour enough cleansing solution into small glass for one bandage change.
3. Place paper towel on tray.
4. Using tongs, remove cotton balls and Q-tips from jars and place on paper towel.
5. Place gauze squares on paper towel (enough to cover wound).
6. Cut four strips of adhesive. Adhesive should extend 1 1/2 inches beyond the bandage on each side (Picture 5).
7. Lightly stick ends of tape to the edge of the tray.
8. Add one plastic bag and rubber band to tray for the soiled bandage.
9. Carry tray to the area where you plan to change your child's bandage.

(continued)

3 Changing a Gauze Bandage

HOW TO CHANGE THE BANDAGE

1. Gently but firmly remove the old bandage. If bandage sticks to wound, moisten it with clean cool water to loosen.
2. Put old bandage in plastic bag.
3. Wash your hands.
4. Clean wound with Q-tips moistened with cleansing solution (Picture 6).
5. Moisten cotton balls with cleansing solution. Clean around outside of wound.
6. Place used cotton balls and Q-tips in plastic bag.
7. Look at the wound to see if it is healing. The wound should heal from the deepest part. The sides should begin to come together.
8. Place gauze squares on the wound. Put the adhesive around the edges of the gauze (Picture 7).
9. Put the lids back on the jars and bottle of cleansing solution.
10. Using the rubber band, close the end of the plastic bag containing the old bandage and used supplies. Discard in the trash.
11. Store tray of items out of children's reach.

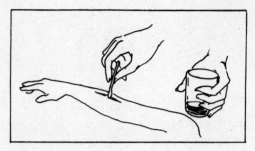

Picture 6 Cleaning the wound.

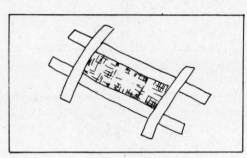

Picture 7 Tape gauze securely.

WHEN TO CALL THE DOCTOR

You should call your doctor (phone: _____) or the clinic (phone: _____) if the wound does not seem to be healing.

SIGNS THAT THE WOUND IS NOT HEALING

- Increased drainage from the wound
- Swelling
- Increased redness around the wound
- Change in odor of the drainage
- Skin around wound feels hot to touch
- Child has temperature above 101° by mouth or above 102° by rectum

Call your doctor if any of these signs occur.

(continued)

MONTGOMERY STRAPS

Adhesive tape causes skin irritation when removed
many times. If the dressing is going to be changed
many times, you can make "Montgomery straps" with
adhesive tape. These straps hold the dressing in
place (Picture 8). You do not need to remove
Montgomery straps each time you change the
bandage unless they become soiled.

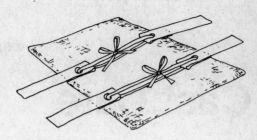

TO MAKE MONTGOMERY STRAPS

1. Cut four pieces of adhesive tape into 6- to
   8-inch lengths.
2. Fold one end of tape under, 1 inch (the tape
   will stick to itself).
3. Cut a hole in each folded end, 1/2 inch from
   the fold (Picture 8).
4. Apply adhesive end to your child's body. Put
   two on each side of the wound (Picture 8).
   (These straps are placed beside the wound, not
   over the wound.)
5. Put a piece of gauze or clean shoe strings
   through the holes in the adhesive tape.
6. Tie the strings snugly over the center of the
   bandage (Picture 8).
7. When changing the bandage, take the ties out
   of the straps before removing the bandage or
   cleaning the wound.

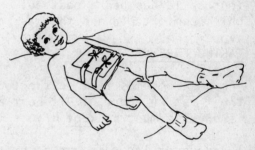

Picture 8 Montgomery straps
hold bandage in place.

Let's talk about...

Cast Care

Your child has had a cast put on. There are some things you need to do to keep the child comfortable and the cast clean.

TAKING CARE OF THE CAST

The cast becomes firm to the touch in 10-15 minutes after it is put on. But, during the first 24 hours, it is soft and can be easily dented or cracked. After the cast is dry, it must be <u>kept</u> dry or it will crack and crumble.

- An arm or leg cast can be protected during bathing with a plastic bag. Do not lower the cast into water. It may be easier for your child to have a sponge bath while the cast is on.
- If the cast becomes soiled, it can be cleaned with a damp wash cloth and a cleanser. If the area you cleaned is large, expose it to the air or sunlight to dry the plaster. Do not put clothing over the cast until it dries.
- The hose of a hair dryer may be used to blow cool air into the cast. (Set temperature of hair dryer on "cool.") This may be used to relieve itching or to dry the cast. (Severe itching may be relieved by medication which your doctor may prescribe.)

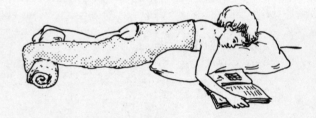
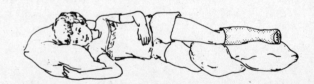

Picture 1 Support cast on pillows or blanket roll. Turn every 2-3 hours.

SKIN CARE

- If your child has a large cast, changing your child's position is important. This will prevent constant pressure on any one skin area. Turn the child about every 2 hours during the day and as often as you can at night. It also helps to put the child's casted arm or leg up on a pillow (Picture 1).
- Check the child's skin every day. Press skin back around all cast edges, and carefully look and feel for reddened areas or sores.
- A reddened area should be rubbed with a small amount of alcohol or lotion.
- Do not allow the child to stick any object under the cast. This may injure the skin.

(continued)

EXERCISE

If exercises are needed, they will be taught
by our hospital physical therapist.

ACTIVITY

If your child must remain in bed, you will
need to plan for play activities he will
enjoy.

• Books, records, and tapes can be borrowed
  from the library.
• Encourage the child's friends to visit.
• A reclining lawn chair can be used as a
  daytime bed. This type of chair can
  easily be moved to different parts of
  the house for a change of scenery.
• Some children with casts can go to school
  (with the doctor's permission). If the
  child has to stay home, call the school
  principal to plan for schooling at home.

TO "PETAL" THE CAST

Petaling the cast protects your child's
skin from the rough edges of the cast.

To petal the cast, wait until the cast is
dry. Cut several 2-inch pieces of adhesive
tape, making one end rounded. Then apply to
the cast edges as shown in Picture 2.

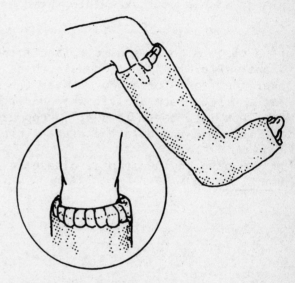

Picture 2 Petal the cast to protect
skin from rough edges.

WHEN TO CALL THE DOCTOR

Contact the Orthopedic Clinic (phone:_____), Emergency Room (phone:_____),
or your doctor (phone: _____):

• If child complains of tingling and/or numbness of toes or fingers
• If toes or fingers are cold to the touch or appear blue
• If toes or fingers become swollen
• If child often complains of pain
• If a foul smell from the cast or if staining occurs that was not present when
  the child went home. This may be a sign of a pressure sore and should be checked
  by the physician.

(continued)

3 Cast Care

SPECIAL HINTS FOR CARE OF A SPICA CAST

If your child has a spica cast and is not toilet trained, a diaper must be used to protect the cast.

A disposable diaper should be used if possible (Picture 3). This diaper may need to be cut smaller to fit properly. The diaper should be tucked into the cast (Picture 3).

If a cloth diaper is used, place folded diaper (Picture 3) with double thickness over the front for a boy or over the back for a girl. Place plastic wrap under diaper and tuck into cast. This will keep urine off the cast and hold the diaper in place.

If you have any questions, please call _____.

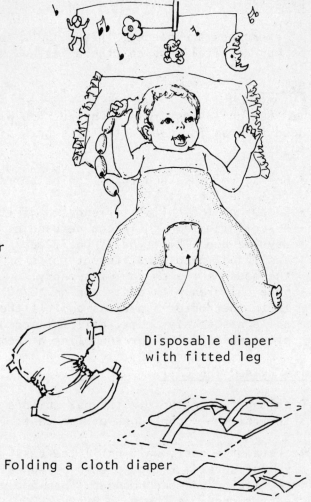

Disposable diaper with fitted leg

Folding a cloth diaper

Picture 3 Diaper tucked into a spica cast.

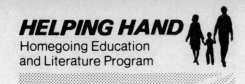

HELPING HAND
Homegoing Education
and Literature Program

Let's talk about...

Crutch Walking

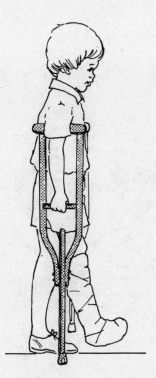

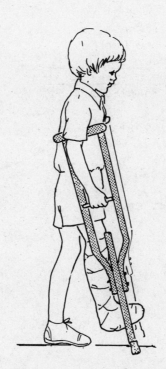

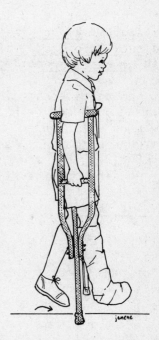

Stand straight, shoulders relaxed. Hold crutches under arms. Hold hand-grips. Keep elbows slightly bent. Keep casted leg out in front.

Move crutches forward slightly ahead of good foot while keeping your balance on your good leg.

With crutches firmly on the floor, push down on hands and hop forward on good leg.

SPECIAL TIPS

- <u>Never lean on underarm pieces.</u> This can cause nerve damage. Always push down with hands.
- <u>To go upstairs</u> - Keep casted leg and crutches on ground. Push down with hands and hop up onto step with good leg. Straighten good leg and bring casted leg and crutches up.
- <u>To go downstairs</u> - Face stairs. Put crutches and casted leg on lower step. Push down with hands. Hop down to step on good foot.
- Make sure you have rubber safety caps on the bottom of the crutches. These keep you from slipping.

If you have any questions, please call _____.

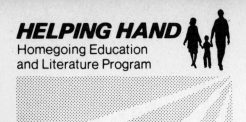

HELPING HAND
Homegoing Education
and Literature Program

Let's talk about...

Ear Irrigations (Washings)

Child's Name: _____

Age: _____

Irrigate _____ ear(s) _____ time(s) a day.

Your child has an ear infection. The pus (drainage) caused by bacteria (germs) must be washed out. Your child's ear may be very sore, and he may not want you to wash it out. But, if this is not done, he may have poor hearing or other illness later on.

YOU WILL NEED

Bottle of medication
Glass jar
Pan of warm water
Bulb syringe
Towel
Small pan with cover

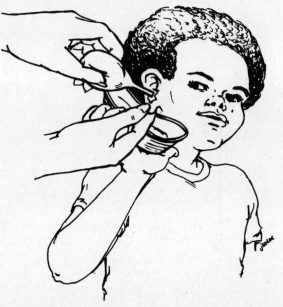

Picture 1 Wash out ear gently.

WHAT TO DO

1. Wash your hands.
2. Read the label on the medication bottle.
3. Make the solution following the directions on the bottle.
4. Pour the amount of solution needed into the jar.
5. Place the jar in a pan of warm water. Let solution become warm.
6. Fill bulb syringe with the warm solution.
7. Test temperature by dropping 2 drops on your wrist. It should be warm (not hot or too cold).
8. Have a person hold your child if necessary.
9. Place towel around child's shoulders to catch drips.
10. Hold small pan under child's ear.
11. Hold your child's ear lobe. For a child under 3 years, gently pull down and back. For a child 3 years or older, gently pull up and back (Picture 1).
12. Gently squeeze the bulb syringe and let solution flow into and out of the ear.
13. Repeat this until solution runs clear.
14. Gently dry outside of ear with towel.
15. Your child may return to play.

(continued)

HOW TO CLEAN THE EQUIPMENT

1. Flush used solution down the toilet.
2. Wash bulb syringe, glass jar, and small pan in soapy water. Rinse and place in pan.
3. Cover items with water and bring to a boil.
4. Put cover on pan and boil for 10 minutes.
5. Let cool.
6. Drain water.
7. Leave items in covered pan until next treatment.
8. Be sure to clean equipment after each treatment.

If you have any questions, please call _____

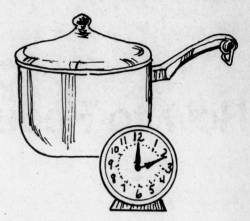

Picture 2 Boil equipment for 10 minutes.

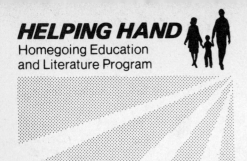

HELPING HAND
Homegoing Education
and Literature Program

Let's talk about...

How to Reduce a Fever

A fever is a rise in body temperature above
normal. If your child looks flushed, his
skin is hot, and he is restless, he may
have a fever. Take your child's temperature.
If the temperature is above 103° by rectum,
the temperature must be lowered to normal.
One way to help the fever to come down is
to give the child a sponge bath in a tub.
The child will cry and will not want you to
sponge him. But, continue the sponging
because it is important to bring down the
temperature.

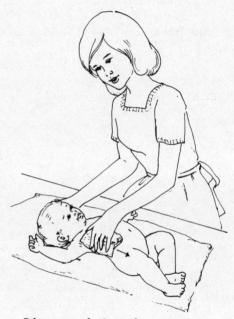

Picture 1 Gently stroke
child's skin.

YOU WILL NEED

Child's bath tub for infant
Regular bath tub for older child
Clean wash cloths
Towels

WHAT TO DO

1. Fill the bath tub with 2 inches of water that is warm to your wrist.
2. Remove the child's clothing. Place child in tub or on a padded surface.
3. Wet and partially wring out a wash cloth.
4. Sponge child's body with the wash cloth. Use long soothing strokes over face,
   neck, arms, chest, back, and legs. Rub slightly. Sponge water on chest and
   back. (Picture 1).
5. Sponge child for 20 minutes.
6. Remove child from tub and cover him with a light blanket.
7. Wait 30 minutes.
8. Take child's temperature.
9. If the temperature is still high, repeat sponging until the temperature is
   101° rectally.
10. If child starts to shiver, stop sponging. When shivering stops, warm the
    water and put child back in tub or on padded surface.
11. Dress your child so he is comfortable for the temperature of the home.
12. NEVER LEAVE CHILD ALONE WHEN TAKING TEMPERATURE OR REDUCING FEVER.

(continued)

OTHER INFORMATION

- To help to keep the temperature normal, give clear liquids. Have the child drink as much water and juice as he will take.
- Your child may have _____ baby aspirin, every _____ hours, or _____ every ____ hours. Give this only as directed by a doctor.
- Call your doctor or the Emergency Room if the temperature remains over _____° by rectum or _____° by mouth.
- Call your doctor or the Emergency Room if he vomits medicine or fluids _____ times.

If you have any questions, please call _____ .

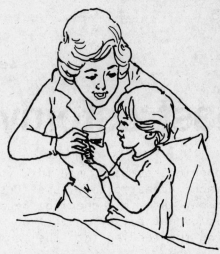

Picture 2 Give him his favorite drink.

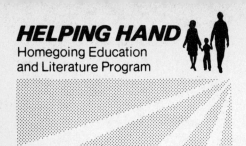

Let's talk about...

Gastrostomy Tube Feeding

An opening has been made into your child's stomach. A gastrostomy tube (G-tube) has been put into this opening. Because your child cannot eat by mouth, you will be giving the feeding into the stomach through the G-tube.

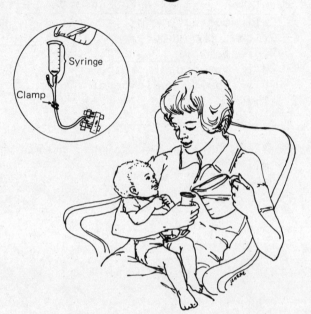

YOU WILL NEED

Ascepto syringe
Measuring container with pouring spout
Formula or blended mix as prescribed by
  your doctor
Clamp or rubber band
Glass of water
Paper towels
Tray

PREPARING TO FEED YOUR CHILD

1. Wash hands.
2. Pour correct amount of feeding into measuring container. Place container of feeding in pan of warm water.
3. Allow feeding to reach room temperature.
4. Change baby's diaper if necessary. Wash your hands again.

Picture 1 Hold baby while feeding.

FEEDING YOUR CHILD

- If child is an infant, hold your baby in the curve of your arm (cuddling position), and keep his head raised (Picture 1).
- If your child is older, put him in a high chair or seat.
- If child cries during the feeding, stop feeding until he is quiet and comforted.

HOW TO FEED

1. Drop 2 or 3 drops of the feeding on the inside of your wrist. It should feel warm, not hot.
2. Put the tip of the syringe into the open end of the G-tube (Picture 1).
3. Hold the tip of the syringe no higher than your child's shoulder.
4. Clamp the tube if it is open.
5. Pour feeding into the syringe (Picture 1). Unclamp the tube.
6. Keep adding more feeding as the syringe empties. To prevent air from getting into the stomach, do not let the tube run dry.
7. After all the feeding is in the stomach, add 1/2 ounce of water. The water clears the formula from the tube and prevents it from clogging.
8. Remove the syringe. Close the clamp or fold the end of the catheter over and secure with a rubber band unless you are instructed to keep it open.
9. Fasten G-tube to child's clothing with a safety pin.

(continued)

AFTER THE FEEDING

1. If your child is an infant, bubble (burp) after feeding. A small infant should be burped after every 2-3 ounces. Sit infant on your lap. Support baby by placing your hand on his chest and your fingers under his chin. Pat his back until air comes up.
2. If you put him to bed right after feeding, place baby in bed on his right side. This allows the feeding to follow the normal course of the intestinal tract.
3. Raise the head of the bed 6 or 8 inches by placing pillows under the mattress.

CLEANING THE EQUIPMENT

1. Rinse syringe, spoon, and measuring container with cold water. Wash in soapy water. Rinse and dry.
2. Place paper towel on tray.
3. Replace items on tray.
4. Cover with paper towel.
5. Store in cupboard.

OTHER INFORMATION

- You will be instructed by the doctor whether to leave the tube clamped or unclamped.
- If vitamins are ordered, use liquid vitamins and drop them into tube with the formula.
- Never change baby's formula or give more than your doctor ordered.
- If your child's appetite is not satisfied, ask your doctor for advice on increasing feeding.
- Always keep another sterile G-tube and syringe in your home. Some suppliers do not carry child-size supplies. If necessary, you can get an extra tube from Children's Hospital.
- If child's abdomen becomes distended (stomach puffs up), unclamp the tube. Wait 1 hour. If the abdomen is still puffed up, call your doctor (phone: _____) or Children's Hospital Emergency Room (phone: _____) for advice.
- If the tube comes out, place a gauze square over the opening. Place a clean folded diaper over that to absorb the stomach contents. Take your child to your doctor or an emergency room to have the tube replaced. You should do this in time to give the next feeding. Take the extra tube with you.
- When you feel ready, your surgeon or nurse may teach you to replace the tube.

If you have any questions, please call _____.

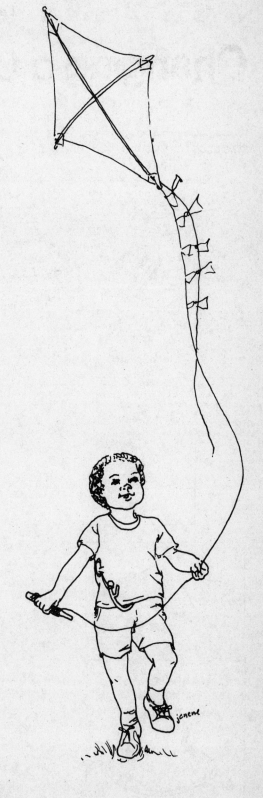

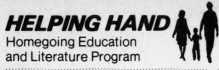
Let's talk about...

Changing a Gastrostomy Tube

Your child has a gastrostomy (gas-TRAH-sto-me) tube. This tube is a feeding tube that goes into the child's stomach. You will need to change your child's gastrostomy tube (G-tube) every 4-6 weeks. If the tube comes out, put in a new one within 4 hours.

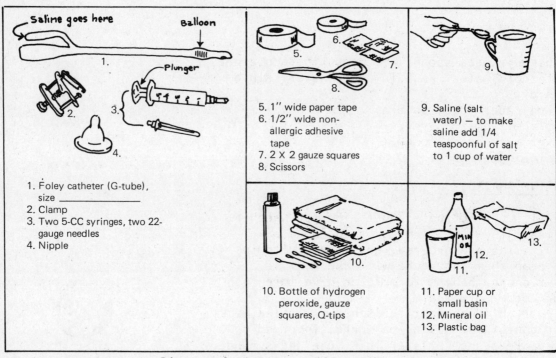

Saline goes here   Balloon

Plunger

1. Foley catheter (G-tube), size _____
2. Clamp
3. Two 5-CC syringes, two 22-gauge needles
4. Nipple

5. 1" wide paper tape
6. 1/2" wide non-allergic adhesive tape
7. 2 X 2 gauze squares
8. Scissors

9. Saline (salt water) — to make saline add 1/4 teaspoonful of salt to 1 cup of water

10. Bottle of hydrogen peroxide, gauze squares, Q-tips

11. Paper cup or small basin
12. Mineral oil
13. Plastic bag

Picture 1 What you will need.

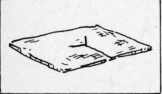

Picture 2

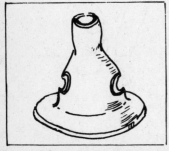

Picture 3

PREPARING THE MATERIALS

1. Wash your hands.
2. Cut to center of a gauze square to make an opening for the G-tube (Picture 2).
3. Cut four pieces of paper tape 3 to 5 inches long.
4. Cut one piece of adhesive tape 2 inches long.
5. Cut hole in the end of the baby bottle nipple large enough to slip G-tube through (Picture 3). Cut a smaller hole on each side of the nipple. This allows air to circulate. The nipple may be used until it starts to get soft and sticky.

(continued)

TO REMOVE THE G-TUBE

1. Open the clamp. Let stomach contents drain into cup or basin (Picture 4).
2. Put the needle into closed end of G-tube (Picture 5).
3. Pull back on the plunger of the syringe to remove the saline in balloon.
4. Gently loosen the bandage.
5. Gently remove G-tube and bandage. Place old G-tube and bandage into plastic bag for disposal.
6. Hold gauze over opening to absorb stomach contents.
7. Gently rub a little mineral oil into old adhesive tape marks. This helps them come off when washed.
8. Wash skin around opening with soapy water. Rinse and dry well.

TO PUT IN A NEW G-TUBE

1. Put G-tube with attached nipple into the stomach opening. Be sure balloon is below the skin line. When the stomach contents come up the tube you will know the G-tube is in the stomach (Picture 6).
2. Fill syringe with _____ cc of fresh saline.
3. Inject saline into closed end of the G-tube to blow up balloon (Picture 6). The balloon keeps the tube from coming out.
4. Gently pull on G-tube to make sure it is securely in place.
5. Clamp the G-tube.
6. Place 2 X 2 gauze around G-tube (Picture 7).
7. Push nipple down so it touches the gauze firmly.
8. Tape nipple to gauze and to skin with paper tape on all four sides (Picture 8).
9. Tape G-tube at top of nipple with adhesive to keep nipple in place (Picture 8).

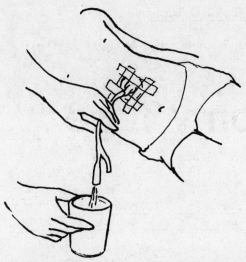

Picture 4

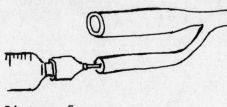

Picture 5

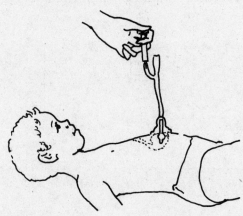

Picture 6

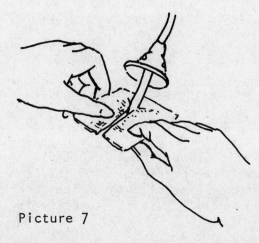

Picture 7

(continued)

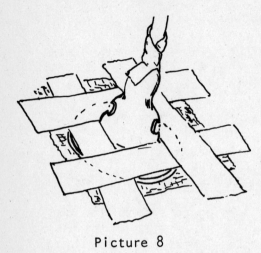

Picture 8

CARE OF THE SKIN AROUND G-TUBE

The skin around the G-tube must be washed every day.

1. Gently clean skin around G-tube with Q-tips moistened with mixture of half water and half peroxide.
2. After the skin is dry, put a clean 2 X 2 gauze square around the G-tube (Picture 7).
3. Tape the nipple down over the bandage (Picture 8).
4. <u>Be sure to keep the skin clean and the bandage dry, or the skin may become red and irritated.</u>

If you see bleeding or drainage around the tube, call the clinic (phone: _____) or your doctor (phone: _____) for advice.

HELPING HAND
Homegoing Education
and Literature Program

Let's talk about...

Having an I.V.

You are going to have an intravenous (in-tra-VEE-nus) or "I.V.". Water with medicine in it will be put into your body through a tube.

WHEN THE I.V. IS PUT IN

First, the nurse or doctor will tie a rubber band around your arm or foot. This will make your veins easier to see.

After your arm is very still she will wash your skin with a cotton ball dipped in a cleaner.

Next, she will put a small needle into your vein. It will stick a little and will hurt at first, but if you hold still, it won't take very long.

Then the nurse or doctor will put tape over the needle and a soft board under your arm or foot. She will put pieces of tape around your arm and around the board to hold it in place.

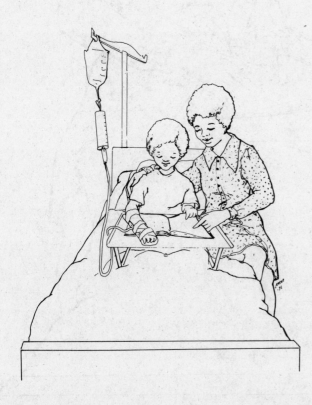

This needle is hooked up to a long plastic tube. The tube is connected to a plastic bag that hangs on a pole. This plastic tube carries the water from the bag into your arm or foot.

You will be able to sit up and do things with your other hand while you have an I.V.

WHEN THE I.V. IS TAKEN OUT

When you don't need the I.V. any more, the nurse will take off the tape and will take the needle away. Taking off the tape will feel like taking off a band-aid. Taking out the needle will feel like a little pinch.

There will be a tiny mark where the needle was. The nurse will put a band-aid over this to keep it clean. The mark will soon go away.

Your arm or foot will feel a little stiff. This will get better when you move it around.

If you have any questions, be sure to ask your nurse or doctor.

(Turn the page for a picture to color.)

(continued)

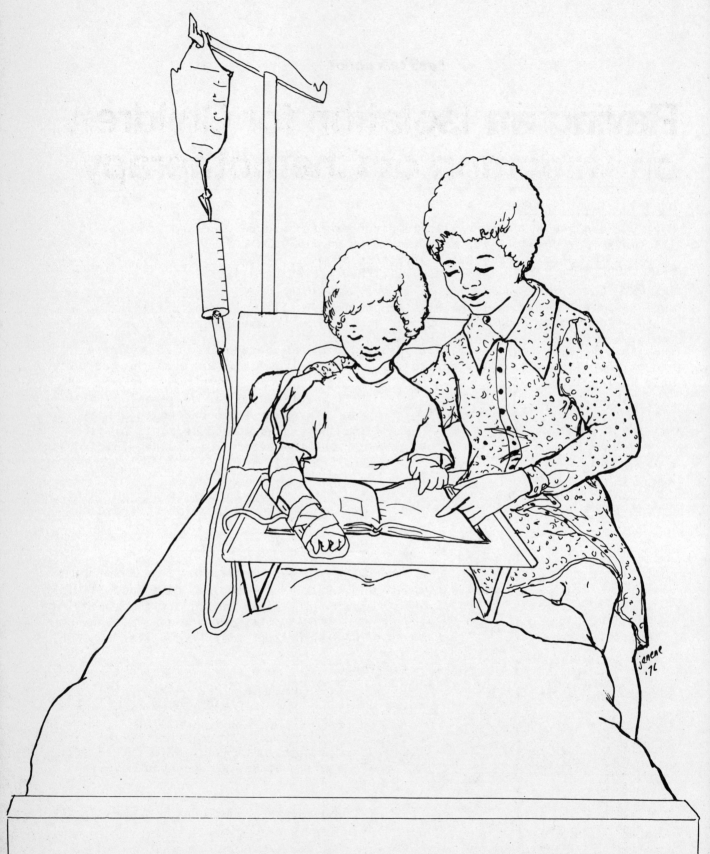

"I can still read a book or play while I have an I.V."

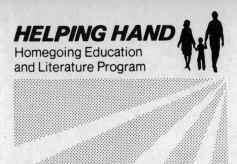

HELPING HAND
Homegoing Education
and Literature Program

Let's talk about...

Protective Isolation for Children on Radiation or Chemotherapy

Your child has been placed in a room by himself. The door has a "protective isolation" sign on it. This means that other people entering the room will need to carry out certain rules. These rules are made to protect your child as much as possible against infection.

Radiation therapy or chemotherapy lowers your child's natural immunity (resistance) against infection. While his resistance is low, his body cannot fight off germs and viral infections as well.

There are some things we can do to help protect against infection.

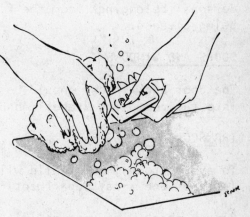

Picture 1 Handwashing is a must!

HANDWASHING

Parents, hospital workers, and visitors must wash their hands when entering the room (Picture 1).

USE OF MASKS AND GOWNS

- Hospital personnel will wear masks and clean gowns when caring for (touching) your child. They will wear only a mask if they do not have to touch the child.
- Parents do not need to wear masks and gowns. We assume you will not spread any "new germs" to your child that he has not already been exposed to at home.
- Your child should wear a mask whenever he leaves the room.

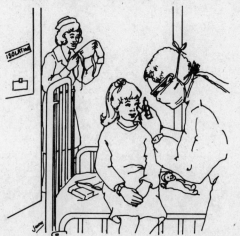

VISITORS

Please check with the nurse for visiting rules. Not more than two visitors should be in the room at one time. Visitors who have colds, flu, skin diseases, or sickness of any kind should not be in the same room with your child.

Picture 2 Masks help to protect you from germs.

(continued)

2 Protective Isolation for Children on Radiation or Chemotherapy

PLAY

While your child is in the room alone and in need of protection, play and being with people is still necessary.

Toys and craft items are available from the patient activities therapist. The child's favorite toy from home will help to give him comfort in a hospital room.

CLEANING

So Housekeeping personnel can thoroughly clean your room, please remove all personal belongings from the floor. If possible, step outside the room while it is being cleaned.

DOORS AND WINDOWS

The door and windows should be kept closed to prevent airborne bacteria from coming into the room. The drapes can be pulled back if your child wants to see outside.

TRANSPORTATION

To avoid crowds, your child will be transported to other areas of the hospital (such as the X-ray Department) at nonbusy times when possible.

Please check with your child's nurse before taking him for a walk or ride in the hall or to other areas of the hospital.

If you have any questions, be sure to ask your nurse or doctor.

HELPING HAND
Homegoing Education
and Literature Program

Let's talk about...

Postural Drainage

Child's Name: _____

Postural drainage is a way for you to help your child to get rid of extra mucus in his lungs. Too much mucus can block the air passages in the lungs. Giving postural drainage to your child at home helps to keep extra mucus from building up.

HOW DO THE LUNGS WORK?

We breathe in air (inhale) through our nose and mouth (see Picture 1). The air goes through the windpipe (trachea) and into the large airways of the lungs (bronchi). Then it goes into the small airways (bronchioles) and to the air sacs (alveoli).

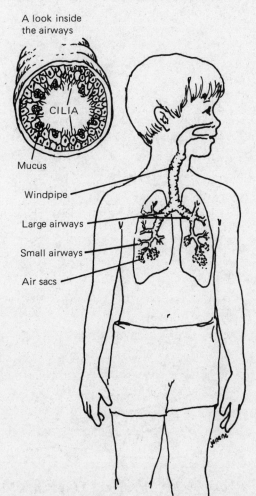

A look inside
the airways

CILIA

Mucus

Windpipe

Large airways

Small airways

Air sacs

Picture 1 This is the way the lungs look inside the body.

The air sacs in the lungs do important work. The oxygen, which we need to live, goes from the air sacs into the blood. The carbon dioxide goes from the blood into the air sacs and out into the air when we breathe out (exhale).

WHAT IS MUCUS?

All the parts of the lung have a protective mucous lining. The mucus that covers the lining catches tiny pieces of dirt, dust, and other particles from the air we breathe. These particles would irritate the lungs or cause infection if they stayed in the lungs.

HOW DOES THE MUCUS GET OUT OF THE LUNGS?

All the parts of the air passages are lined with tiny hairs called cilia. The cilia act like an escalator and carry the mucus and particles up to the windpipe to be coughed out or swallowed.

WHAT HAPPENS IF THERE IS TOO MUCH MUCUS?

Normally, there is just the right amount of mucus in the lungs. But when the lungs become irritated or infected, large amounts of thick mucus are made. This happens because the lungs are working extra hard to get rid of the infection or irritation.

(continued)

2 Postural Drainage

This extra mucus can block the air passages. If air passages are blocked, the air cannot move in and out of the air sacs. Then we do not get enough oxygen in our blood.

Extra mucus can also stop the cilia from working. If cilia do not work, we have to help the lungs get the mucus out. This is why postural drainage is done.

HOW IS POSTURAL DRAINAGE DONE?

Postural drainage helps to move the extra mucus into the windpipe where it can be coughed up more easily. There are 4 steps: positioning, clapping, vibrating, and coughing.

<u>1. Positioning</u>: The child should be positioned so the part of the lung to be drained is higher than any other part of the lung (see pictures on pages 4-5). Being in a comfortable position makes the treatment more effective and easier for both you and the child. You can use a pillow to give more comfort. Always have the child's knees and hips bent to help the child to relax and to make coughing easier. A small child can be placed on your lap for the "head down" position (see pictures). An older child can lie head down on a padded board.

If your child will need to have postural drainage over a long period of time, ask your nurse about a postural drainage table.

<u>2. Clapping</u>: To clap, cup your hands by bending them at the knuckles. Hold the thumb against the index finger. Keep fingers together to form a cup (Picture 2). Now clap your hands, first one and then the other, on the areas of the chest or back (as in pictures on pages 4-5). Do the clapping fairly fast. The rate of clapping should be comfortable - not so fast that the person clapping gets too tired. The clapping should be firm so the mucus in the lungs will be moved. A shirt or lightweight towel should be used over the area. During the clapping, the child should breathe normally.

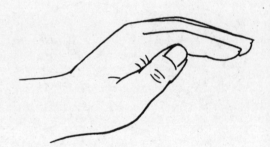

Picture 2 Hold hand like this to form a cup.

Explain to the child before you start that the clapping will make a noise like a galloping horse, or drums in a parade. Clapping, when done correctly, does not hurt. However, it is very important that your child does not think of it as punishment.

<u>3. Vibrating</u>: After the clapping, vibration is done over the same area of the lung. To do the vibration, stiffen your shoulder and arm so your whole shoulder, arm, and hand vibrates (like shivering) (Picture 3). The vibration should be done with gentle pressure on the area.

Have the child take a regular breath. Vibrate as the child exhales (breathes out) completely. Vibration should be repeated for five exhalations. If the child can, have him say "SSSS" when he breathes out.

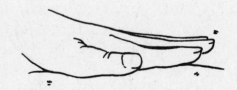

Picture 3 Hold hand like this to vibrate.

(continued)

4. Coughing: After the mucus has been loosened by clapping and vibrating, have the child cough and spit out as much mucus as possible. Coughing is started in the position you are using. The child may then sit up if necessary.

PUTTING IT ALL TOGETHER

1. Place the child in position #1 (see pictures on pages 4-5). Clap for 1 minute and vibrate five times.
2. Ask your child to cough. (Your child may not be able to cough up something after each position.)
3. Then, clap for another minute in this same position, vibrate five times again, and encourage coughing.
4. Now go on to the next positions and do the same thing (see pictures).

OTHER INFORMATION

- The chart is marked for your child. Give your child postural drainage at these times: _____.
- Plan to give this treatment before the child eats. (The positioning may cause vomiting or stomach discomfort if there is food in the stomach.)

If you have any questions, please call _____.

(continued)

POSTURAL DRAINAGE

STEP 1: UPPER LOBES — APICAL POSTERIOR SEGMENTS

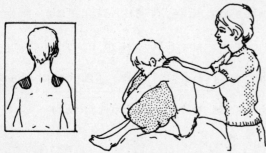

Sit and lean forward over pillow; clap on shoulders on both sides.

STEP 2a: UPPER LOBES — APICAL & ANTERIOR SEGMENTS, FOR SMALL CHILDREN UNDER 6 YEARS OLD

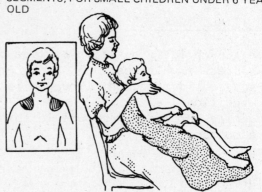

Sit and lean back against pillow; clap over the collar bone.

STEP 2b: UPPER LOBES — APICAL & ANTERIOR SEGMENTS FOR CHILDREN OVER 6 YEARS OLD & ADULTS

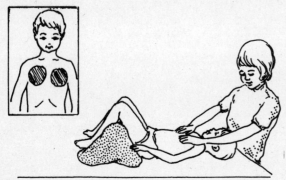

Lie flat on back with pillow under knees; clap just below the collar bone.

STEP 3: RIGHT UPPER LOBE — POSTERIOR SEGMENT

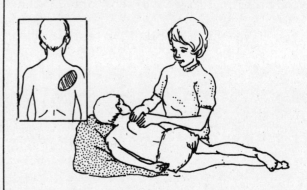

Lie on left side; place pillow in front from shoulders to hips and roll slightly forward; clap over the right shoulder blade.

STEP 4: LEFT UPPER LOBE — POSTERIOR SEGMENT

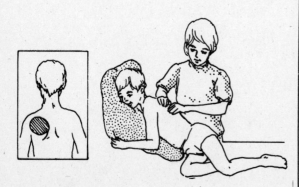

Lie on right side, chest elevated 45°, place pillow in front from shoulders to hips and roll slightly forward; clap over left shoulder blade.

STEP 5: LOWER LOBES — APICAL SEGMENTS

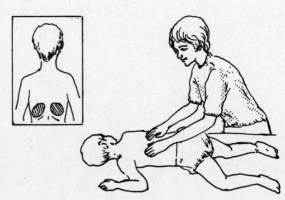

Lie flat on stomach; clap over lower ribs.

STEP 6: LEFT LOWER LOBE — LATERAL BASAL
SEGMENT, HEAD & CHEST DOWN 45°

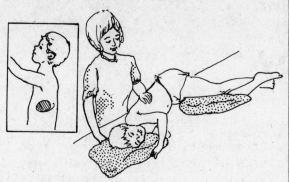

Lie on right side; knees bent; pillow under head and knees;
clap at lower ribs.

STEP 7: LEFT UPPER LOBE — LINGULAR SEGMENT

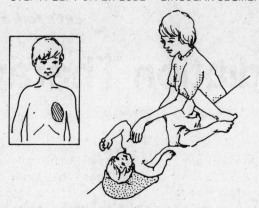

Lie on right side; clap over the left nipple.

STEP 8: LOWER LOBES — ANTERIOR BASAL
SEGMENTS — HEAD & CHEST DOWN 45°

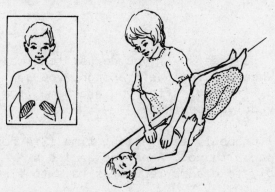

Lie on back; pillow under knees; clap over lower ribs.

STEP 9: RIGHT MIDDLE LOBE, HEAD & CHEST DOWN
45°

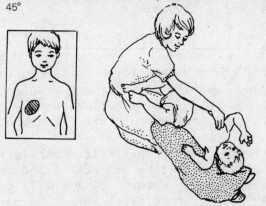

Lie on left side; place pillow behind child from shoulders to
hips and roll back on it. Clap over the right nipple.

STEP 10: RIGHT LOWER LOBE — LATERAL BASAL
SEGMENTS, HEAD & CHEST DOWN 45°

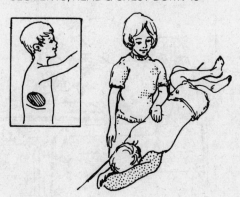

Lie on left side; knees bent; pillow under head and knees;
clap at lower ribs.

STEP 11: LOWER LOBES — POSTERIOR BASAL
SEGMENTS, HEAD & CHEST DOWN 45°

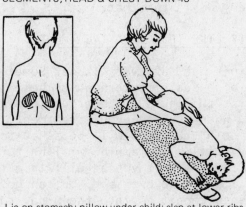

Lie on stomach; pillow under child; clap at lower ribs.

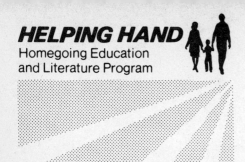

HELPING HAND
Homegoing Education
and Literature Program

Let's talk about...

Radiation Therapy

Radiation therapy is a special kind of x-ray treatment. It is different from regular x-rays because it does not take pictures of what is inside you. Instead it uses high-energy rays (like the sun's rays, except you cannot see them). These rays get rid of the cells in your body that are making you sick.

Your doctor has talked with a doctor who is trained to give x-ray treatments. He is called a radiologist. Together they have decided that you can be helped by these special x-ray treatments.

WHERE YOU WILL HAVE THESE TREATMENTS

You will go to University Hospital for your treatments. If you do not feel well at first, you might go there in an ambulance. When you feel well enough, you can ride there in a cab. A volunteer or nurse will go with you. After you are home from the hospital, your mother or father can probably drive you there.

Your first visit to University Hospital will probably take a long time (3-4 hours). Your parents will take your chart and go along with you. A person called a dosimetrist will measure you and will probably take some regular x-rays to find the exact spot where treatment is to be given. Little lines or marks will be put on this part of your body with ink. You should try not to wipe off these marks when you wash yourself, so the exact spot can be found every day after that.

WHAT IT IS LIKE TO HAVE A TREATMENT

The machines used are very large. Sometimes you will also see computers which help the radiologist to figure out how much radiation you need. When you have your treatment, you will lie on a table and will be asked to stay very still. The machine will be turned on, and it won't hurt you at all. In a few minutes, it will be over and you can go. Your parents cannot go into the x-ray room with you, but they can see you on a television outside the room (Picture 1).

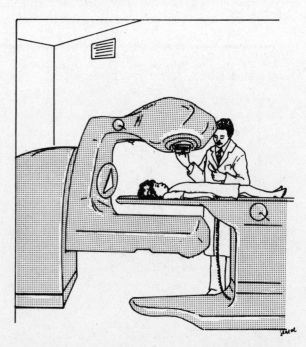

Picture 1 Having a treatment.

After the first day, you may have five treatments a week for several weeks.

(continued)

OTHER INFORMATION

- It is a good idea not to eat anything for a few hours before and after your treatment. This is because the radiation sometimes makes people sick to their stomach. Some people do not get sick at all.
- Everyone having radiation therapy should eat well-balanced, nutritious meals.
- You should check with the radiologist before taking any medicine or before using any ointments or mouth washes.
- Keep the area being treated away from heating pads, sunlamps, direct sunlight, or very cold temperatures.
- You will probably have blood counts (finger sticks) at Children's Hospital to see if you are getting the right amount of radiation. If your blood count is low, your doctor might have you wait a day or so before having another treatment, and you will be put on isolation to protect you from other people's germs. If you are staying in the hospital, hospital workers will wear masks over their faces and gowns over their clothes when they take care of you.

If you have any questions, please talk with your nurse or doctor, or call _____.

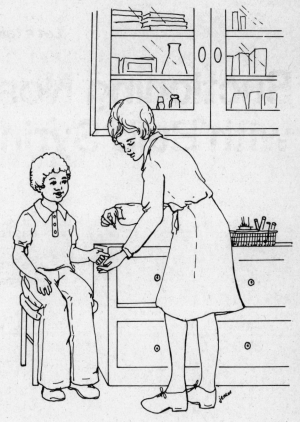

Picture 2 Having a blood count.

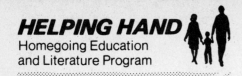

Let's talk about...

Suctioning Nose with Bulb Syringe

Suctioning mucus out of your baby's nose makes it easier for him to breathe and to eat.

Before suctioning, you should thin the mucus with normal saline (salt water) nose drops.

YOU WILL NEED

1 cup warm water   Small blanket roll
Kitchen measuring spoon   Nose droppers
Salt   Tissues
Clean jar with cover   Bulb syringe

TO MAKE THE SALINE NOSE DROPS

1. Fill 1 cup with warm (not hot) tap water.
2. Add 1/2 level teaspoon of salt.
3. Stir to dissolve the salt.
4. Keep this salt water in a clean, covered jar.

HOW TO PUT NOSE DROPS INTO CHILD'S NOSE

1. Roll up a small blanket and place under baby's shoulders (Picture 1).
2. Using nose dropper, drop _____ drops of saline into each nostril.
3. Hold your baby in this position for about 2 minutes. This will give the saline enough time to thin the secretions. Then suction.

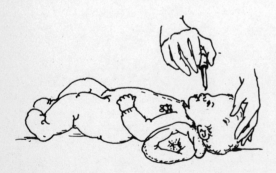

Picture 1 Put saline nose drops in baby's nose.

(continued)

TO SUCTION (See Picture 2)

1. Suction your baby's nose <u>before</u> feeding. (If you suction it after the baby has been fed, the saline and suctioning may cause vomiting.)
2. Squeeze the air out of the bulb (Step 1).
3. Gently place the tip of the bulb into a nostril (Step 2).
4. Let the air come back into the bulb. The suction will pull the mucus out of the nose and into the bulb (Step 3).
5. Squeeze mucus out of bulb onto a tissue.
6. Suction the other nostril the same way.
7. Gently wipe off the mucus around the nose with tissues to prevent skin irritation.

AFTER SUCTIONING

Wash the cup, dropper, and bulb syringe in cool soapy water. Squeeze the bulb several times to clean out the mucus. Rinse with clear water.

If you have any questions, please call _____.

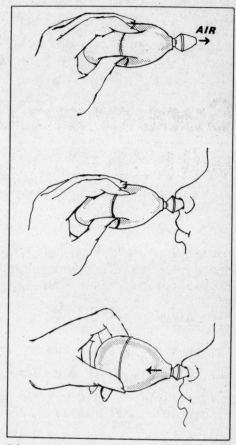

Picture 2 How to suction baby's nose.

HELPING HAND
Homegoing Education
and Literature Program

Let's talk about...

Care of a Sutured Wound

Your child has a wound that needed sutures (stitches). The care of the wound depends on the size and location of the injury and on the type of stitches used. Please follow these directions in caring for the wound at home.

MEDICATIONS

Your child was given the following medications:

☐ DPT, ☐ DT, ☐ tetanus immune globulin

A prescription was given for medicine to take at home: _____.
Please tell your family doctor that these medications have been given.

BANDAGES

☐ No bandage used.
☐ Keep bandage on until doctor removes it.
☐ Keep bandage on for 24 hours, then remove
   it.
☐ Change bandage every _____ hours.

CLEANING THE WOUND

☐ Do not disturb or clean the wound.
☐ Starting 24 hours after injury, clean
   wound gently with Q-tips using a hydrogen
   peroxide solution (half water and half
   hydrogen peroxide). Do this twice a day.
   This will remove crusts, reduce scarring,
   and make removal of stitches easier.

SUTURES (STITCHES)

☐ The stitches will not need to be removed. They will come out themselves. This may
   take several weeks.
☐ The stitches should be removed in _____ days. You have an appointment in the
   Surgery Clinic on (date): _____ at (time): _____.
☐ Call your family doctor for an appointment to remove the stitches.

(continued)

WATCH FOR THESE SIGNS OF INFECTION

- Increasing redness around wound
- Increasing pain
- Increasing tenderness
- Discharge or drainage from wound
- Increased swelling
- Foul odor from wound
- Fever

OTHER INFORMATION

- To change wet or dirty bandages, moisten old bandage with cold water and remove gently.
- Sometimes when you clean a wound you may loosen the knot on the stitches. If one or two become untied, don't worry, but proceed gently. If the wound opens, see your doctor as soon as possible.

If you have any questions, please call your family doctor (phone: _____), the Surgery Clinic (phone:_____), or the Emergency Room (phone:_____).

HELPING HAND
Homegoing Education
and Literature Program

Let's talk about...

Taking a Temperature

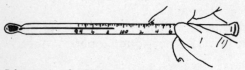

Picture 1 This temperature
reading is 98.6°, which is the
normal reading.

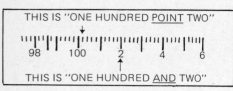

THIS IS "ONE HUNDRED POINT TWO"

98   100   2   4   6

THIS IS "ONE HUNDRED AND TWO"

Picture 2 To read a thermometer: The space between the
short marks is 0.2° (two
tenths of a degree). The space
between the large marks is 1°
(one degree).

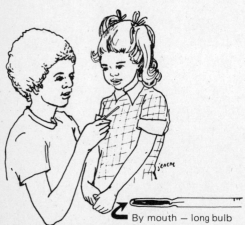

By mouth — long bulb

Picture 3

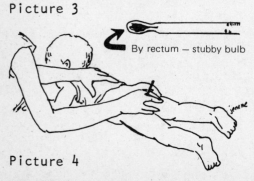

By rectum — stubby bulb

Picture 4

READING A THERMOMETER

1. Check to make sure the bulb of the thermometer
   is not broken or cracked.
2. Hold the thermometer at eye level. Turn it
   until you see the scale markings on the top
   and the numbers on the bottom (Picture 1).
   Bring it down slightly below eye level and
   turn it slowly. You will see a shining band.
3. Read the number at the end of the band. This
   is the temperature (Picture 2).
4. If the mercury is above 94°, shake it down by
   grasping the thermometer firmly and snapping
   the wrist sharply. Read the thermometer.
5. General rule for age: If the child is newborn
   to 6 years, take temperature by rectum. If he
   is 6 years and over, take the temperature by
   mouth if child is cooperative.

TO TAKE AN ORAL TEMPERATURE (BY MOUTH)

1. Use a thermometer with a long bulb (Picture 3).
2. Place thermometer under the child's tongue.
   Tell child to keep lips firmly closed but not
   to bite it.
3. Leave thermometer in place for 3 minutes. Read
   it.

TO TAKE A RECTAL TEMPERATURE (BY RECTUM)

1. Use a thermometer with stubby bulb (Picture 4).
2. Place infant on stomach. Put vaseline on bulb
   of thermometer (Picture 4).
3. Put thermometer 1 inch into rectum. Hold in
   place for 3 minutes. Remove it and read it.

CARE OF THE THERMOMETER

To clean a thermometer, draw it through a soapy
cotton ball or tissue. Rinse in cool water. Store
it in a safe place, out of the reach of children.

REMEMBER: You are placing a piece of glass into
your child's body. Never leave the child alone
while taking his temperature.

If you have any questions, please call _____.

(continued)

Read the Thermometer

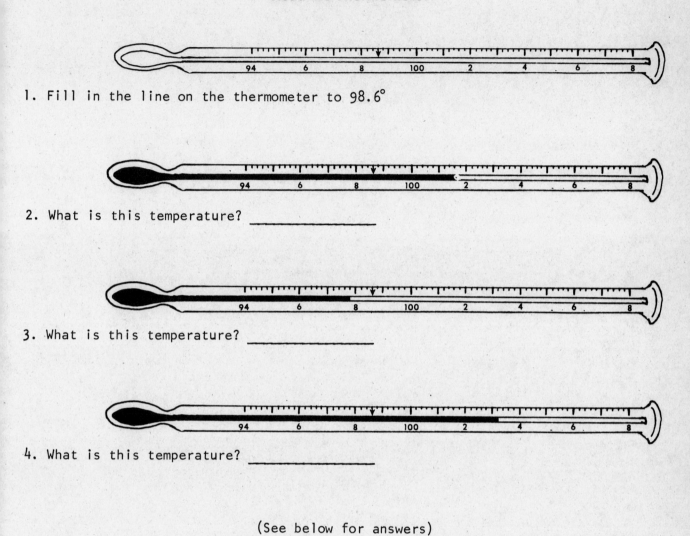

1. Fill in the line on the thermometer to 98.6°

2. What is this temperature? _____

3. What is this temperature? _____

4. What is this temperature? _____

(See below for answers)

----

1. This is ninety eight point six degrees.

2. 101.6° (one hundred and one point six degrees)
3. 97.8°   (ninety seven point eight degrees)
4. 103.2° (one hundred and three point two degrees)

HELPING HAND
Homegoing Education
and Literature Program

Let's talk about...

Care of a Child with a Tracheostomy

Child's Name: _____

CONTENTS

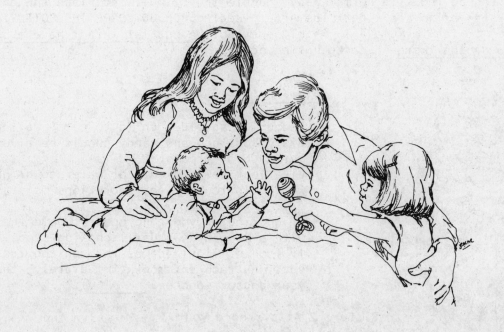

(continued)

2 Care of a Child with a Tracheostomy

DAILY CARE

Now that your child has a tracheostomy
("Trach"), he is a little different than
other children. But he is only different
in the way he breathes and "talks." He now
breathes air directly into his windpipe
rather than through his nose (Picture 1).
For a while he will not be able to talk
because the air he breathes does not go
through the vocal cords.

You may feel afraid when you first start
taking care of your child on your own. This
is normal. Keep in mind that you are
helping your child to breathe. Things will
become easier after you get used to doing
the suctioning and "trach" care. The
following information will help you.

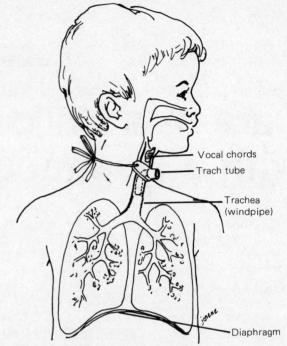

Picture 1 Air goes through the "trach"
and into the lungs.

PARENT-CHILD RELATIONSHIP

It is important to treat your child like a normal child. It is important not to
overprotect him, or to treat him as if he is sick. If you do, the child will
feel different than other children and may become overdemanding. This child is
"special" only in the way he breathes. Help others also to understand this.

FEEDING

Infants

Your baby can be fed as a normal baby. Bubble (burp) well and place the child in
an infant seat or on his right side after feeding. DO NOT PROP THE BOTTLE. Be
careful not to let formula drip into the trach. Do not let infant have a bottle
unless you can be there in case choking occurs.

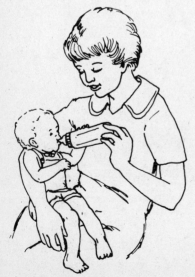

Older Child

- Encourage an older child to eat a well-balanced
  diet. Soda pop and candy should be given only
  for special treats.
- Give your child plenty of water to drink. This
  will help to keep the secretions moist, not
  dry.
- If choking or vomiting occurs, hold the child
  with his head down until choking stops.
- If food or liquid comes through the trach,
  suction trach and mouth immediately, then call
  your doctor (phone: _____).

Picture 2 Always hold your
baby while feeding him.

(continued)

BATHING

You may bathe your child in a tub if you like, but do not allow water to get into the trach. Give the child time for playing in the water. NEVER LEAVE YOUR CHILD ALONE IN THE TUB.

CAUTION: Do not use powders or aerosol sprays in the same room with your child. Particles and fumes can get into the lungs through the trach. This will cause a "burning feeling" and breathing problems.

SKIN CARE AROUND THE TRACH

- Gently wash the skin around the trach using a Q-tip and half-strength hydrogen peroxide (half water and half hydrogen peroxide). Be careful not to let water get into the trach. Rinse skin well with plain water. Gently pat dry. Do this every day.
- If there is a rash, drainage, or unusual odor around the trach opening, call your doctor for advice.
- While holding the trach, check the ties to make sure the knot is secure. The ties may become dirty, but do not change or tighten them unless your doctor tells you to do so.

DENTAL HYGIENE

Infant

- Mouth care begins around 6 months of age, when the first teeth come in.

- Cleanse inside of baby's mouth with a clean gauze dipped in salt water (1/4 teaspoonful of salt to 1/2 cup of water) (see Picture 3). Do this at least twice a day.
- Do not let baby go to bed at night with a bottle. The milk or juice film on the teeth can cause cavities.

Older Child

- At 1 1/2 years, start brushing the child's teeth every day.

- Around 5 years of age or earlier, let him start brushing his own teeth. This will not always be done well. You will need to give him lots of help.
- By the time he is 6 or 8 years old, start teaching the use of dental floss. By the time he is 11 or 12 years old, he can do it well on his own.
- The first dental examination should be done at 3 years of age.

CLOTHING AND BEDDING

- You do not need to buy special clothing for your child.
- Turtle necks or clothing that cover the trach opening should not be worn.
- Necklaces, strings, fuzzy clothing, fuzzy blankets, and stuffed animals should be avoided. Tiny beads or fibers from these articles can get into the trach and make it hard for the child to breathe.

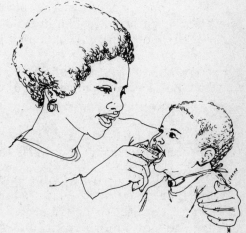

Picture 3 Keep inside of baby's mouth clean.

(continued)

4 Care of a Child with a Tracheostomy

PLAY

- Encourage normal play activity for the child's age.
- Remove any thin objects or small parts from play area. Your child might put these objects into the trach.
- Outdoor play is fun for the child too. You must cover the trach to prevent cold air and dust from entering the lungs (Picture 4). You may cover the trach with a disposable mask like those worn in surgery, or a trach mask lined with gauze that has been moistened with saline. A scarf tied loosely around the neck works well too.
- Children should avoid contact sports such as football or soccer.
- A child with a trach should NEVER go swimming until after the trach has been removed permanently.

COMMUNICATIONS

At first, your child will not be able to talk to you. This is because the air from the lungs does not pass through the vocal cords. It is important for his growing up that you talk to him, read stories, and name pictures. He will learn to "talk" fairly soon after the trach is in place.

Infant

- Encourage an infant to make sounds by placing your finger on the trach opening for a few seconds at a time.
- Tie a bell on the child's ankle so the infant can "call" for you when you're needed.

Older Child

- An older child will learn to place his first finger over the trach opening and talk. It will become automatic to place his finger on the opening to talk and to take it off to breathe. This may take a while to learn. Your child may also learn to cover the trach opening with his chin. The words will not be as clear, but it is easier for the child because both hands are free.
- Your child must have a way, other than talking, to "call" for you when you're needed. Some of the ways are:

Young Child - Tie bells to child's shoes; attach horn to tricycle (see Picture 4).

Older Child - Keep paper and pencil at child's bedside. If child is in another room and the trach becomes blocked, your child can throw a toy to get your attention. A bell or squeeze toy can also be given to the child.

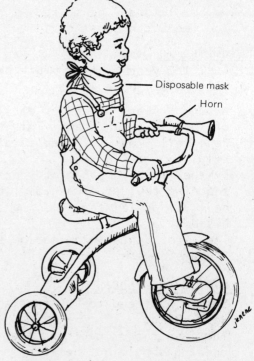

Disposable mask

Horn

Picture 4 Protect the child while he is playing outside.

(continued)

BABYSITTERS

A child with a trach needs to be watched closely 24 hours a day. Plans must be made so the parents can have proper rest. Therefore, it is best to teach another person how to care for the child. Your child will be less fearful if this is a person he knows and trusts and if this person knows his care very well.

WHEN TO CALL THE DOCTOR

- If food or liquid comes through the trach
- If there is a rash, drainage, or unusual odor around the trach opening
- If there are streaks of blood in the mucus

OTHER SAFETY TIPS

- Animals with fine hair should not be inside the home. Hair can float and get into the trach.
- Keep the home as free from lint and dust as you can.
- Do not use powders, chlorine bleach, ammonia or aerosol sprays in the same room with your child. Particles and fumes can get into the lung through the trach. This will cause a "burning feeling" and breathing problems.
- Always carry a hand aspirator, spare trach tube, and scissors with you when you are away from the home. Things may happen to the trach when you are shopping, riding in a car, or doing other normal activities.
- The child should not be around anyone who smokes cigarettes, cigars, etc. Smoke will irritate the child's lungs.

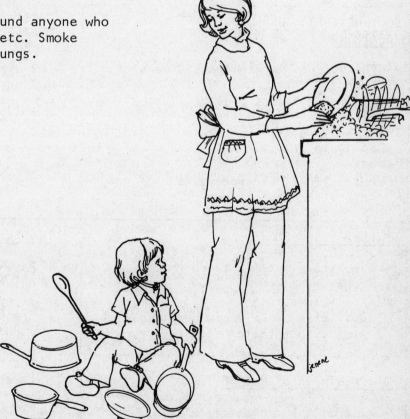

Picture 5 Talk to your child often.

(continued)

EQUIPMENT PREPARATION AND CARE

The following is a list of equipment you will need for the care of your child. The items marked with an asterisk (*) should be obtained from Children's Hospital.

Equipment Checklist

EQUIPMENT NEEDED FOR SUCTIONING AND MAKING SALINE

* ☐ Electric portable suction pump and instruction manual
* ☐ 2 5-ft. pieces of rubber tubing
* ☐ 2 Y-connectors
* ☐ 24 red rubber catheters, size ____
* ☐ Catheter marked with tape (for model only)
* ☐ 10-cc syringe
  ☐ 3 quart-size jars (large mouth) with lids
  ☐ 2 narrow mouth bottles
  ☐ Tongs
  ☐ Bottle brush
  ☐ 1 large pan with lid (for sterilizing equipment)
  ☐ 2 2-quart pan with lids

  ☐ Funnel
  ☐ Measuring cup
  ☐ Drinking glass
  ☐ Paper cups (5 oz. size)
  ☐ Measuring spoon
  ☐ Tray
  ☐ Clock or watch
  ☐ Drinking water
  ☐ Salt (table)
  ☐ Paper towels
  ☐ Facial tissues
  ☐ Baking soda (for suction pump jar)
  ☐ Permanent marker
  ☐ Tape (adhesive or masking)

EQUIPMENT FOR CONTINUOUS MIST TREATMENT

* ☐ Heavy duty air compressor machine
* ☐ Nebulizer jar
* ☐ Tubing - 2 sets plus drip bag
* ☐ Trach mask (with ties)
  ☐ Sterile distilled water
  ☐ A-33 Solution
    OR
  ☐ Mild liquid detergent and distilled white vinegar

FOR TRACH TUBE WITH INNER CANNULA

  ☐ 2 small jars with lids
  ☐ 1 bottle sterile saline
  ☐ 1 bottle hydrogen peroxide
  ☐ Sterile pipe cleaners
  ☐ Cellophane or adhesive tape

EMERGENCY EQUIPMENT

* ☐ One spare sterile tracheostomy tube: type _____ size _____
* ☐ Portable suction device: DeVilbiss or De-Lee mucus trap with catheter size _____

MISCELLANEOUS EQUIPMENT

  ☐ Paper masks for trach
  ☐ Scissors (for cutting trach ties if necessary)
  ☐ Flashlight and extra batteries (to use if electricity goes off)
  ☐ 2 ground adaptors (if home does not have grounded electrical receptacle)

EQUIPMENT FOR SKIN CARE

  ☐ 1 bottle hydrogen peroxide
  ☐ Q-tips

(continued)

How to Prepare Equipment for Use (Sterilizing)

All equipment used for trach suctioning must be very clean (sterilized) before it is used. The following information will guide you in preparing the equipment.

YOU WILL NEED

2 quart-size jars with lids   Bottle brush
1 narrow-mouth bottle   Large pan with lid
Tongs   Tray
Catheters   Paper towels
10-cc syringe

WHAT TO DO

1. Wash your hands.
2. Wash items in soapy water and rinse (Picture 6).
3. Using 10-cc syringe, force soapy water through catheters several times. Rinse with clear water in same way.
4. Place clean items in a large pan.
5. Cover items with water.
6. Bring water to a boil, then cover pan with lid.
7. Boil 10 minutes (start timing after boiling begins). (Note: Do not let the pan boil dry. If the catheters stick to the pan, they will be damaged.)
8. Remove pan from heat.
9. Let cool to room temperature.
10. Remove tongs from water, touching only the handles.
11. Using tongs, lift jars and empty the water.
12. Using tongs, place boiled catheters in the sterile jar (Picture 7).
13. Label jar with catheters "clean."
14. Place tongs inside a clean folded towel.
15. Label the other jar "used."
16. Label bottle "ready for use."
17. Place lids on jars.
18. Put jars, bottle, and wrapped tongs on clean tray covered with paper towel (Picture 8).

Always have sterile catheters available. When sterile catheter supply gets low, sterilize used catheters.

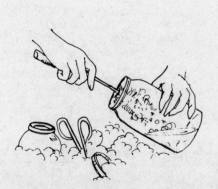

Picture 6 Wash equipment before sterilizing.

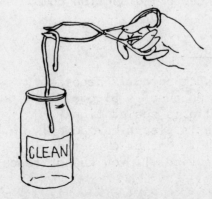

Picture 7 Carefully place catheters in jar.

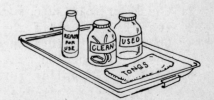

Picture 8 Put jars, bottle, and tongs on tray.

(continued)

How to Make Saline (Boiled Salt Water)

YOU WILL NEED

Drinking water
Table salt
Measuring cup
Measuring spoon
2 2-quart pans with lids
1 quart size jar and lid
Funnel

WHAT TO DO

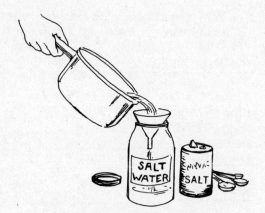

Picture 9 Pour sterile saltwater into jar.

1. Wash your hands.
2. Wash pans, spoon, funnel, jar, and lid in soapy water and rinse.
3. Fill pan with 1 quart (4 cups) plus 1/4 cup of water.
4. Add 2 level teaspoonfuls of salt to water.
5. Bring to a boil. Cover pan.
6. Boil gently for 10 minutes (start timing after boiling begins).
7. Place bottle, lid, and funnel in other pan. Cover with water.
8. Bring to boil. Cover pan, boil 10 minutes.
9. Let both pans cool to room temperature.
10. Remove jar from pan. Do not touch inside of jar.
11. Pour cool saline into jar using funnel.
12. Place lid on jar. Label jar "salt water."

Care of the Suction Equipment

TO CLEAN SUCTION JAR AND TUBING

1. Once a day, remove jar, tubing, and y-connector from the suction pump. Empty the jar. Wash them in soapy water and rinse.
2. Fill the jar with 1/4 cup of tap water and 1 teaspoonful of baking soda.
3. Replace the jar on the suction pump.
4. Check to make sure lid of suction pump is on tight.
5. Connect tubing and y-connector to suction pump.
6. Turn on pump to make sure it works.

IF SUCTION PUMP DOES NOT WORK

1. Use hand aspirator for suctioning if necessary.
2. Check to make sure suction pump is plugged in.
3. Test jar to see if the lid is sealed tight.
4. Check to make sure there is electrical power.
5. Check instruction manual for other directions.
6. Call your supplier for advice. If you cannot reach the supplier, call _____.

(continued)

How to Give Mist

To keep the mucus in the lungs thin and moist, give your child periods of continuous mist at home. This is done by placing the mist collar on the child during naptimes and at bedtime. You will know that he is receiving enough mist if the mucus remains thin. If the mucus gets thick, you should give the child more mist. Giving the moist air makes his breathing easier.

Try to keep bedtime and naptime as normal as possible. Continue to read stories, play music, or do whatever has been the normal routine.

YOU WILL NEED

Heavy duty air compressor machine
Nebulizer jar
Corrugated tubing (4 lengths of tubing with 2 bags)
2 trach masks
Sterile, distilled water - 1 gallon
Cleaning solution (either mild detergent and white vinegar or A-33)
2-gallon container with lid

WHAT TO DO

1. Fill nebulizer jar with sterile water to the line on the jar.
2. Attach the nebulizer jar to the air compressor.
3. Connect the trach mask ("mist collar") to the tubing with the bag in place (corrugated tubing to bag to corrugated tubing) and attach this to the nebulizer.
4. Turn on the machine and look for the cloud of mist from the trach mask.
5. Place the trach mask over the child's trach tube and fasten it with the ties.

TO CLEAN THE MIST EQUIPMENT

Once a day:
1. Empty the nebulizer jar.
2. Rinse the nebulizer jar, trach mask, tubing, and drip bag with tap water.
3. Clean all the pieces of equipment using either the detergent and vinegar solutions or A-33.
4. After cleaning, refill the nebulizer with sterile distilled water and put it back on the compressor. (To make sterile distilled water, boil distilled water for 10 minutes and let it cool to room temperature.)

If You Use Detergent and Vinegar Solutions

1. Wash nebulizer jar, trach mask, drip bag, and tubing in mild detergent and water. Rinse with tap water.
2. Soak all equipment for 10 minutes in white distilled vinegar solution (add one part vinegar to four parts distilled water).
3. Take equipment out of solution, shake it off, and air dry.
4. Throw used solution away.
5. You may soak equipment in 70% rubbing alcohol for 10 minutes instead of in vinegar solution.

(continued)

If You Use A-33 Solution

A-33 is a special solution that kills bacteria and mold spores which may harm the child with a tracheostomy.

1. Mix 2 ounces of A-33 concentrate with 1 gallon of tap water.
2. Store in covered container large enough to hold both the solution and equipment (about 2-gallon size). Make new A-33 solution once a week.
3. To clean mist equipment, soak nebulizer, trach mask, drip bag, and tubing for 10 minutes in A-33 solution. Rinse with tap water.
4. Take equipment out of solution, shake it off, and air dry.
5. The same solution can be used for 1 week.

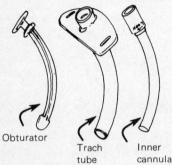

Obturator   Trach   Inner
              tube   cannula

Picture 10 Parts of a trach tube. (Obturator is used ONLY for putting the trach tube in.)

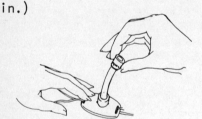

Picture 11 Removing the inner cannula

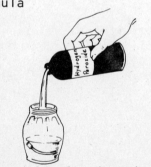

Picture 12 Cleaning the inner cannula

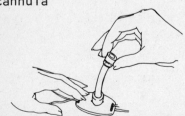

Picture 13 Putting inner cannula back into trach

How to Clean the Inner Cannula

If the trach tube has an inner cannula, it will need to be cleaned (Picture 10).

YOU WILL NEED

2 small jars with lids
Hydrogen peroxide
Sterile pipe cleaners
Bottle of sterile saline
Adhesive tape

WHAT TO DO

1. Wash your hands.
2. Unlock and remove inner cannula (Picture 11). (Leave the trach tube in place.)
3. Suction mucus out of trach tube.
4. Place inner cannula in jar.
5. Pour hydrogen peroxide over inner cannula (Picture 12).
6. Remove two sterile pipe cleaners from package.
7. Brush inner cannula with pipe cleaners and hydrogen peroxide.
8. Look through inner cannula to be sure all mucus has been removed.
9. Place inner cannula in the other jar. Pour sterile saline over inner cannula. Shake off extra saline.
10. Place inner cannula back into trach tube (Picture 13).
11. Lock inner cannula securely in place.
12. Fold over end of package that contains pipe cleaners. Seal with small piece of adhesive tape.
13. Throw away used hydrogen peroxide, saline, and used pipe cleaners.
14. Wash jars and lids with soapy water. Rinse. Boil 10 minutes in covered pan. Cool. Remove from pan. Put lids on jars and store until next use.

(continued)

OTHER INFORMATION
- Store bottle of hydrogen peroxide in cupboard away from light.
- Store hydrogen peroxide out of child's reach. Do not use it if it is not clear. Do not use it does not foam when cleaning cannula.
- Purchase a month's supply of pipe cleaners. Take these to the Central Sterile Supply Department of the hospital and have them sterilized.

SUCTIONING YOUR CHILD

The purpose of tracheostomy suctioning is to remove mucus from your child's trach and windpipe. You may feel afraid when you first start doing the suctioning. This is normal. Try to remember you are not hurting your child, you are helping him to breathe. Try to keep your mind on what you are doing, rather than on how he is acting. Each time it will become easier for you to do.

When to Suction

In the beginning, you will need to suction your child about every _____ hours around the clock. After that, suction as the child needs it.

Encourage the child to cough. This helps to get the excess mucus out of the lungs.

Later on, if your child is old enough, he will start learning to suction himself.

You can see, feel, and hear signs that your child needs to be suctioned (Picture 14).

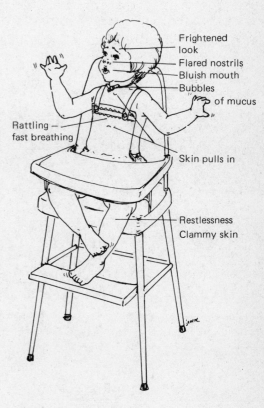

Picture 14 Signs that the child needs to be suctioned.

WHAT YOU WILL SEE
- Your child may become restless and cannot be calmed by cuddling or rocking.
- He may have trouble breathing. He may breathe faster.
- The hollow in his neck may "pull in."
- The skin below the breast bone may "pull in."
- He may have a "frightened look" on his face.
- An infant may have difficulty sucking.
- There may be bubbles of mucus at the trach opening.
- The color around his mouth may look pale, bluish, or dusky.
- His nostrils may flare out.
- If you see any of these signs, suction out the mucus.
- Sometimes you will see streaks of blood in the mucus. This happens even though you are careful. Call the doctor if it becomes worse.

WHAT YOU WILL FEEL AND HEAR
- Touch the child's chest and back with the flat of your hand. You may feel a "rattling."
- You may also hear the rattling in his chest.
- If you feel or hear any of these signs, suction out the mucus.

(continued)

How to Suction

YOU WILL NEED

Electric portable suction pump
Tubing
Y-connector
Jar of sterile catheters, labeled "clean"
Jar for used catheters, labeled "used"
Bottle labeled "ready for use"
Sterile tongs (wrapped in clean towel)

Paper cup of normal saline
8-oz. glass of clean water
Marked catheter
Tissues
Large safety pin
Clock or watch

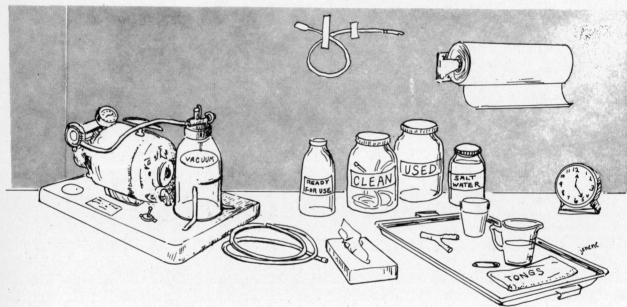

Picture 15 Assembling the suction equipment.

PREPARING EQUIPMENT FOR USE

1. Wash your hands.
2. Assemble equipment needed (Picture 15).
3. Attach tubing to suction machine bottle.
4. Secure tubing with safety pin to keep it from falling on floor.
5. Attach y-connector to tubing.
6. Using sterile tongs, pick sterile catheter out of "clean" jar.
7. Place tip of catheter into "ready for use" sterile bottle (Picture 16).
8. Attach open end of sterile catheter to y-connector.

(Note: Post pages 12 and 13 on your wall for quick reference.)

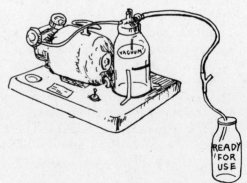

Picture 16 Have catheters ready for use at all times.

(continued)

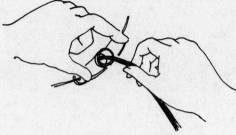

Picture 17 Hold trach tube when putting in catheter.

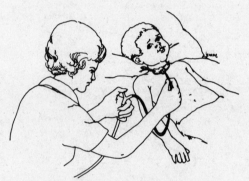

Picture 18 Put thumb over y-connector to make vacuum.

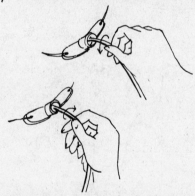

Picture 19 Twirl catheter between fingers as you suction.

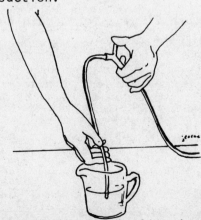

Picture 20 Draw saline into tubing to clean out mucus.

TO SUCTION

1. Wash your hands.
2. Pour small amount of saline into cup.
3. Remove catheter from "ready to use" bottle. Do not let the tip of the catheter touch anything but the trach.
4. Hold trach with your hand to keep it steady (Picture 17). Dip the tip of the catheter into the cup of sterile saline to moisten it.
5. Put sterile catheter into child's trach as far as shown on the marked catheter.
6. Remove your hand from the trach and place your thumb over the open end of the y-connector to make a vacuum (Picture 18).
7. Start pulling catheter out. Twirl catheter between thumb and index finger to keep catheter from sticking to the trachea (Picture 19).
8. Draw saline from cup through tubing to clean mucus out of catheter (Picture 20).
9. Repeat suctioning until your child breathes easily. <u>Do not leave catheter in longer than 7 seconds</u>. It will cause your child to feel as if he is suffocating.
10. Allow rest periods between suctioning. The length of time will depend on your child's strength.

AFTER SUCTIONING

1. Draw plain water through catheter and tubing to clean out mucus (Picture 20).
2. Turn off motor of suction pump.
3. Throw away used saline and paper cup.
4. Put used catheter into jar labeled "used."
5. Using sterile tongs, pick sterile catheter out of "clean" jar.
6. Place tip of sterile catheter in bottle labeled "ready for use" (Picture 16).
7. Attach open end of sterile catheter to y-connector.
8. <u>Every 24 hours sterilize "ready for use" bottle</u>. Have another sterile bottle ready to use.

(continued)

14 Care of a Child with a Tracheostomy

CHILDHOOD ILLNESS

As with any child, your child may become ill. It is important that you be aware of the signs of illness or infection.

<u>WHEN TO CALL THE DOCTOR</u>

If you notice any of the signs of illness, infection, or breathing problems in your child, call your doctor (phone: _____).

<u>Signs of Illness or Infection</u>

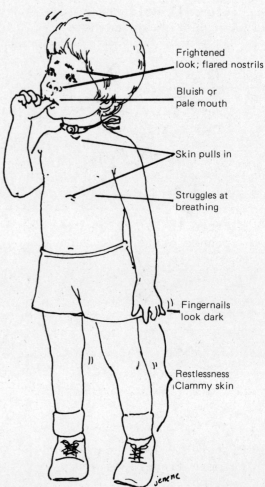

- If child has fever (rectal temperature above 101°F or whatever your doctor advises)
- If child is coughing up yellow or green mucus
- If child coughs up pure blood in the mucus
- If the mucus changes from a "bad" odor to a foul odor
- If pulse rate is over _____ and has not decreased in half an hour

<u>Signs of Breathing Problems</u>

- If breathing becomes different than is usual for the child
- If your child works or struggles at breathing even when sitting quietly
- If your child becomes pale and sweaty
- If the skin below the ribs pulls in
- If the skin below the sternum (breast bone) pulls in
- If the skin around the trach tube pulls in
- If the lips turn darker or duskier or if the fingernails look dark

Call the Emergency Squad (Phone: _____) if these signs occur and <u>are not relieved by suctioning.</u>

Picture 21 Signs of breathing problems.

(continued)

HOW TO COUNT RESPIRATIONS (BREATHS PER MINUTE)

1. Count respirations while child is as quiet as possible.
2. Count one respiration each time the child breathes in.
3. Lay your hand gently on child's chest.
4. Begin counting respirations when the second hand of your watch is at 12. Count for 1 full minute.
5. Write down number of respirations so you will have this information for the doctor.

HOW TO COUNT A CHILD'S PULSE (HEART BEAT)

1. Count the pulse (heart beats) while child is as quiet as possible.
2. Lay your finger tips against the pulse area on the neck just below the angle of the jaw (Picture 22).
3. Press lightly.
4. When you feel the pulse, begin counting beats.
5. Count for 1 full minute. (If the pulse is regular, you may take it for 30 seconds and multiply by 2.)
6. Write down the pulse rate.

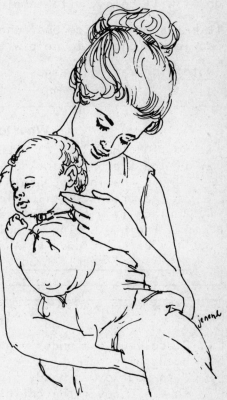

Picture 22 Counting the child's pulse.

IMMUNIZATIONS

Make sure your child's immunizations are kept up to date. The following chart will be helpful to you.

Average ages when healthy infants and children should receive immunizations:

AGE*	TYPE OF IMMUNIZATION GIVEN
2 months	DPT and polio
4 months	DPT and polio
6 months	DPT and polio
15 months	Measles, rubella, mumps
18 months	DPT and polio booster
4-5 years	DPT and polio booster
14-16 years	DT (adult) booster and then every 10 years
Adult	Tuberculin skin test

*The ages when immunizations are given may vary with each doctor.

(continued)

EMERGENCY CARE

If an emergency happens, you must be ready to act. Knowing <u>what</u> to do and <u>how</u> to do it will help you to remain calm and to be prepared.

It helps to practice emergency care on a doll with a "trach opening." You and other people you choose to help with your child's care should practice these procedures.

(<u>Note</u>: You can post pages 16 and 17 on a wall for quick reference.)

What to Do if Your Child Stops Breathing

1. SUCTION THE TRACH AT ONCE.
2. If the trach is blocked with mucus and you cannot suction the mucus out, remove the inner cannula and suction again.
3. If the trach is still blocked, cut the ties and pull the trach tube out.
4. Replace it with the extra trach tube.
5. Tie the new strings snugly and securely.
6. If your child does not breathe when the trach tube is clear of mucus, give <u>artificial respiration</u>.

How to Give Artificial Respiration

1. Place your arm under your child's neck so his head falls back.
2. With your other hand, pinch the child's nose shut and cover the child's mouth (Picture 23).
3. Seal your lips around the trach opening. Blow just hard enough to make the child's chest rise.
4. Remove your mouth and allow the chest to fall.
5. Breathe into your child's trach _____ times per minute.

If stomach contents come up into your child's mouth, wipe out all the contents you can, then suction mouth and trach at once.

If necessary, have someone call the emergency or rescue squad. DO NOT LEAVE THE CHILD ALONE.

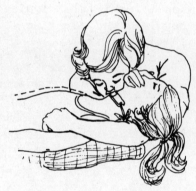

Picture 23 Giving artificial respiration

```
IMPORTANT PHONE NUMBERS

Emergency Squad: _____
Information for the squad (your address):
_____
Doctor(s): _____
_____
Emergency Room: _____
E.N.T. Clinic: _____
Nursing Unit: _____
Suction Pump Supplier: _____
Local Drug Store: _____
Community Health Nurse: _____
Other: _____
```

Complete this list of phone numbers, copy it, and tape it up by your phone(s).

(continued)

What to Do if the Trach Tube Comes Out

Before you leave the hospital, you will be taught how to put the trach tube back in if it comes out. Your best safeguard is to review mentally what you will do and to practice what you have been taught.

Always carry a spare trach tube and scissors with you when you are away from the home. Emergencies can happen when you are shopping, riding in a car, or doing other normal activities.

IF TRACH TUBE COMES OUT COMPLETELY

1. Get the spare trach tube and remove the inner cannula.
2. Put ties onto the trach tube.
3. Put the obturator into the trach tube (Picture 24). The obturator will guide the trach tube in. (The end is rounded to protect the inside of the windpipe.)
4. Hold the trach tube so that it curves downward (Picture 25).
5. Gently ease the trach tube and obturator into the opening in the child's neck. Do not force it.
6. If the trach tube does not go in easily, pull back 1/4 inch. Try to ease it in by turning it slightly from side to side.
7. When the trach tube is in place, remove the obturator immediately (Picture 26).
8. Tie the ties securely.
9. Observe your child closely for any breathing problems.
10. Suction as needed.
11. Replace and lock inner cannula.

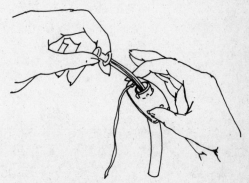

Picture 24 Put the obturator into the trach tube.

IF YOU ARE UNABLE TO GET THE TRACH TUBE BACK IN

1. Stay with the child and have someone call the emergency squad.
2. Be calm. Remember, the trach opening will not close up suddenly.
3. If child is not breathing, give artificial respiration (mouth to trach opening).

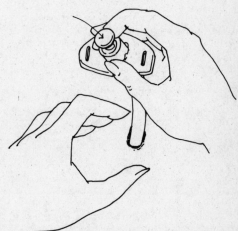

Picture 25 Gently ease the trach tube into the opening in the child's neck.

IF TRACH TUBE COMES OUT 1 INCH OR LESS

1. Gently slide the same trach tube back in.
2. Make sure the ties are tied securely.
3. Suction as needed.
4. Try to find out why it came out so you can prevent it from happening again.

WHEN TO CALL THE DOCTOR

Your doctor will want to know if your child stopped breathing or if his trach tube came out. Be sure to call the doctor after the child is breathing well on his own.

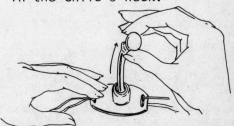

Picture 26 Remove obturator immediately after trach tube is in place.

Let's talk about...

Your Child's Urinary Diversion

Your child has had an operation that has changed the way he urinates (passes water). He now has a small stoma or ostomy (opening) on his tummy where the urine comes out. The medical term for your child's ostomy is _____.
This change may be for a short length of time, for several months, or for years. Your child will wear a small appliance over the stoma to collect the urine so he can do the things other children do. The appliances for the stoma are small and cannot be seen under normal clothing. Only you, your child, and your doctors and nurses will know your child has an ostomy. Your child will be able to eat, to drink, bathe, and to play much the same as before the operation.

It is very important that you show your child that you love and accept him and his stoma. By your gentle touch and tender loving care, he will know that he is a very important part of the family. Your feelings and reactions will determine how your child feels and reacts to his new stoma. Let your actions and expressions reassure him that he is loved and wanted.

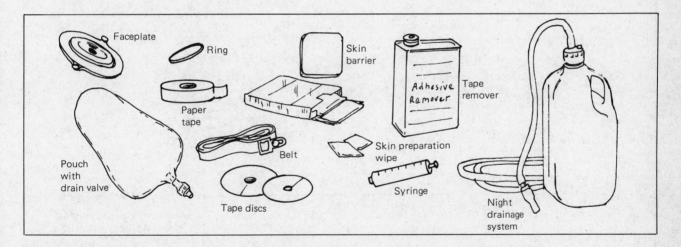

YOU WILL NEED

Faceplate
Pouch with drain valve
Ring
Tape disc
Cotton balls
Gauze pads
Belt
Paper tape
Wash cloth
Hand towel
Mild soap

Funnel or syringe
Measuring cup
White distilled vinegar 4%-5%
Scissors
Overnight drainage system
Tape remover
Liquid detergent

OPTIONAL

Skin preparation wipe
Skin barrier

(continued)

Putting the Appliance Together

1. Begin by washing your hands. Lay the faceplate on a flat surface with the round groove upward. (It might be helpful to tape the faceplate to a table top.)

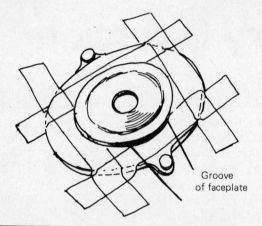

Groove of faceplate

2. Fit the pouch onto the groove of the faceplate. Begin at the bottom and work upward. The pouch will stretch a little bit to fit into the groove.

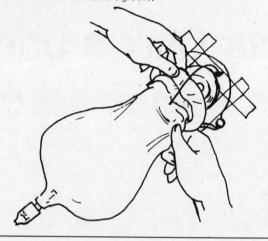

3. Next, put on the ring. Thread the pouch, drain end first, through the ring.

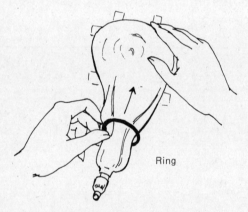

Ring

4. Slide the ring into the groove of the faceplate between the pouch and its cuff. You will have to stretch the ring a little to make it fit. This ring holds the pouch to the faceplate. It must be tight to insure a good seal.

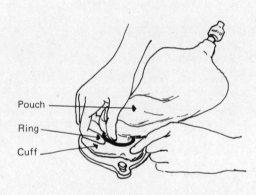

Pouch

Ring

Cuff

5. Now your reusable appliance is put together. It is helpful to have two complete appliances — one to wear and another ready to use.

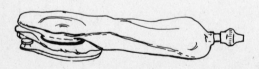

Faceplate + pouch + ring = appliance

6. Before applying the appliance, a tape disc must be put on. Lay the appliance on a flat surface with the faceplate up. Peel off the paper on one side of the tape disc.

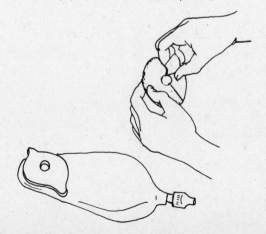

(continued)

7. Turn the sticky side toward the faceplate. Center the opening of the tape disc over the hole in the faceplate. Starting at the opening for the stoma, carefully press the tape disc to the faceplate.

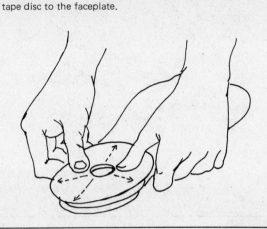

8. Remove the paper from the other side of the tape disc. Lay appliance aside.

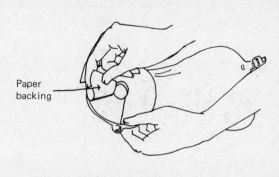

Paper backing

Applying the Appliance

1. Empty your child's pouch into the toilet or a container. Then, have your child lie down flat on his back.

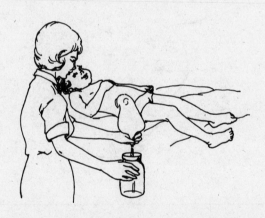

2. Unhook the belt from the faceplate.

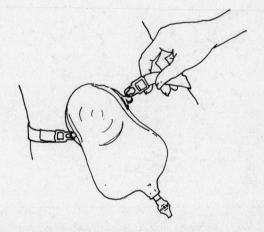

3. To remove the faceplate from your child's body, gently push the skin away from the upper edge of the tape disc. Pull off appliance. Lay it aside.

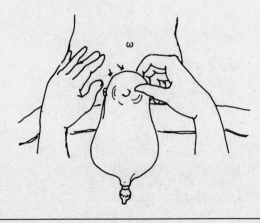

4. Clean the stoma and skin around it with a soft wash cloth and mild soapy water. Rinse well. Pat dry.

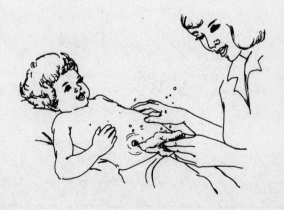

(continued)

5. If there is an extreme build-up of adhesive on your child's skin, remove it with a cotton ball soaked with tape remover. Wash the skin well with soap and water, rinse, and pat dry. Tape remover must be <u>completely washed and rinsed off</u> to prevent skin burn.

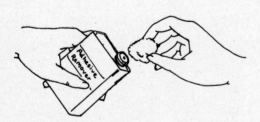

6. Hold a gauze pad or soft cloth on the stoma to keep draining urine off the skin. Skin must be completely dry if the tape disc is to stick well. If you are using a skin preparation, put it on now and allow it to dry.

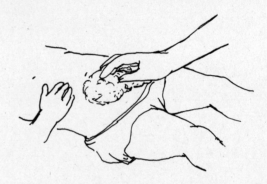

7. If you are using a skin barrier, cut a hole in the skin barrier that is the same size and shape as the stoma. Trim down the outer edge of the skin barrier so that it is the same size as, or slightly smaller than, the tape disc.

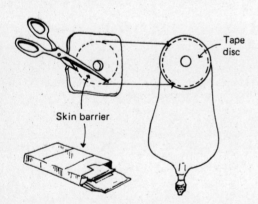

8. Apply the skin barrier to clean, dry skin by centering it over the stoma and applying gentle pressure. Put a gauze pad back on the stoma to collect drainage.

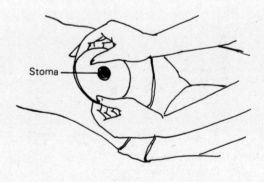

9. Center the opening of the appliance over the stoma and press in place. Be sure that the drain valve is at the bottom of the appliance or at an angle that is easy to drain. Belt tabs should be in a position to hook to the belt. Hold appliance in place for a few seconds.

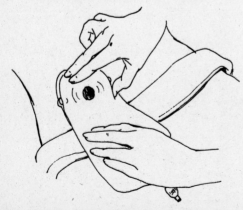

10. Put four pieces of paper tape on the edges of the appliance (avoid the belt tabs). The tape will look like a picture frame.

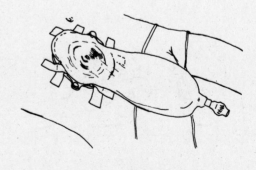

(continued)

11. Attach the belt to the belt tabs and adjust the belt to fit the child. It should not be tight.

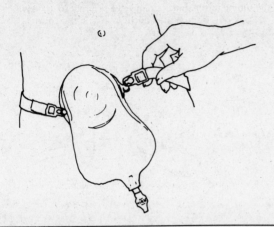

12. Brush any exposed tape disc with a cotton ball to keep tape from sticking to your child's clothing.

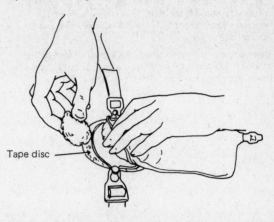

Tape disc

13. Check to make sure the drain valve at the bottom of the pouch is closed.

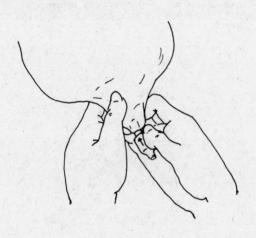

14. Now give TLC (Tender Loving Care) — you've both done a good job.

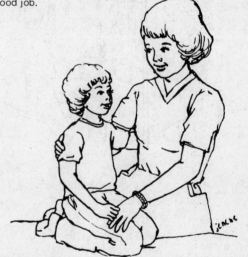

Bathing the Stoma

1. Every other day a solution of 1/3 cup white vinegar and 2/3 cup warm tap water should be put into the bottom of the pouch to prevent urine crystals from forming on the stoma.

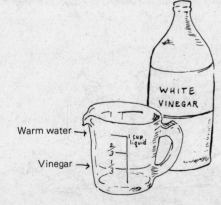

Warm water

Vinegar

WHITE VINEGAR

2. Make sure the drain valve is open before putting the vinegar solution in the pouch. You may use a funnel or syringe to add the solution. Have your child lie down for 20 minutes or so to allow time for the vinegar solution to bathe the stoma. After 20 minutes, empty the pouch and close the drain valve.

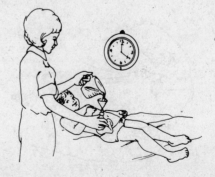

(continued)

Night Drainage

1. Special systems are available so that your child's pouch will empty at night by itself. This lets both of you get the rest and sleep you need. These drainage systems can be used all day as well.

   When using a drainage system, the tubing should be free of kinks. The drainage bottle and tubing should always be lower than the stoma so urine flows freely.

2. Use a system designed for your child's pouch. Connect the tubing to the pouch drain valve securely so urine will not leak out. Be sure the pouch drain is in the "open" position.

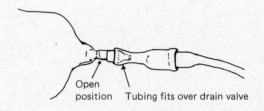

Open
position   Tubing fits over drain valve

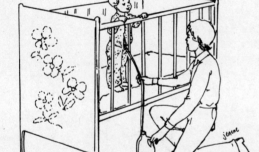

3. When you disconnect the night drainage system from the pouch, be sure to return the drain valve to the "closed" position.

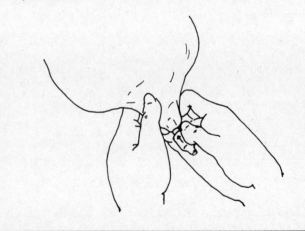

Cleaning The Equipment

1. Remove the soiled tape disc before cleaning the appliance.

2. To clean the drainage system, use a syringe and force soapy water or vinegar through the tubing. Rinse well. Wash and rinse bottle at least every other day. Wash and rinse soiled appliance each time it is changed.

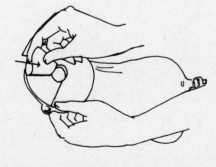

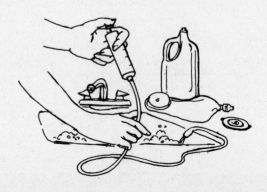

(continued)

SPECIAL TIPS

- Allow yourself enough time to put on the appliance. If you try to work too fast, you may not get a good seal, and the appliance will need to be changed more often.
- The best time to change the appliance is in the morning before your child begins to drink fluids.
- When pouch becomes half full, it should be emptied.
- Remove appliance every 3 or 4 days. If the appliance leaks, it should be changed right away to keep the urine from breaking down the skin around the stoma.
- One faceplate will last for several months.
- Pouches can be used for about 14 days. Pouches should be discarded after this time or sooner if they become stiff, crackly, or if they have an odor.
- Use normal clothing for your child. The appliances are small and can't be seen. Avoid very tight belts.
- Bathing will not harm your child's stoma. You may bathe your child with his appliance on or off. Use mild soap for bath time. Avoid bubble bath and bath oil in the bath water. These could harm the stoma.
- Your child should be able to romp and to play just like other children, but contact sports should be avoided.

DIET TIPS

- Have your child drink plenty of fluids such as water, weak tea, Kool-Aid, and cranberry juice to keep the urine as clear as possible.
- Your child should not eat asparagus. This causes a bad odor in the pouch.

WHEN TO CALL THE DOCTOR (Phone:_____)

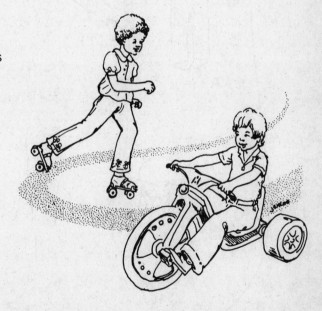

- If skin around stoma becomes red
- If urine becomes cloudy
- If there is more mucus than usual
- If odor suddenly is noticed in urine
- If there is far less urine than usual
- If child has pain in lower back (where kidneys are)
- If you notice a sudden change in the length or color of the stoma (Some bleeding of the stoma is expected, especially when the pouch is changed. A lot of red drainage in the pouch should be reported to your doctor.)

FOLLOW-UP APPOINTMENTS

- Faceplates are checked every few months after surgery by the doctor or ostomy nurse. Stoma sizes often change.
- When you return for check-ups with your child, bring supplies so the pouch can be changed.

If you have any questions, please call _____.

(continued)

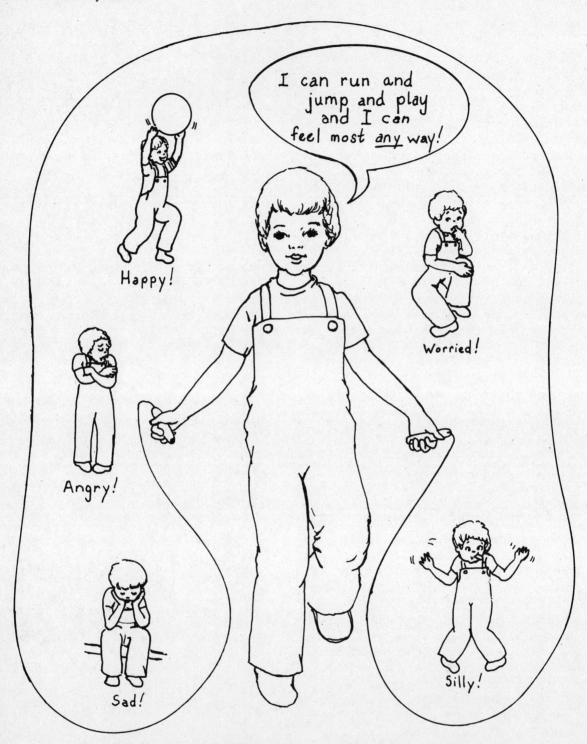

Your nurse will mark the spot where your child's stoma is. Your child may wish to color this picture to show you how he feels.

section 3
Diagnostic Tests

HELPING HAND
Homegoing Education
and Literature Program

Let's talk about...

Atropine Drops for Eye Exam

Your child will be having a special eye exam at his next visit. Please put atropine eye drops in both of the child's eyes each day <u>for 3 days just before the examination</u>.

```
Child's Name: _____
Appointment:
 Date: _____
 Time: _____
```

You will be given a prescription for the eye drops. Take it to the pharmacy to get it filled before leaving the hospital today, or get it filled in a drug store. The prescription may be filled anytime before the first day you are to use it.

If you know you will not be able to keep the appointment, do not start the drops.

To change the appointment, please call _____.

<u>WHAT TO DO</u>

1. Wash your hands. Read the label on the bottle.
2. Have the child sit with his head tilted back.
3. Gently pull the lower eyelid down and forward to make a little pocket (see Picture).
4. Carefully put 1 drop of Atropine in each eye. (Do not let dropper touch the eye or any other surface.)
5. Put 1 drop in each eye 3 times a day. (Suggested times: 8 A.M., 2 P.M., 8 P.M.)
6. Do this for the 3 days before the eye exam (date) _____
(date) _____ (date) _____.
Do not use the drops on the day of the exam (date) _____.

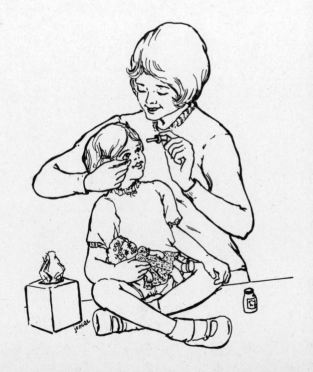

<u>WHAT TO EXPECT</u>

The pupils (dark part of the eye) will become larger after the eye drops are put in. Your child will not be able to read or to do close work because things will look blurred to him. The blurring will last a week or 2 and will not harm the eyes. Bright lights or sunlight may bother your child's eyes. The use of sunglasses will help when the child is in bright light.

(continued)

CAUTION

- Put the medicine away each time you use it. Store it out of the reach of children.
- Do not use the drops for any other purpose.
- Throw the unused medicine away by pouring it down the sink when the 3 days are over.
- If your child should need medical care for any reason, it is important to tell the doctor or nurse that he has been getting atropine drops.

SCHOOL

Your child may attend school. Tell the teacher that his vision will be blurred for 7 to 10 days. He may not be able to read or to do close work during this time.

If you have any questions, please call _____.

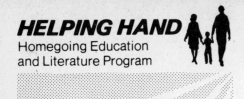

Let's talk about...

Having a Barium Enema

A barium enema is given so x-ray pictures can be taken of your child's bowel.

TO PREPARE FOR THE TEST

_____

_____

_____

_____

_____

_____

_____

_____

Child's Name: _____
Appointment:
  Date: _____
  Time: _____
Please bring your child to:
☐ Line 5 at Clinic Registration Desk
   (first floor)
☐ Emergency Room Desk

HOW THE TEST IS DONE

An enema of white solution will be given to your child. Some water will be put into his "bottom" through a tube. He will feel full for a little while.

He will lie on a table. X-ray pictures will be taken with a large camera that hangs from the ceiling. The pictures will show what his bowels look like. The camera will not touch or hurt him.

OTHER INFORMATION

_____

_____

_____

(continued)

AFTER THE TEST

- A normal diet may be given.
- A report will be sent to your doctor.

Call the Radiology Department (phone:_____) if you have any questions or cannot keep the appointment.

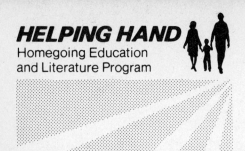

Let's talk about...

Having a Bone Marrow Test

Child's Name: _____
Appointment:
  Date: _____
  Time: _____

Bone marrow is found in many bones of your body. The cells in your blood are made in the bone marrow. A bone marrow test is done to see if the blood cells are being properly made.

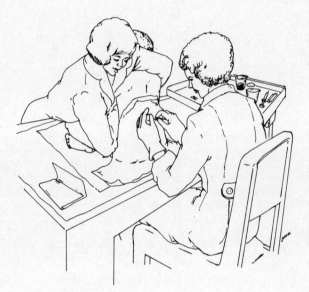

GETTING READY FOR THE TEST

You will be asked to sit or to lie on a table. A person will stand in front of you and hold you. This person will help you stay very still. Holding still will make the test get done faster.

Next, the person doing the test will choose a place usually on your hip or back to take out a drop of bone marrow. These areas are chosen because they are close to the skin. Touch your back and feel how close the bones are to the skin.

Next, this chosen spot is washed with a cotton ball soaked in iodine. The iodine is then washed off with alcohol. This may feel cold to you. After the skin is washed well, some towels will be put around the clean spot where the bone marrow test is going to be done.

THE TEST

A small amount of numbing medicine is put into the skin so the test will not hurt as much. This stings a little bit at first, but soon your skin will begin to feel numb.

After the skin is numb, a tiny drop of bone marrow is pulled up into the syringe. During this part of the test, you may feel pressure or pain for an instant. Then the test is over.

AFTER THE TEST

The bone marrow that has been taken out is put on slides and looked at under a microscope to see how your blood cells are made.

If you have questions, please ask your nurse or doctor.

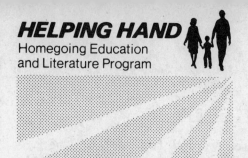

Let's talk about...

Cardiac Catheterization

A cardiac catheterization (CAR-dee-ack cath-e-ter-i-ZA-shun) means to pass a catheter (thin tube) through the blood vessels and into parts of the heart. A solution is then put into the tube, and it flows into the heart. This shows a picture of your heart on a screen like a TV screen. The doctor can look at these pictures and tell how your heart is made and how it is working.

> Child's Name: _____
> Appointment:
> Date: _____
> Time: _____

GETTING READY FOR YOUR TEST

Plans have been made for you to have a heart test. This will be done in the Cardiology (car-dee-ALL-o-gee) Department. On the morning of the test you will not have breakfast. After the test is over and you are fully awake, you will be given clear liquids to drink. Before you leave your room to go to Cardiology, you will be given some medicine by injection (shot). This will make you sleepy. You will then be put on a cart and pushed to Cardiology.

WHAT YOU WILL SEE

In Cardiology, you will be put on a long table. There will be a big camera over it. This hangs from the ceiling, but does not touch you. On the wall you will see monitors that look like TV sets. The workers that do the test will be dressed in blue clothes. Their hair will be covered with blue paper hats. Some will wear masks that cover their mouths and noses. This is to keep germs that might be on the worker away from you. When their masks are on, you will only see their eyes.

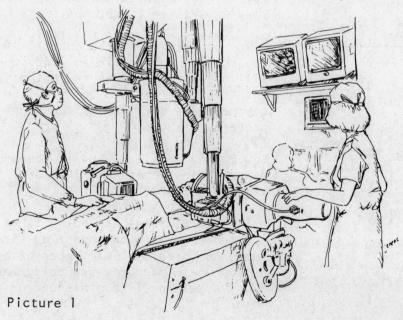

Picture 1

(continued)

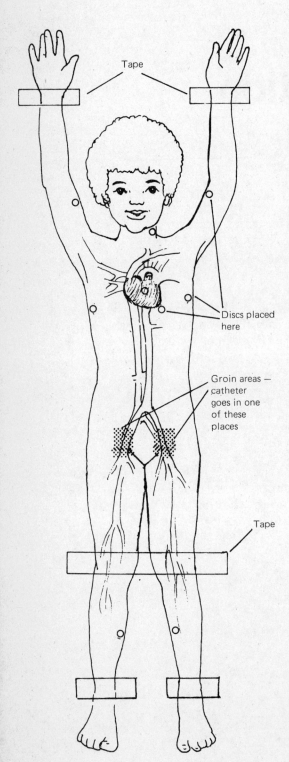

Tape

Discs placed here

Groin areas — catheter goes in one of these places

Tape

Picture 2 Preparing for the test

PREPARING YOUR BODY FOR THE TEST

You will feel very sleepy, and for part of the time you will go to sleep. Small drops of lotion will be put on your arms and legs. Small discs (circles of plastic or metal) will be put on your skin and held in place by bracelet-like straps. Wires from these discs lead into a machine. Adhesive tape will be put over your wrists and ankles. A piece of tape will be put across your knees. This is to keep you from moving around while you are asleep. The skin around both groin areas (where your legs join your body) will be cleaned with a brown solution. This will feel cool. This brown solution will be wiped off with cotton balls.

Your body will be covered with cotton towels except in the groin areas. The towels will be held in place with four clips. You will hear a soft clicking sound when they fasten the towels together with the clips.

You will be covered from the knees down with a cloth bed sheet.

Small pieces of gauze will be placed over your eyes. This will protect your eyes from bright lights when pictures are being taken.

HAVING THE TEST

A small amount of numbing solution will be injected into the skin of your groin. You will feel a little prick and burning feeling. This will last only 10 to 15 seconds.

Next, you will feel the doctor's fingers touching the skin on your groin to find your pulse and then a little pressure when the catheter (tube) is put in. This tube is used to carry the white solution to the heart so it makes the heart show up on the pictures.

You may fall asleep, but if you are awake and want to know something, just ask. Your questions will be answered.

While the pictures are being taken, you can feel the table you are on move from side to side and back and forth. You will hear cameras making motor noises while pictures are being taken. It will sound something like a blender or cake mixer motor.

(continued)

Medicine will be injected into your blood to make the pictures of your heart and blood vessels show up. This will make you feel warm all over for a little time.

When the picture-taking part of the test is over, you will have a little more to go.

Next, you will have a phonocardiogram (fo-no-CAR-dee-o-gram). This test records the sounds your heart makes.

Little microphones (mikes) will be placed in different places on your chest and groin area.

When your heart beats, the sounds will be written down on a piece of paper.

Next a vectocardiogram (vec-toe-CAR-dee-o-gram) will be done. This test takes Polaroid pictures of the electrical forces in the heart. Sticky discs will be placed on your chest, arms, legs, neck, and back. You will hear clicking sounds when the camera snaps the picture.

AFTER THE TEST

Everything will be taken off that was put on your body. A bandage will be put on your groin where the tube was put in. The bandage is put on to keep any blood from coming out of the place where the tube was put in.

You will still feel sleepy. You will be put on a cart and taken back to your room.

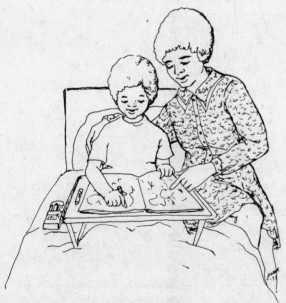

Picture 3 You must stay in bed for 24 hours after the test.

WHAT HAPPENS IN THE NEXT 24 HOURS

You _must_ stay in bed for 24 hours. This allows time for the place on your groin to start healing. You will use the bed pan or urinal in bed instead of walking to the bathroom. When you are fully awake, you will be given something to drink. A nurse will come in often to check your bandage and listen to your heart.

The cardiologist (heart doctor) will study all the pictures and what is written on the papers that evening or the next day to find out how your heart is working. Then the heart doctor will talk to your parents about the test before you go home.

While you are resting after the test, you may color the picture on the next page.

If you have any questions, be sure to ask your doctor or nurse.

(continued)

WHAT DO YOU SEE?

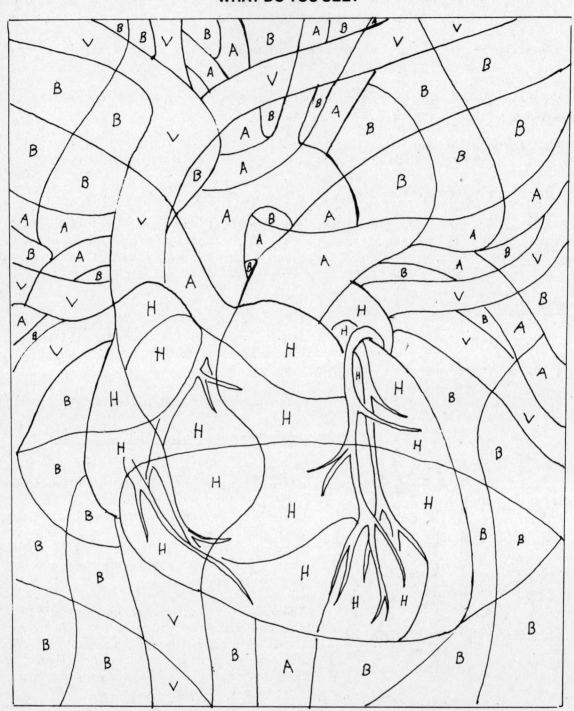

H is for Heart.   To see what your heart looks like, color the H spaces RED.

A is for Artery.   Arteries carry blood from your heart to your body. Color A's ORANGE.

V is for Vein.   Veins carry blood back to your heart. Color V spaces BLUE.

B is for Body.   Color B spaces YELLOW. See how your heart looks inside your body.

HELPING HAND
Homegoing Education
and Literature Program

Let's talk about...

Having a CT Scan

A CT Scan (Computed Tomography) is a type of x-ray that takes pictures of your child's brain or abdomen (tummy). It does not hurt or touch him. The only thing he has to do is lie very still while the pictures are being taken. On the day of the scan, do not give any food or water for 4 hours before the test.

```
Child's Name: _____
Appointment:
  Date: _____
  Time: _____
If your child is an Outpatient, please
bring child to:
☐ Line 5 Clinic Registration Desk
   (first floor)
☐ Emergency Room (first floor)
☐ Neurology Clinic (fourth floor)
```

HOW THE SCAN IS DONE

Your child may be given some medicine in the vein to make him sleepy. He will feel a little stick, but if he holds still it will last only a few seconds.

If your child is having a brain scan, any metal hair clips or wigs will be removed. If your child has thick, long hair, it will be covered with a cotton cap. Parents will be asked to wait in the waiting room.

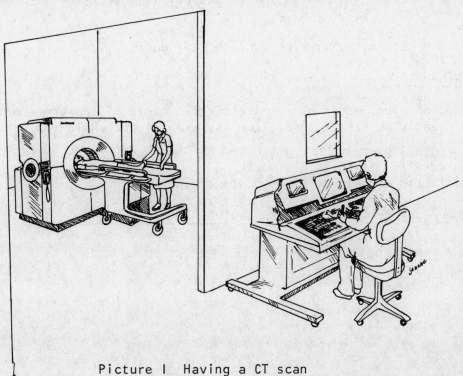

Picture 1 Having a CT scan

(continued)

2 Having a CT Scan

The child will be placed on a padded table. A strip of adhesive tape will put across his forehead and attached to the table on each side to help him hold his head still. If a scan of your child's abdomen is being taken, his arms may be strapped above his head so they are not in the picture.

Sometimes the technician will cover the child's eyes with a piece of gauze. A light strap will be put across his body and fastened to the table to keep him from moving.

The technician will move the table so that the child's head or abdomen is just inside the opening of the machine (Picture 1). Then the technician will go into another room to start the x-ray machine. The technician will stay in the other room to run the machine, but will always be able to see the child through the window and talk to the child through an intercom system.

The x-ray machine moves around the part of the body being scanned and makes a whirring sound. As it moves, x-ray beams are sent out. These beams are picked up by the x-ray detectors. They are measured and collected in the memory of the computer. The computer prepares a picture of the section of the body on a film.

The child must hold his head and body very still until the motor stops running. The technician will be watching the TV screen to see that the picture is being taken correctly.

Your child may ask the technician any questions he wants to know before and after the test.

AFTER THE TEST

Your child will be returned to you in the waiting room. He may be sleepy or groggy if medicine was given.

The report of the x-ray will be sent to your doctor.

OTHER INFORMATION

If the doctor gives medicine to make certain parts of the brain or abdomen show up clearly on the pictures, you may expect your child to:

· feel warm all over
· have a metallic taste in his mouth
· feel a little nauseated (sick to stomach)

If you have any questions, please call _____.

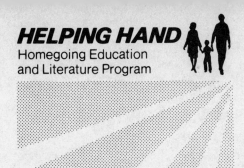

HELPING HAND
Homegoing Education
and Literature Program

Let's talk about...

Having a Cystogram

A cystogram (SIS-toe-gram) is an x-ray picture of the urinary bladder. By looking at the picture, the doctor can tell how big the bladder is and how it is working.

TO PREPARE THE CHILD FOR THIS TEST

1. Explain the test to your child.
2. Your child may eat and drink before the x-ray.

```
Child's Name: _____
Appointment:
  Date: _____
  Time: _____
Please bring your child to:
 ☐ Line 5 at Clinic Registration Desk
    (first floor)
 ☐ Emergency Room Desk
```

THE TEST

Your child will be asked to lie on the examination table. A soft rubber tube (catheter) will be placed into the child's bladder. This may hurt a little bit, but the child should try to relax. After the tube is in place, you will take your child to the X-ray Department.

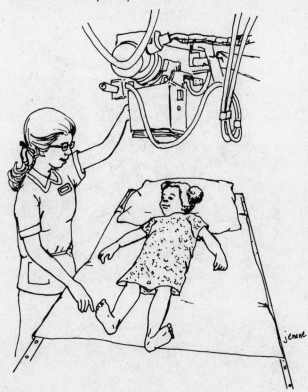

A dye will be placed into the bladder through the tube. This will not hurt the child. While the bladder is taking up the dye, x-ray pictures will be taken. When your child has a feeling of fullness and an urge to urinate (pass water), the catheter will be removed. X-rays will be taken as the child empties his bladder of urine.

AFTER THE TEST

• Your child may have burning on urination (passing water). This may last a few hours. Have the child drink more liquids.
• A report will be sent to your doctor.

If you need to change the appointment, or if you have any questions, please call
_____.

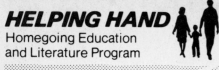
Let's talk about...

Having an E.C.G.

The electrocardiogram (ee-lek-tro-CAR-dee-o-gram) is a recording of your child's heart beats.

HOW THE TEST IS DONE

First, your child's shirt and shoes are taken off. Then he lies down quietly on a bed. He must not wiggle his fingers or toes. If he does, the test might not come out right.

Child's Name: _____
Appointment:
  Date: _____
  Time: _____
Please bring your child to:
☐ Line 5 at Clinic Registration
  Desk (first floor)
☐ Emergency Room Desk

The E.C.G. technician puts dots of lotion (like hand lotion) on six areas of the chest. The lotion is also put on small flat discs. These discs are placed on the child's arms and legs and are held in place by a soft strap. Each disc is connected to a wire that leads to the E.C.G. machine.

The technician turns on the machine. She touches the six chest areas with a soft rubber ball. When the ball touches the chest, it picks up electrical impulses of the heart.

Wires also carry impulses from the arms and legs to the machine. The machine writes these impulses on a piece of paper. The test takes about 5 minutes, if the child holds very still.

AFTER THE TEST

The doctor will read the graph or tracing from the machine. This report will be sent to your doctor or clinic.

If you need to change your appointment, or if you have any questions, please call the E.C.G. office (phone:_____).

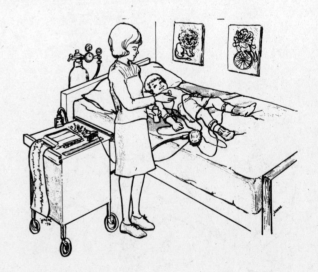

(Turn the page for a picture to color.)

(continued)

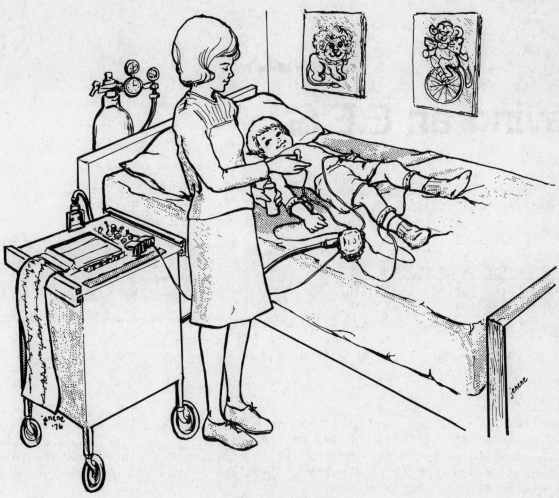

Having an E.C.G.

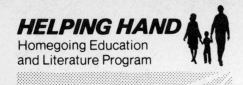

HELPING HAND
Homegoing Education
and Literature Program

316

Let's talk about...

Having an E.E.G.

The electroencephalogram (e-lek-tro-en-SEF-ah-lo-gram) or E.E.G. is a recording of the electrical activity of the brain. It records your child's brain waves. The E.E.G. is painless and safe.

Child's Name: _____

Appointment:

  Date: _____

  Time: _____

Please bring your child to:

☐ Line 5 at Clinic Registration Desk (first floor)

☐ Emergency Room Desk

TO PREPARE THE CHILD FOR THE TEST

1. Explain the test to the child.
2. Shampoo the child's hair well.
3. Comb and brush the hair neatly. If hair is long, put it into a ponytail or tie it back.
4. Do not use any hair spray or hair dressing.
5. Do not tease the hair.

THE TEST

Your child will be shown what will happen. Moist discs (called electrodes) are placed on areas of the child's head. Cotton balls hold the electrodes and wires in place. The child is asked to lie very still with his eyes closed and try to relax. The machine records the faint electrical impulses of the brain on the graph paper. This test takes about 45-50 minutes.

AFTER THE TEST

A doctor will read the graph (or tracing). His report will be sent to your doctor or clinic.

If you cannot keep the appointment, or if you have any questions, please call the E.E.G. laboratory (phone:_____).

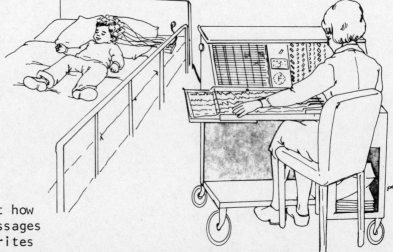

The discs pick up messages about how your brain is working. These messages are sent to the machine which writes them down.

HELPING HAND
Homegoing Education
and Literature Program

Let's talk about....

Having a Gallbladder Test

During a gallbladder test, an x-ray
picture is taken of the gallbladder.
The doctor can tell how big the
gallbladder is and how it is working by looking at the picture.

MEDICATION

You have been given a prescription for
medication. Take this to your drug store
and buy the medication before the test.
This medicine makes the gallbladder show
in the x-ray pictures.

```
Child's Name: _____
Appointment:
  Date: _____
  Time: 8:30 A.M.
Please bring your child to:
□ Line 5 at Clinic Registration
  Desk (first floor)
□ Emergency Room Desk
```

THE DAY BEFORE THE TEST

1. Give your child a light supper between 4:00 and 6:00 P.M., the evening before
   the x-ray. We suggest fruit, fruit juice, vegetables (canned without fat or
   butter), and bread with jelly only. <u>Give no milk.</u> Your child should <u>not</u> have
   fatty foods like potato chips, meat, or fried foods.
2. At 6:00 P.M., have your child take the tablets,
   one at a time, with water. If the child vomits
   the tablets, call your doctor.
3. Do not allow the child to chew gum, eat food,
   or smoke after the medicine has been taken.
   Your child may have small amounts of water
   until midnight. <u>After midnight, do not give
   your child food or water until after the test.</u>
4. Explain the test to your child.

THE TEST

Your child will lie down on an x-ray table. He
will be asked to lie very still. X-ray pictures
will be taken with a large x-ray camera. These
special cameras take pictures of how your body
looks inside. The x-ray pictures do not hurt.

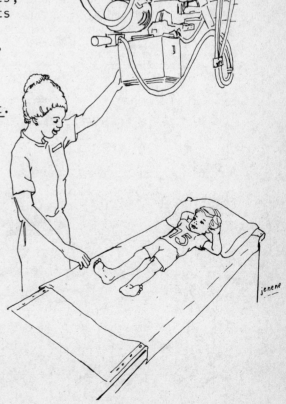

AFTER THE TEST

Your child will be ready to go home and may eat
a normal diet. Your doctor will be told the
results of the x-ray.

If you need to change the appointment or if you
have any questions, please call _____.

HELPING HAND
Homegoing Education
and Literature Program

318

Let's talk about...

Having a Glucose Tolerance Test

A glucose tolerance test (GTT) measures how much sugar there is in the blood. The blood tests show how the body uses this sugar.

<u>ON THE DAY BEFORE THE TEST</u>

Child's Name: _____
Appointment:
  Date: _____
  Time: _____
Please bring your child to:
☐ Line 5 at Clinic Registration
  Desk (first floor)
☐ Emergency Room Desk
(Be prepared to spend 3-4 hours at the hospital.)

• A baby under 6 months of age should be given the last bottle of formula at 2 A.M. the morning of the test day. Do not give anything by mouth after 2 A.M. except water.
• A child 6 months or older should be given a light meal the evening before the test day. This meal consists of fruit, orange juice, toast, crackers, or cookies. No other food or liquids should be given until the test is completed. Do not give anything by mouth after midnight, except water.
• The night before the test your child should get a good night's rest.
• If your child eats food by mistake after midnight, call the clinic lab (phone:_____) and make a new appointment.

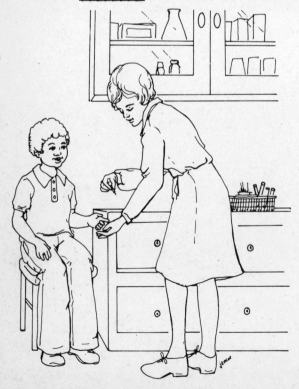

<u>THE TEST</u>

A technician will give your child sugar water to drink. Then he will prick the child's finger several times so the blood samples can be taken. This will be done at the end of 15, 30, and 45 minutes, and 1, 1 1/2, and 2, and 3 hours. If your child vomits (throws up) anytime before or during the test, please tell the nurse.

<u>AFTER THE TEST</u>

• The child will be hungry after the test, and his finger will be a little bit sore.
• An infant should be given a bottle.
• A child should be given a regular lunch.
• Later, your doctor will tell you the results of the test.

If you have to change the appointment or if you have any questions, please call _____.

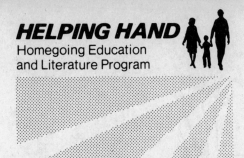

HELPING HAND
Homegoing Education
and Literature Program

Let's talk about...

Having an I.V.P.

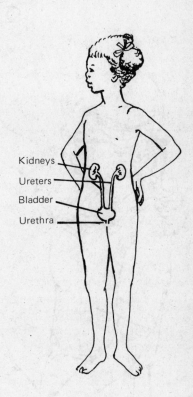

Kidneys
Ureters
Bladder
Urethra

```
Child's Name: _____
Appointment:
  Date: _____
  Time: _____
Please bring your child to:
  ☐ Line 5 at Clinic Registration Desk (first
    floor) at 7:30 A.M.
  ☐ Emergency Room Desk at 7:30 A.M.
```

The purpose of an intravenous pyelogram
(in-tra-VEE-nus PIE-el-o-gram) or I.V.P. is to
look at the size and function of the kidneys and
urinary tract by taking x-ray pictures.

TO PREPARE THE CHILD FOR THIS TEST

1. Do not give your child food or water after
   midnight the day before the x-ray examination.
   Infants may have a bottle at 2 A.M.
2. Explain the test to the child.

THE TEST

A clear dye will be injected into the child's vein through a needle. This is
usually done in the arm. The dye is taken up by the kidneys. This makes the kidneys
show up on the x-ray film.

AFTER THE TEST

• Your child will be ready to go home.
• A doctor will read the x-ray. His report will be sent to your doctor or clinic.

If you need to change the appointment or if you have any questions, please
call _____.

(Turn the page for a picture to color.)

(continued)

2 Having an I.V.P.

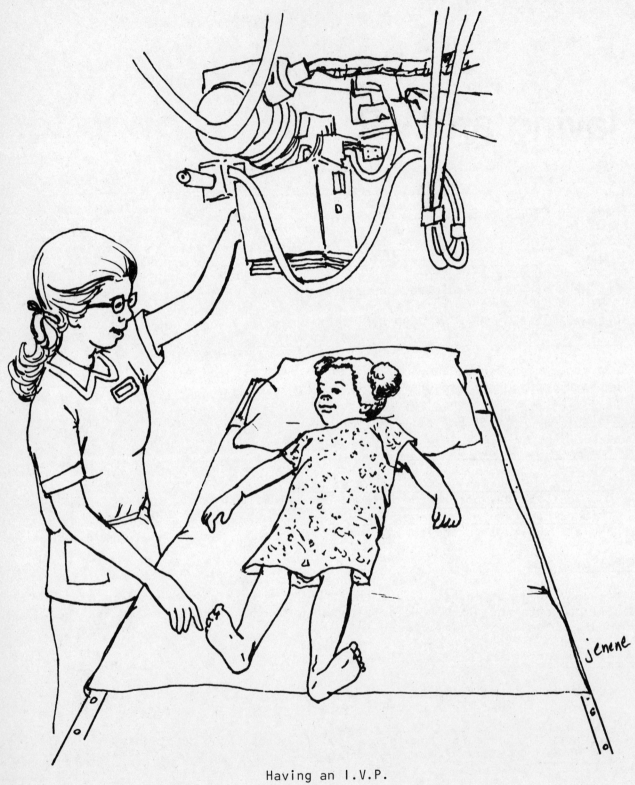

Having an I.V.P.

HELPING HAND
Homegoing Education
and Literature Program

Let's talk about...

The Nuclear Medicine Laboratory

Your doctor has made plans for your child to have a_____ scan in the Nuclear (NU-klee-ar) Medicine Laboratory. This is a standard test used to help to diagnose your child's illness.

Child's Name: _____
Appointment:
  Date: _____
  Time: _____
Please bring your child to:
☐ Line 5 at the Clinic Registration Desk (first floor)
☐ Emergency Room Desk

TO PREPARE THE CHILD FOR THE TEST

- Do nothing special to get ready for this test, unless your doctor gives you special instructions. Explain the following information to your child.
- Your child may have food while he is waiting for pictures to be taken, unless the doctors say not to.

HAVING A SCAN

Your child will lie down on a table or cart under a scope. Next, your child will be given an injection (shot) of a very small amount of radioactive medication. This has been measured, and it is safe. It will hurt a little, but not very much if the child holds his arm still. After that, several pictures will be taken of your child lying in different positions. He must hold very still. This test will take at least _____ hours. After the test, your child may return to normal activity.

If you have any questions, please call _____.

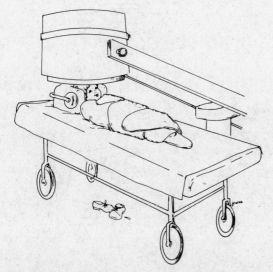

Picture 1 This is the camera. It is big and heavy, but it is safely balanced, and it barely touches the child.

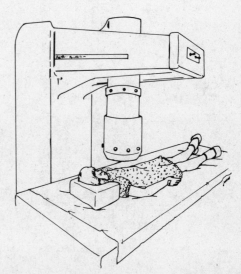

Picture 2 This is the "scanner." It moves slowly across the body as pictures are taken.

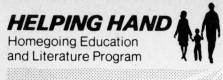

HELPING HAND
Homegoing Education
and Literature Program

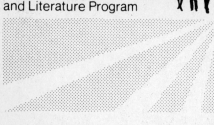

Let's talk about...

Having an X-Ray

An x-ray machine takes pictures of the inside of the body. It doesn't hurt.

HOW THE PICTURE IS TAKEN

An x-ray machine is a large camera which hangs from the ceiling. Your child will be asked to sit or to lie down on the end of the table and to hold very still. A parent or aide will hold the child. A technician will focus the camera and will take the picture.

Child's Name: _____
Appointment:
 Date: _____
 Time: _____
Please bring your child to the X-ray Department at the west end of the new building (first floor).

AFTER THE X-RAY

You will be asked to wait a short while in the waiting room until the picture is developed.

Then the technician will tell you to return to your clinic or to your doctor.

Your doctor will tell you what your child's x-ray picture shows.

If you need to change the appointment, or if you have any questions, please call the X-ray Department (phone:_____).

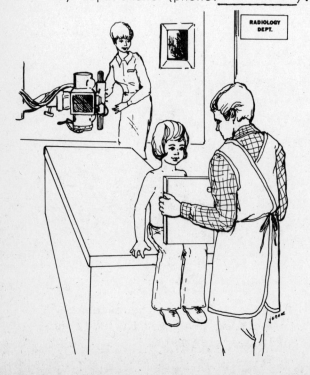

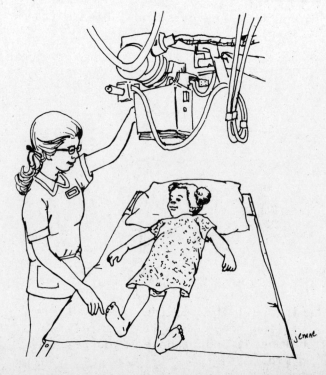

section 4
Child Care/ Health Information

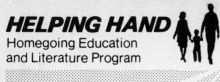

HELPING HAND
Homegoing Education
and Literature Program

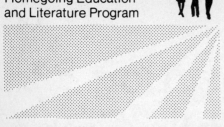

Let's talk about...

Bathing Your Baby

A mild soap bath three or four times a week will help to keep your baby clean and free from skin rashes and chafing. A plain water bath can be given on other days or if your baby is hot and "sweaty." This is a fun time for your baby. Kicking and moving about without clothes on is pleasant. It is a good time to talk to baby and to let him learn to make sounds.

SAFETY TIPS

Here are some safety tips to remember when you give the bath:

- Gather all the things you will need <u>before</u> you start giving the bath.
- The temperature of the room should be 75-80° to keep the baby from chilling. Avoid drafts.
- The bath water temperature should be slightly above 100° to prevent chilling or burning. If you do not have a bath thermometer, test the water with your elbow. When you put your elbow in the water, it should feel warm, not hot.
- Always keep a firm hold on baby after lathering. Soapy bodies are slippery.
- <u>Never leave your baby alone during the bath, not even "for a second."</u>

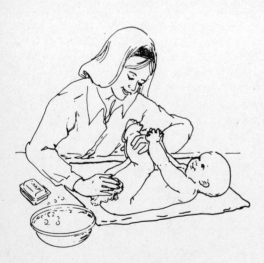

Picture 1 Bathing baby on a pad

YOU WILL NEED

Clean basin or tub
2 bath towels
Soft wash cloth
Shirt or gown, stretch sleeper
Manicure scissors or clippers
Pad
Cotton receiving blanket
Clothes bag for soiled linen

Keep the Following Items on a Tray

Jar of cotton balls
Mild soap
Pitcher of warm water if bath area is not near
   sink
Pin holder
Safety pins
Comb and hair brush

(continued)

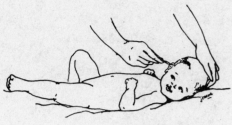

Picture 2 Cleaning outer ear
with a cotton twist

BATHING YOUR BABY

Your baby may be bathed on a pad until he is old
enough to sit up. Make a bath pad by putting a
clean towel on top of a folded blanket.

1. Wash your hands.
2. Fill the wash basin with about 3 inches of
   warm water. Test for correct temperature.
3. Arrange all items within easy reach.
4. Make two cotton twists. To make them, take
   small pieces of cotton. Roll pieces between
   your palms.
5. Undress your baby.
6. Place him on the pad (Picture 1).
7. <u>Face</u>: Using a soft wash cloth, wash the face
   with clear water.
8. <u>Eyes</u>: Wash eyes gently with moist cotton ball.
   Start at inner corner and wash toward ears.
   Use a fresh ball for each eye.
9. <u>Ears</u>: Wash the outer part of the ear with
   moist cotton twists (Picture 2). Use a clean
   twist for each ear. Pat dry with bits of dry
   cotton ball. Do not use Q-tips inside baby's
   ears.
10. <u>Hair and scalp</u>: Pick up your baby. Support
    his head in your hand and his back with your
    forearm (Picture 3). Rest baby's buttocks on
    your hip. Holding your baby this way gives
    him a sense of security.

    Wet baby's head with clear water. Make a
    soapy lather with your hands. Apply a small
    amount of soap lather to his head, including
    the "soft spot." Rub gently in a circular
    motion. Hold baby's head over basin. Rinse
    soap off with water using cupped hands or
    a wet wash cloth. When all the soap is off,
    pat his head gently with towel to dry.
11. <u>Body</u>: Place baby back on the pad. Make a
    soapy lather with your hands. Start at the
    baby's neck and lather baby's entire body.
    Make sure you clean in the skin folds and
    between fingers and toes. Rinse soap off with
    a wet wash cloth. Dry baby with a soft towel.

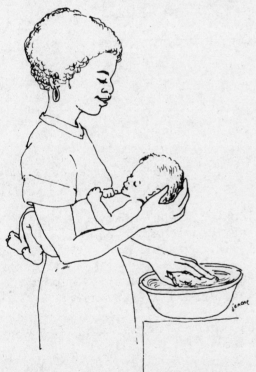

Picture 3 Holding your baby
securely

(continued)

12. <u>Genital area</u>: If your baby is an uncir-
    cumcised boy, pull back the foreskin
    that is over the head of the penis.
    Wash gently with soapy water. Rinse with
    clear water from the pitcher. Dry. Pull
    the foreskin back over the head of the
    penis. Do this every time you bathe
    your baby. Natural secretions collect
    under the foreskin. The skin may become
    red and irritated. The penis of a
    circumcised boy should be gently washed,
    rinsed, and dried.

    If your baby is a girl, spread the labia
    (folds of the genitals) apart. Wash
    gently front to back with soapy water.
    Rinse, dry.

AFTER THE BATH

Dress baby. Brush and comb hair. Put baby
in a safe place. Clean the basin. Put items
back on tray and store it out of children's
reach.

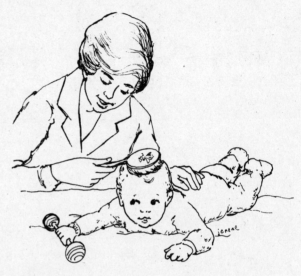

Picture 4 Brushing away old skin

<u>Nails</u>: Clean baby's fingernails and toe
nails. Clip the nails with manicure scissors
as needed. If the fingernails are not kept
short, the baby may scratch his face.

SPECIAL SCALP CARE

If your baby's scalp becomes dry, scaly, or "dirty looking," apply baby oil after
the shampooing. Leave it on until the next day. The next day shampoo baby's hair,
then brush the hair and scalp well to remove old skin (Picture 4).

If the scalp still does not look clean, keep doing this every day until it looks
normal. Wash the brush and comb with soapy water, rinse, and dry every day.

If you do this several times and the scalp still does not look normal to you, you
may want to ask your child's doctor what to do about it.

If you have any questions, please call _____.

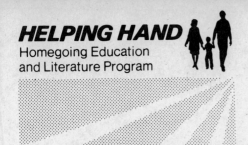

HELPING HAND
Homegoing Education
and Literature Program

Let's talk about...

Birth Control Pills-5 Day Start

Name of Pill: _____

Taking birth control pills is a good way to prevent pregnancy. But birth control pills only work if you take one every day.

HOW TO TAKE THE PILLS

1. Wait until your menstrual period starts before starting your first package of birth control pills.
2. Take your first pill on the fifth day of your menstrual period (see chart).
3. Then take one pill every day.
4. When you have taken all 28 pills in your package, begin a new package the next day. Make sure you always have enough pills at home so you do not run out.
5. Do not stop taking the pills during your monthly period.
6. You must take one pill every day to keep from getting pregnant. Try to take the pills about the same time every day.
7. If you forget to take one pill, take it as soon as you remember. This means that you may need to take two pills in one day. For example, take one as soon as you remember and one at your regular time on the same day. If you miss two or more pills in a row, please call the Teenage Clinic (phone:_____). They will tell you what to do.

ADDITIONAL PROTECTION

Your birth control pills will not keep you from getting pregnant until you have been taking them for 10 days. During that beginning period you should use some additional means of birth control (condoms, contraceptive foam, cream, or jelly) at the time of sexual intercourse.

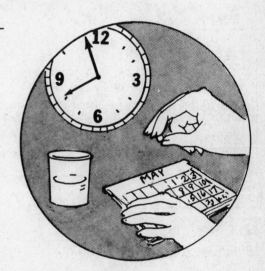

Take a pill every day.

IF YOUR PERIOD BEGINS ON	START TAKING PILLS ON
Sunday ⟶	Thursday
Monday ⟶	Friday
Tuesday ⟶	Saturday
Wednesday ⟶	Sunday
Thursday ⟶	Monday
Friday ⟶	Tuesday
Saturday ⟶	Wednesday

(continued)

2 Birth Control Pills—5 Day Start

COMMON SIDE EFFECTS

During your first two packages of 28 pills, you may develop common side effects, such as breast tenderness, upset stomach, mild headache, small weight gain or a small amount of bleeding (spotting) between periods. If these side effects continue during your third package of pills, please call the clinic but <u>do not stop taking your pills.</u>

CAUTION

- Store all medicine out of children's reach.
- Store in locked cupboard when possible.
- Give medicine only as ordered by your doctor.
- When medicine is no longer needed, flush it down the toilet.
- If a sick child accidentally takes too much of this medicine, it can make him very sick. Call your doctor (phone:_____), the Poison Control Center (phone:_____), or the Emergency Room (phone:_____) if this happens.

WHEN TO CALL THE DOCTOR

Call the clinic (phone:_____) or your doctor (phone: _____) immediately if you have:

- Severe headaches
- Pains in your chest or legs
- Shortness of breath
- Blurred vision

If you are not sure how to take your pills, or if you have any other questions, call the Teenage Clinic (phone:_____).

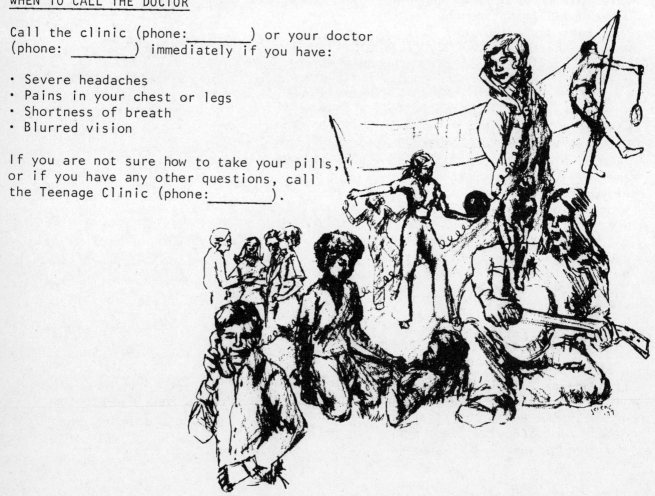

Let's talk about...

Birth Control - Using a Diaphragm

A fairly safe way to prevent an unwanted pregnancy is to use a diaphragm (cap) while having sexual intercourse (sex). The diaphragm is sealed in place over the cervix of the uterus with a gel that destroys sperm (Picture 1). You must use the diaphragm carefully.

WHEN TO PUT IN THE DIAPHRAGM

Put the diaphragm in <u>before</u> you are going to have sexual intercourse.

HOW TO PUT IN THE DIAPHRAGM

1. Rinse off the diaphragm with water if it has been stored in corn starch.
2. Gently dry it with a soft cloth.
3. Hold it up to the light and look for holes. If there are holes in it, it will not work. So, you will need to get a new one before having sex.
4. Put a teaspoonful of gel into the diaphragm (Picture 2).
5. Carefully spread the gel around the rim and inside surface of the diaphragm. Then place it on a clean surface.
6. Wash and dry your hands to remove gel.
7. Get into a squatting position. Relax and take your time.
8. Using your longest finger, find the cervix of your uterus. It will feel like the tip of your nose.
9. Squeeze the diaphragm into a long narrow shape (Picture 3).
10. Put the diaphragm into your vagina, far enough to cover the cervix.
11. Feel around the rim to make sure it covers the cervix and is securely in place.

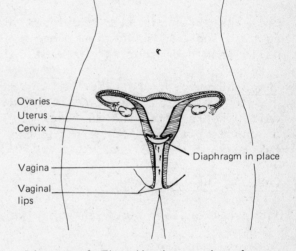

Ovaries
Uterus
Cervix
Diaphragm in place
Vagina
Vaginal lips

Picture 1 The diaphragm in place

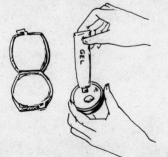

Picture 2 Spread the gel all over the diaphragm.

HOW LONG SHOULD THE DIAPHRAGM BE LEFT IN PLACE?

Leave the diaphragm in place for at least 6 hours after the last sex act. It takes 6 hours for the gel to destroy the sperm.

(continued)

2   Birth Control—Using a Diaphragm

WHEN TO ADD MORE GEL

- You will need to put in more gel before having sex if the diaphragm and gel have been in place more than 2 hours.
- Fill the applicator with gel. Put it all the way into the vagina. Push the gel in. Remove applicator (see Picture 4).
- Use an applicatorful of gel after each sex act.

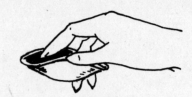

Picture 3 Squeeze the diaphragm into a long narrow shape.

HOW TO REMOVE THE DIAPHRAGM

Hook the outer rim with the index finger. Pull down to loosen the suction. Remove. Your fingernails should be short to prevent injury.

DOUCHING

Wait 6 hours after the last sex act, if you want to douche. It takes 6 hours for the gel to destroy the sperm.

CARE OF THE DIAPHRAGM

1. Wash the diaphragm with soapy water after each use.
2. Rinse and dry well.
3. Hold it up to the light to see if there are holes. Also fill it with water to see if it leaks.
4. If it is free of holes, powder it with corn starch and store in a container.
5. If you need a new diaphragm, call your doctor for an appointment.

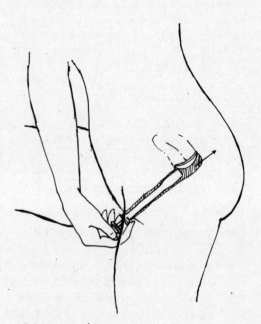

Picture 4 Put in more gel with applicator.

OTHER INFORMATION

- You may go about your normal activities with the diaphragm in place. Check to make sure it is in place after having a bowel movement.
- If you have a large weight gain or loss, you should talk with your doctor. It may be necessary to be fitted for a new diaphragm.

If you have any questions, please call _____ .

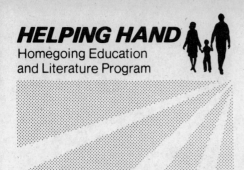

HELPING HAND
Homegoing Education
and Literature Program

Let's talk about...

Birth Control-How to Use Foam

Contraceptive vaginal foam is used to destroy the man's sperm when having inter-course (sex). This foam must be put into the vagina 30 minutes or less before <u>each</u> act to avoid an unwanted pregnancy. When a woman uses foam, her partner should use a condom (rubber). Foam by itself is a "risky" method.

<u>HOW TO USE THE FOAM</u>

1. Foam must be put into the vagina 30 minutes or less before each sex act.
2. Shake the foam can well before each use. Place the can upright. Remove the cap.
3. Place the applicator over the top of the can and gently tilt it (Picture 1). Use only enough pressure to allow the foam to slowly fill the applicator.
4. Fill the applicator completely. Remove applicator from can.
5. Put the applicator into the vagina as far as it will go (Picture 1). Then pull it back an inch so it does not press against the back of the vagina.
6. Press applicator plunger all the way in. Then remove the applicator.
7. Fill the applicator again and repeat steps 5 and 6.
8. Put in another applicator of foam before repeating intercourse.

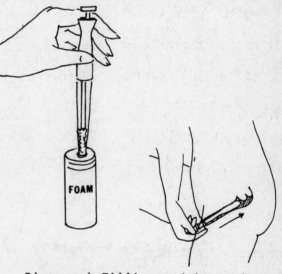

Picture 1 Filling and inserting applicator of foam

<u>HOW TO CARE FOR THE APPLICATOR AND FOAM CAN</u>

• Take applicator apart after each use. Wash with warm soapy water. Rinse well. Do not boil.
• Store foam at room temperature.
• Store out of reach of children.

<u>OTHER INFORMATION</u>

• When you hear a sputtering sound and the applicator fills very slowly with foam, you will know the foam can is almost empty. Keep an extra can ready to avoid running out of supplies.
• Foam may be obtained at your local pharmacy without a prescription.
• Douching is not necessary. But, if you wish to douch, wait at least 6 hours after having sex. This gives the foam time to work. Use only warm water for douching.

If you have any questions, please call the Teenage Clinic (phone:_____).

Let's talk about...

Birth Control-Using an IUD

The intrauterine (in-tra-U-ter-in) device (IUD) is made of plastic or copper and is placed inside the uterus (womb) by the doctor. It is a fairly good way to prevent pregnancy but cannot be worn by every woman. If your doctor has prescribed it for you, there are some things you should know.

Your IUD will work only if it stays in the right place.

TO MAKE SURE YOUR IUD IS IN PLACE

1. Check to be sure your IUD has not come out. This should be done about once a month, especially after your menstrual period.
2. To check your IUD, wash your hands, then get into a squatting position.
3. Put your middle or index finger into your vagina and reach as far back as you can. You will feel a soft bump like the end of your nose. This is the tip of the uterus. Feel around this bump for the string of your IUD (Picture 1).

4. If you can feel the string, your IUD is in the correct position. If you cannot feel the string, or if you feel any of the hard part of your IUD, call the nurse in the Teenage Clinic (phone: _____).
5. Each time you remove a sanitary napkin or tampon during your period, you should look to be sure that your IUD is not caught on it.
6. Most IUD's that come out do so either during or before your first monthly period. We suggest that you use another method of birth control (contraceptive foam, cream, jelly, or condoms) with your IUD until after your first monthly period.

ACTIVITY

You may continue to swim, to use tampons, and to do all other activities which you did before your IUD was put in.

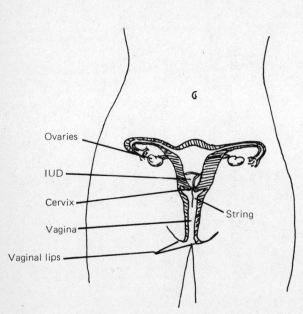

Ovaries

IUD

Cervix

Vagina

Vaginal lips

String

Picture 1 IUD in place

(continued)

WHAT ABOUT BLEEDING AND CRAMPING?

After you have your IUD put in, you can expect to have a longer monthly period for the first two periods. You may have more bleeding during these two periods. You may also have a few days of "spotting" between your first few periods as your body becomes adjusted to your IUD. This is normal.

If you have cramps after your IUD is put in, you may take aspirin or the medication you usually take for monthly cramps. If you are having cramps immediately after your IUD is inserted, you may lie down and place a heating pad or warm water bottle on your abdomen.

WHEN TO CALL THE DOCTOR

If any of the early IUD danger signals occur, call the Teenage Clinic (phone: _____) immediately.

Early IUD Danger Signs

• Abdominal pain
• Heavy vaginal bleeding
• Fever or chills
• Vaginal discharge with a bad odor

If you have any questions about your IUD, call the Teenage Clinic (phone:_____).

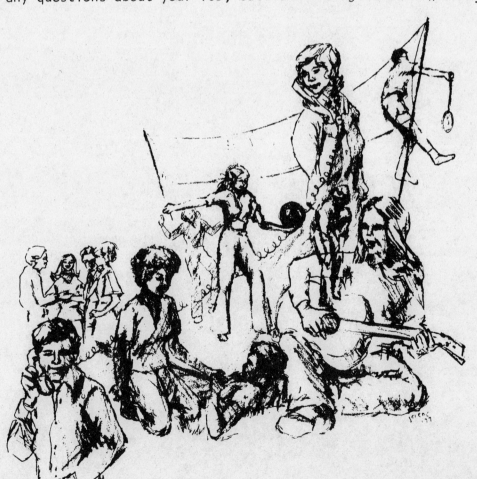

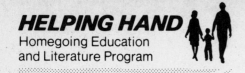

HELPING HAND
Homegoing Education
and Literature Program

Let's talk about...

Body Outline:
Infant/Toddler, Female

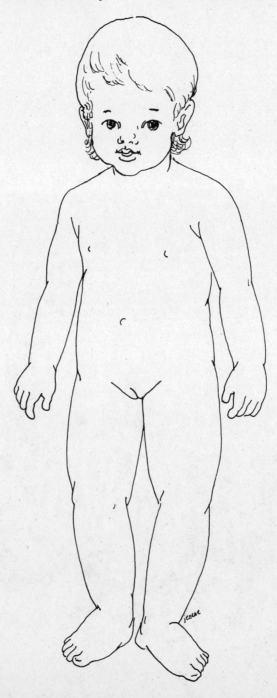

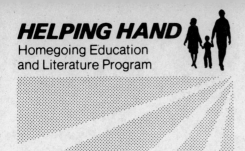

HELPING HAND
Homegoing Education
and Literature Program

Let's talk about...

Body Outline: Infant / Toddler, Male

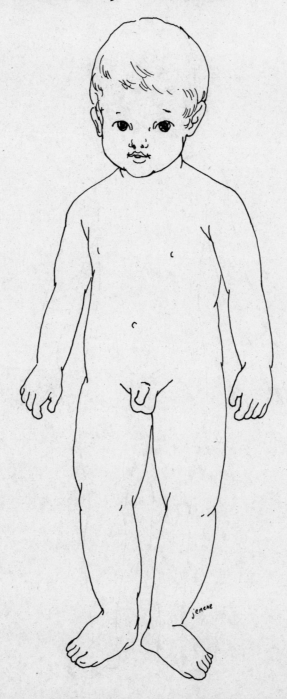

HELPING HAND
Homegoing Education
and Literature Program

Let's talk about...

Body Outline:
Preadolescent, Female

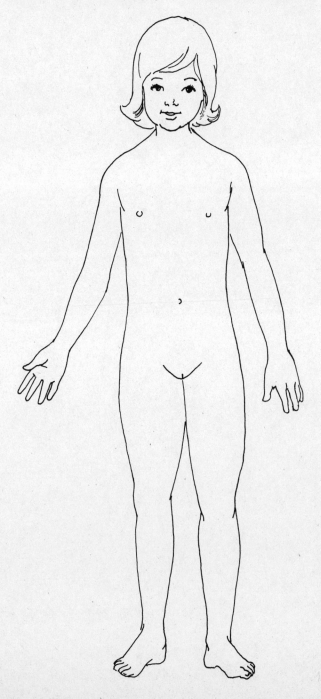

HELPING HAND
Homegoing Education
and Literature Program

Let's talk about...

Body Outline: Preadolescent, Male

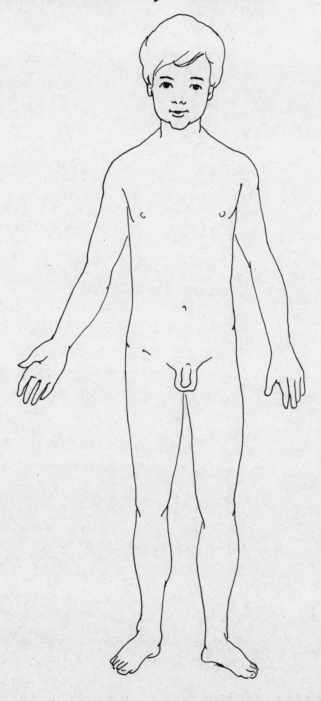

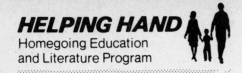

HELPING HAND
Homegoing Education
and Literature Program

Let's talk about...

Body Outline:
Adolescent, Female

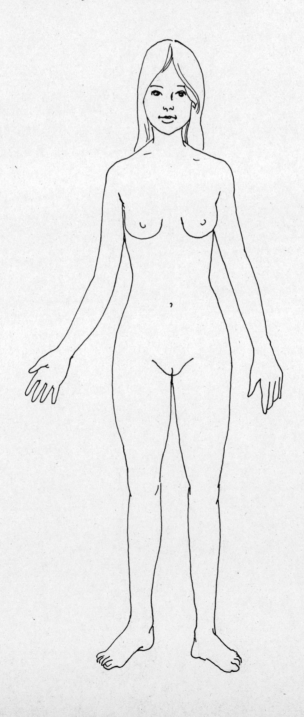

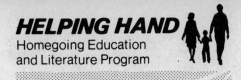

HELPING HAND
Homegoing Education
and Literature Program

Let's talk about...

Body Outline:
Adolescent, Male

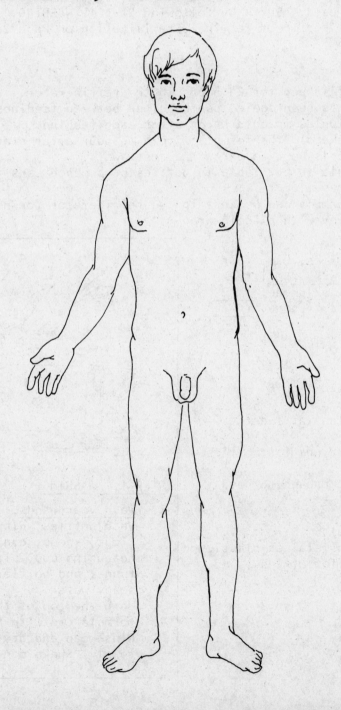

HELPING HAND
Homegoing Education
and Literature Program

Let's talk about...

Preparing Baby's Formula

There are several ways to prepare formula. The methods explained here are the Aseptic Sterilization Method and the Terminal Sterilization Method. Either method may be used. Begin by following Step 1. WASHING, then continue with either Aseptic or Terminal Sterilization on Page 2.

SPECIAL TIPS

- Prepared formula will keep for 24 hours in the refrigerator.
- Boiled water that has been cooled can be given between feedings.
- Wash bottles and nipples in cold water after each feeding.
- If baby does not take all the formula within an hour after starting to give the bottle, it is best to throw the rest away.
- Ready-to-feed formula is available in bottles or 8-ounce cans and is best to use when traveling.
- An opened can of formula can be kept in the refrigerator for not more than 24 hours. Cover with plastic wrap.

If you have any questions, call your doctor (phone: _____), the Department of Dietetics (phone: _____), or nurse (phone: _____).

YOU WILL NEED

- ☐ Formula (concentrated liquid) - as ordered by doctor
- ☐ 8 oz. nursing bottles (at least 8 bottles)
- ☐ Nipples, discs and rings for bottles
- ☐ Bottle brush
- ☐ Pan with lid (large enough to hold 8 bottles)
- ☐ Measuring cup
- ☐ Pitcher (quart-size)
- ☐ Large, long-handled metal or plastic (not wooden) spoon for mixing
- ☐ Funnel
- ☐ Tongs
- ☐ Can opener

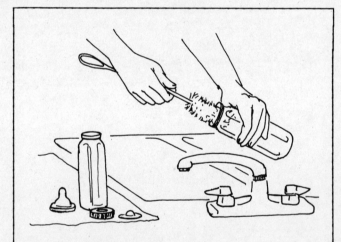

STEP 1. WASHING

1. Wash your hands.
2. Wash bottles, nipples, discs, rings, spoon, can opener, measuring cup, pitcher, tongs, funnel and bottle brush in hot soapy water.
3. Wash the top of the concentrated formula can with hot soapy water. Rinse can and dry with clean towel. Shake can well.

(continued)

NOTE: Use either Aseptic or Terminal Sterilization Method - not both

☐ ASEPTIC STERILIZATION METHOD

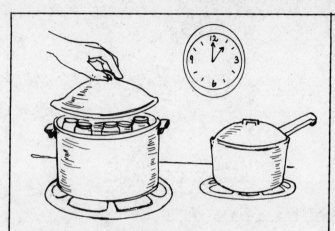

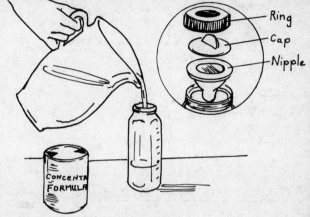

Ring
Cap
Nipple

STEP 2. STERILIZATION

1. Put bottles, nipples, discs, rings, spoon, can opener, measuring cup, tongs and funnel on a rack or clean cloth in the bottom of a large pan. Fill with water, cover pan and place over heat.
2. In another pan, put _____ ounces of water to make sterile water. Cover pan and place over heat.
3. After water in both pans starts to boil, let boil for 5 minutes.
4. Before removing lid, allow to cool.

STEP 3. PREPARING BOTTLES

1. Measure _____ ounces of sterile water and pour into quart-sized pitcher.
2. Measure _____ ounces of CONCENTRATED LIQUID FORMULA. Add to sterile water. Mix well with spoon.
3. Pour _____ ounces of this formula into each of _____ bottles.
4. Using tongs, place nipples upside down on bottles. Cover with discs and rings.
5. Place in refrigerator until it is time to feed your baby. Use within 24 hours.

(continued)

☐ TERMINAL STERILIZATION METHOD

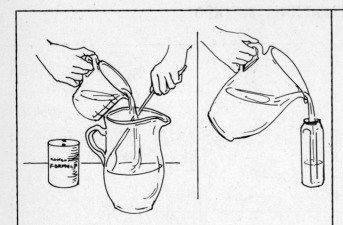

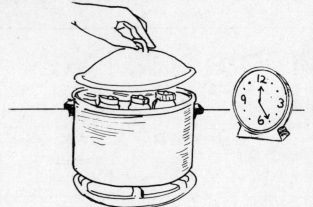

STEP 2.   PREPARING BOTTLES

1. Measure _____ ounces of water into a clean pitcher or mixing bowl.
2. Punch 2 holes in the top of the clean formula can with the clean can opener.
3. Add _____ ounces of CONCENTRATED LIQUID FORMULA to water in the pitcher and stir.
4. Pour _____ ounces of formula into _____ clean nursing bottles. Put nipples, discs and rings on nursing bottles loosely.

STEP 3.   STERILIZING

1. Put the bottles on a wire rack or towel in the kettle and add 3 inches of water. Place the kettle over heat.
2. As soon as the water starts to boil, cover kettle with a lid and let boil for 25 minutes.
3. After 25 minutes, remove kettle from heat and let cool. When nursing bottles are cool enough to touch, tighten the rings and put bottles in the refrigerator. Use within 24 hours.

HELPING HAND
Homegoing Education
and Literature Program

Let's talk about...

Immunizations

Immunizations (im-mu-ni-ZA-shuns) are medicines given to protect your child against certain harmful diseases. Immunizations are given by mouth or by injections (shots).

NAMES OF IMMUNIZATIONS	DISEASES IMMUNIZATIONS PROTECT AGAINST
DPT	Diphtheria (a bacterial infection that causes a membrane to form in the throat) Pertussis (whooping cough) Tetanus (lock jaw)
Trivalent Sabin (oral polio) (OPV)	Polio
Rubella vaccine	3-Day German measles
Measles vaccine (rubeola)	2-Week measles (hard measles)
Tuberculin skin test	This is a test to see if your child has Tuberculosis (TB). It is not an immunization.

Immunizations are usually given according to a special schedule. Ages when healthy infants and children should receive immunizations are:

AGE*	TYPE OF IMMUNIZATION GIVEN
2 months	DPT and polio
4 months	DPT and polio
6 months	DPT and polio
15 months	Measles, rubella, mumps
18 months	DPT and polio booster
4-5 years	DPT and polio booster
14-16 years	DT (adult) booster and then every 10 years
Yearly	Tuberculin skin test

*The ages when immunizations are given may vary with each doctor.

(continued)

WHAT TO EXPECT AFTER AN IMMUNIZATION IS GIVEN

Immunizations can cause your child to have a fever. If his temperature is 101° (rectally) or more, give (name of medication): _____
amount: _____. You may repeat this one time 3-4 hours later.

Call the clinic (phone: _____) if the fever lasts longer than 24-48 hours.

YOUR CHILD'S IMMUNIZATION RECORD

You will be given an immunization record for your child. When each immunization is given, your doctor or nurse will write the date on this card. It is important that you keep this record in a safe place.

You will need to take this record with you:

- When the child returns for medical check-ups
- When your child enrolls in school
- If your child is injured and has an open cut
- If you move to a new area and place of medical care

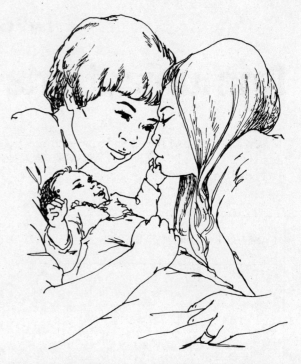

Your child needs your protection.

OTHER INFORMATION

German measles vaccine (rubella) should be given to girls before child-bearing age. If a pregnant woman gets German measles early in her pregnancy, her baby can have birth defects.

If you have any questions, please call _____.

HELPING HAND
Homegoing Education
and Literature Program

Let's talk about...

Rubella Immunization

Rubella (German measles) is an infection caused by a virus. To protect your child from this disease, an injection (shot) of vaccine has been given. This vaccine should protect your child for life.

It is very important that all children receive this vaccine around 15 months of age.

Pregnant women can have a child born with birth defects if they have never had the vaccine and get German measles when pregnant.

WHAT TO EXPECT AFTER THE SHOT

Your child may have a mild fever (under 102°) a few hours after the shot is given. A slight rash, joint pain, and mild fever may happen 7-10 days or even longer after the shot is given.

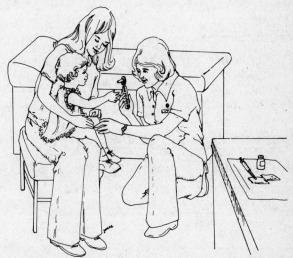

WHAT TO DO

1. If your child has a fever or pain, you may give this medication:

   _____
   amount: _____ .
2. You may repeat this dose one time 3-4 hours later.
3. Do not give medicine more than two times.

Protect your child against German measles.

WHEN TO CALL THE DOCTOR

If your child has other symptoms, or continues to have a fever, they may be due to other causes. You should call the nurse (phone: _____) or your doctor (phone: _____).

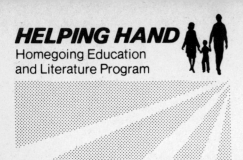

HELPING HAND
Homegoing Education
and Literature Program

Let's talk about...

Rubeola Immunization

Your child has been given a rubeola immunization vaccine to protect him from 2-week "hard" measles.

WHAT TO EXPECT AFTER THE SHOT

- Your child may have a fever, be fussy, or irritable. The fever may begin a few hours after the shot is given, or again up to 30 days later. His temperature may go as high as 103° and sometimes higher.
- He may have a slight rash. The rash may appear from 5-12 days after the vaccine (shot) is given.

WHAT TO DO

1. If your child has a fever, you may give this medication: _____
   amount: _____ .
2. You may repeat this dose one time 3-4 hours later.
3. Do not give medicine more than two times.

WHEN TO CALL THE DOCTOR

If your child continues to have the fever or has other symptoms, they may be due to other causes. You should call the nurse (phone: _____) or your doctor (phone: _____).

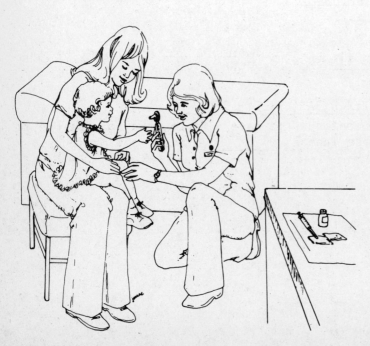

Protect your child against "hard" measles.

HELPING HAND
Homegoing Education
and Literature Program

Let's talk about...

Cleaning the Teeth and Gums

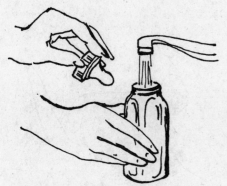

Picture 1 Give baby plain
water to drink at bedtime.

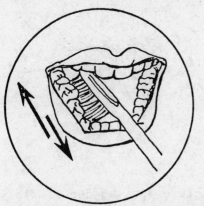

Picture 2 Angle the bristles
against the gum line.

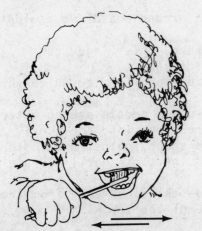

Picture 3 Brush back and
forth.

Healthy teeth and gums are very important to the
health of your child. Teeth must be cleaned to
remove old food and plaque (plak). Plaque is a
harmful layer of bacteria on the teeth that can
cause cavities. To prevent cavities and gum
disease, teeth must be brushed every day.

YOU WILL NEED

A toothbrush small enough to reach every tooth.
 The bristles should be made of soft polished
 nylon with a flat brushing surface.
Toothpaste, or baking soda and salt
Unwaxed dental floss

INFANT MOUTH CARE

· Parents should brush their child's teeth as
  soon as they appear in the mouth. Cleanse your
  baby's mouth with a soft toothbrush dipped in
  salt water (add 1/4 teaspoonful of salt to 1/2
  cup of water). Use a clean gauze dipped in salt
  water if your baby does not like a toothbrush.
· Do not let baby go to bed at night with a
  bottle of formula or juice. The milk or sugar
  in the juice can cause cavities. You may give
  your baby plain water in a bottle at bedtime
  (Picture 1).

TO TEACH BASIC TOOTH BRUSHING

Around 5 years of age or when the child learns to
tie his or her shoes, let him start brushing his
own teeth. This will not always be done well. You
will need to give lots of help.

1. Have your child place the head of the toothbrush along the side of the teeth. Angle the
   bristle tips against the gum line (Picture 2).
2. Move the brush back and forth several times,
   using a gentle "scrubbing" motion (Picture 3).
3. Brush the outer surfaces of each tooth, uppers
   and lowers, keeping the bristles angled against
   the gum line.

(continued)

2 Cleaning the Teeth and Gums

4. Use the same method on all the inside surfaces and chewing surfaces of the teeth, upper and lower.
5. For the inside surfaces of the front teeth, tilt the brush so the bristles point up. Make several gentle back and forth strokes with the "toe" (the front part) of the brush over the teeth and gum tissue.

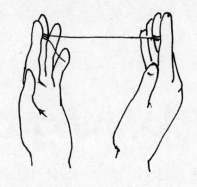

TOOTHBRUSHING TIPS

- A worn-out toothbrush will not clean your child's teeth. Replace the brush often.
- The toothbrush will only clean one or two teeth at a time. Change its position frequently.
- Brush gently and with very short strokes, but use enough pressure so the bristles are felt against the gum.
- Brushing the tongue with the brush will help your child's mouth feel fresh.
- Toothbrushing, like flossing, takes a little bit of time and practice to do properly.
- While it's better to brush after every meal, teach your child to brush (and floss) <u>at least once</u> thoroughly every day, so the plaque build-up is kept under control.
- If you notice any repeated discomfort or bleeding while brushing, consult your dentist.

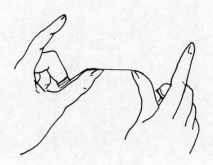

USING DENTAL FLOSS

When your child's teeth come in contact or touch on the sides, you must begin the use of dental floss. By the time he is 11 or 12 years old, he can do it well on his own.

Flossing removes the sticky layer of harmful bacteria called plaque (plak).

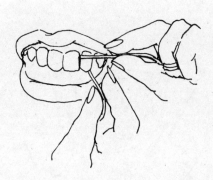

Picture 4 Using dental floss

1. Break off about 18 inches of floss and wind most of it around one of your middle fingers.
2. Wind the rest around the same finger of the opposite hand. This finger can "take up" the floss as it becomes soiled or worn (Picture 4).
3. Use your thumbs and forefingers with an inch of floss between them to guide the floss between the teeth (Picture 4).
4. Holding the floss tightly (there should be no slack), use a gentle sawing motion to insert the floss between the teeth. Never "snap" the floss into the gums! When the floss reaches the gum line, curve it into a c-shape against one tooth and <u>gently slide</u> it into the space between the gum and the tooth until you feel resistance (Picture 4).
5. While holding the floss tightly against the tooth, move the floss away from the gum by scraping the floss up and down against the side of the tooth.
6. Repeat this method on the rest of the teeth.

(continued)

OTHER TIPS FOR HEALTHY TEETH

- Brush teeth every morning and night.
- Brush or rinse with water after eating.
- Have a dental check-up every 6 months.
- Eat crunchy raw fruit and vegetables.
- Drink milk to make strong teeth.
- Only have candy or pop for special treats.
- Drink water instead of pop or sweet drinks if you are thirsty.

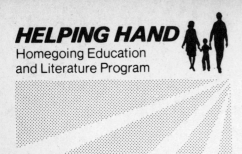

HELPING HAND
Homegoing Education
and Literature Program

Let's talk about...

Going to University Hospital

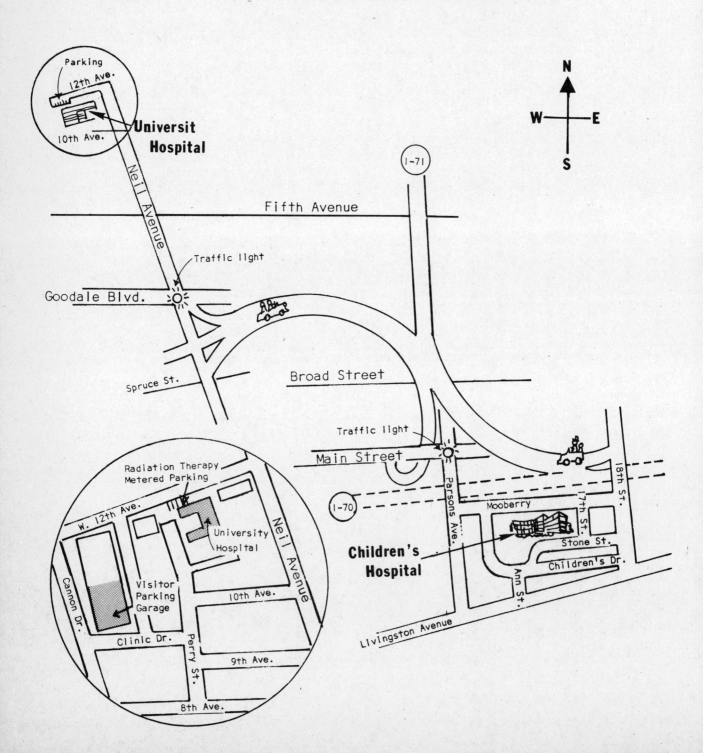

section 5
Medications

HELPING HAND
Homegoing Education
and Literature Program

Let's talk about...

Dosage Schedule for Aspirin and Aspirin-like Medicine

Child's Name: _____
Age: _____

AGE OF CHILD	CHILDREN'S ASPIRIN TABLETS 1 1/4 GR. IN EACH TABLET	LIQUIPRIN	TEMPRA OR TYLENOL DROPS	TYLENOL ELIXIR R (RED) OR TEMPRA SYRUP R (GREEN)
3-6 months	Do not give this to infants	1/4 dropper	0.3 cc	Do not give this to infants
6-12 months	Do not give this to infants	1/2 dropper	0.6 cc	Do not give this to infants
1-2 years	1 tablet	3/4 dropper	0.9 cc	1/2 teaspoonful
2-3 years	2 tablets	1 dropper	1.2 cc	1 teaspoonful
3-4 years	3 tablets	1½ dropper	2.4 cc	1½ teaspoonful
4-5 years	4 tablets (5 grains)	2 droppers	2.4 cc	2 teaspoonfuls
Above 5 years	4 tablets (5 grains)	2 droppers	2.4 cc	2 teaspoonfuls

<u>HOW TO GIVE THE MEDICINE</u>

☐ Give _____ cc's of _____ every _____ hours.

☐ Give _____ teaspoonful(s) of _____ every _____ hours.

☐ Give _____ tablet(s) of _____ every _____ hours.

☐ Give _____ droppers of _____ every _____ hours.

Do not give longer than _____ hours.

<u>NOTE</u>: Use a baking measuring spoon when giving medicine by teaspoon.

(continued)

CAUTION

- Store all medicine out of children's reach.
- Store in locked cupboard when possible.
- Give medicine only as ordered by your doctor.
- When medicine is no longer needed, flush it down the toilet.
- If a child accidentally takes too much of this medicine, it can make him very sick. Call your doctor (phone:_____), the Poison Control Center (phone:_____), or the Emergency Room (phone:_____) if this happens.

If you have any questions, please call _____.

HELPING HAND
Homegoing Education
and Literature Program

Let's talk about...

How to Give Eye Drops

Eye medication has been ordered to treat
your child's eyes. Before you start,
practice by drawing the eye medication
up into the dropper. Squeeze the bulb
and drop one drop back into the bottle,
so you will know how hard to squeeze the
bulb.

Child's Name: _____
Child's Age: _____
Medication: _____
Dose: _____

Explain to your child what you are going to do. Tell your child the medicine
may tingle a little or feel cold. If needed, have another person hold your
child's hands.

<u>WHAT TO DO</u>

1. Wash your hands.
2. Read the label on the bottle.
3. Have the child tip his head back and look up, or lie down and look up.
4. Hold a tissue on the child's cheek under the eye to catch any excess medication.

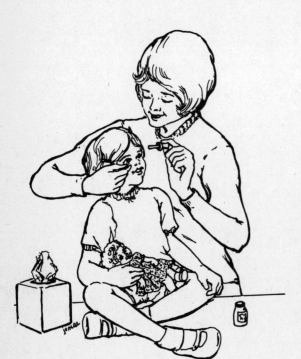

5. Gently pull the lower eyelid down and
   forward to make a little pocket.
6. Put the correct number of drops of
   medication into the eye. Do not
   allow the medication to run into
   the other eye.
7. Release the skin.
8. Have the child gently close his eyes and
   keep his eyes closed for 15 seconds if
   possible.
9. Wipe the extra medication from his face.

<u>CAUTION</u>
- When you have finished, place the
  medication out of the reach of children.
- When medicine is no longer needed, pour
  the remainder down the sink, or flush
  it down the toilet.
- Never use any medicine to treat a
  child's eyes without a doctor's
  prescription.

If you have any questions, please call
_____.

HELPING HAND
Homegoing Education
and Literature Program

Let's talk about...

How to Give an Injection

Sometimes medicine is given by injection (shots) when it cannot be given by mouth. It may be necessary to have someone help you. Explain to the child why the shot must be given. Try to get your child's mind off the shot by giving her a toy or by having her squeeze someone's hand. A child of any age should be allowed to express fear and dislike of the shot.

YOU WILL NEED

Medication
2-cc disposable syringes
25-gauge needles or size _____
Package of 2 X 2 gauze squares
Bottle of rubbing alcohol

2 glass jars with lids
Rubber bands
Small metal file
Cotton balls
Small tray

WHAT TO DO

1. Wash your hands in soapy water. Rinse and dry.
2. Read the label on the medicine.
3. Clean the top of the bottle well with a cotton ball dipped in alcohol.
4. Remove the needle cover from the disposable syringe. Push the plunger back and forth to make sure it moves freely.

To Give The Medicine From a Multiple Dose Bottle

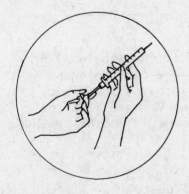 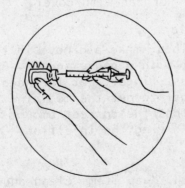 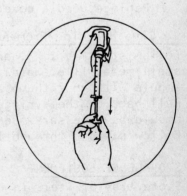

5. Pull air up into the syringe equal to the amount of medicine to be given.

6. Push needle through top of bottle. Push air into the bottle.

7. Turn bottle upside down. Pull the amount of medicine that is to be given into the syringe.

(continued)

2 How to Give an Injection

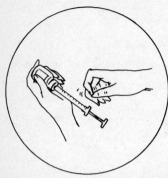

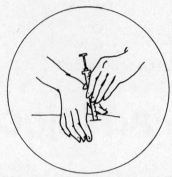

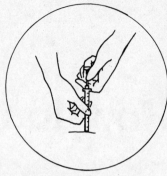

8. Hold syringe pointed up. Tap gently to make air bubbles rise. Gently push on plunger to force air bubbles out. Check syringe again to make sure dosage is correct.

9. Clean skin with cotton ball dipped in alcohol. Pinch up skin where you were taught to give the shot.
10. Hold syringe like a pencil. Slip the needle quickly through the skin at a 90° angle.

11. Pull back on plunger to see if blood appears. If medicine is clear, push plunger all the way into the syringe.

Note: If blood appears discard syringe and repeat steps 3 to 11.

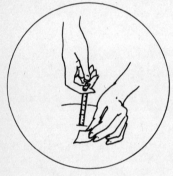

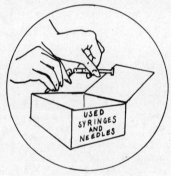

12. Remove needle from injection site. Hold cotton swab over site for a few seconds. Replace needle cover.

13. Break off needle on disposable syringe. Put used syringe and needle in a box or can with cover.

CAUTION: The law states that the syringe must be "rendered inoperable." This means the needle must be broken off and the plunger taken out. This will keep anyone from reusing a disposable syringe.

To Give Medicine From An Ampule

Follow steps 1, 2, 3, and 4. Then, make a groove in the neck of the ampule with small metal file. Hold the top with a gauze square. Snap off the top. Hold the ampule with your thumb and first finger. Put the needle tip into the solution. Pull back on the syringe plunger to get the medicine into the syringe. Tilt the ampule as necessary. Be sure that the correct amount of medicine is in the syringe. Follow steps 8 through 13 for giving the injection.

STORAGE OF EQUIPMENT

Store tray of items in cupboard. Keep items clean and free of dust.

CAUTION: Be sure to keep syringes and supplies out of the reach of children and others who might misuse them.

If you have any questions, please call _____ .

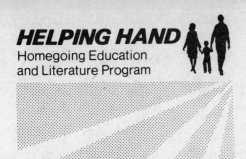

HELPING HAND
Homegoing Education
and Literature Program

Let's talk about...

When to Give Medications

Child's Name: _____
Age: _____
Medication: _____
Dose (Amount): _____

Give this medicine _____ times a day at the times circled on the picture.

6 7 8 9 10 11 12 1 2 3 4 5 6 7 8 9 10 11 12 1 2 3 4 5
Noon   **Midnight**

<u>HOW TO GIVE THE MEDICATION</u>

☐ Take _____ (time) before meals
☐ Take with meals
☐ Take after meals

<u>THIS DRUG IS USED FOR</u>

_____

_____

CAUTION

- Store all medicine out of children's reach.
- Store in locked cupboard when possible.
- Give medicine only as ordered by your doctor.
- When medicine is no longer needed, flush it down the toilet.
- If a child accidentally takes too much of this medicine, it can make him very sick. Call your doctor (phone:_____), the Poison Control Center (phone:_____), or the Emergency Room (phone:_____) if this happens.

(continued)

2 When to Give Medication

<u>WHEN TO CALL THE DOCTOR</u>

Call your doctor (phone: _____) if any of the following symptoms (signs) occur.

1. _____   3. _____

2. _____

HELPING HAND
Homegoing Education
and Literature Program

Let's talk about...

Prednisone

Prednisone (PRED-ni-sone) is a medication in a group known as steroids. The
main purpose of steroids is to help to
reduce inflammation caused by injury
or illness. Prednisone is useful in the
treatment of many illnesses. It is
generally a safe medication when taken with the supervision of a doctor.

| Child's Name: _____ |
| Medication: _____ |
| Dosage: _____ |
| _____ |

Prednisone is similar to hormones (cortisol) or substances produced by the body.
The body's natural production of these hormones may be slowed down for a time by
the use of prednisone. For this reason, it is important that any changes in the
dose should be directed by your doctor. Never stop taking prednisone without first
talking to your doctor. As the dose of prednisone is decreased, the body will
slowly begin to produce more cortisol.

DAILY DOSAGE SCHEDULE

· Your dosage schedule should be directed by
  your doctor. Refer to calendar on page 2.
· If you take prednisone only once a day or once
  every other day, it is best to take it in the
  morning, shortly after arising.
· You should take prednisone with a meal if
  possible.

SIDE EFFECTS

In high doses, some of the side effects (body
changes) from prednisone include increased
appetite and weight gain, puffiness of the face,
increased soft hair, acne, and occasional mood
changes. These are temporary changes which should
go away when the prednisone is stopped. With
long-term use of prednisone, possible side effects
usually not seen are thinning of the bones and
gastritis. Your doctor can usually prevent these
problems by reducing the dose of the prednisone
or by having you use it every other day.

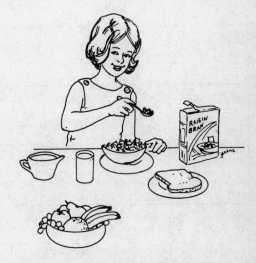

Eat a well-balanced diet.

(continued)

2 Prednisone

DIET

- It is important to eat a well-balanced diet.
- Some people may need extra potassium in their diets. Foods that are high in potassium are bananas, orange juice and oranges, raisins, prunes, dates, tomatoes, melons, squash, lima beans, potatoes, carrots, mushrooms, and milk.
- Your doctor may want you to limit the amount of salt you use while you are taking prednisone. Please follow the instructions you are given.

WHEN TO CALL THE DOCTOR

Call your doctor (phone: _____) if you develop any of these symptoms (signs):

- Stomach pain that is severe or occurs often
- Any infection other than a cold
- Temperature over _____
- Dizziness or weakness
- Blurring of vision
- Severe injury or stress to the body
- Vomiting

OTHER INFORMATION

- Consult your doctor before taking any other medicines or immunizations while on prednisone. You should also tell other doctors or dentists treating you, if you have taken prednisone in the past year.
- We recommend that you wear or carry a medical alert tag or card.

FOLLOW-UP

Your follow-up appointment is on (date): _____ at (time): _____.

Give medicine as directed on this calendar. Month _____ Year _____						
SUNDAY	MONDAY	TUESDAY	WEDNESDAY	THURSDAY	FRIDAY	SATURDAY

HELPING HAND
Homegoing Education
and Literature Program

Let's talk about...

Sodium Valproate "Depakene"

Sodium Valproate "Depakene" is a drug used
for the control of seizures.

Child's Name: _____
Age: _____

GIVING SODIUM VALPROATE

· Give the medication exactly as ordered by the doctor.
· The child should swallow the capsules without chewing to avoid irritation of the mouth and throat.
· If the child vomits all the medicine, give the same dose again <u>one</u> time. If the vomiting continues, call your doctor (phone: _____) or the Neurology Clinic (phone: _____).
· Be sure to get more medicine from the pharmacy <u>before</u> it runs out.
· <u>CAUTION</u>: Do NOT give any form of aspirin. If needed, you may give the child Tylenol or Tempra. Use cold preparations only if it <u>does not</u> contain aspirin.
· If you have a question, call your doctor or pharmacist.

☐ Give Sodium Valproate immediately after meals.

☐ The child should NOT have carbonated beverages (pop), citrus juices or extremely spicy foods at meals when the medicine is given.

Other Information: _____

_____

_____

POSSIBLE SIDE EFFECTS

· Nausea, vomiting
· Indigestion
· Diarrhea
· Stomach cramps
· Sleepiness
· Weight gain or weight loss
· Possible delay in blood clotting
· Itching and skin rash
· Thinning of hair

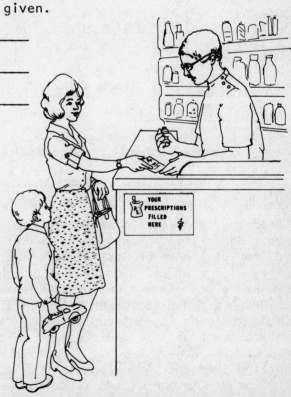

Picture 1 Have prescription refilled before it is all given.

(continued)

2   Sodium Valporate "Depakene"

WHEN TO CALL THE DOCTOR

Call your doctor (phone: _____) or Neurology Clinic (phone: _____):

· if your child has nausea, vomiting or upset stomach
· if drowsiness (sleepiness) becomes very severe
· if seizures increase in number or severity
· if child repeatedly vomits all the medications
· if you are unable to keep your appointment with the doctor

KEEPING A RECORD

Your doctor may want you to keep a record of your child's seizures. You can record this on your calendar at home, or you can use the record system explained below. Bring the record with you when you bring your child for medical check-ups.

☐ Use the record system explained here:

1. Divide each date into enough spaces to record each type of seizure. For example, if the child has two types of seizures, divide the box in half, as in the chart below.

2. Put total number of one type of seizure in one part of the box, and total number of other type of seizure in other part of the box. For example, if a child has 2 myoclonic seizures and 15 staring spells on January 1, you would record it as in the first box.

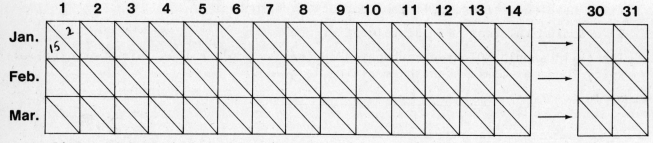

Picture 2 Record the type and number of your child's seizures each day.

FOLLOW-UP APPOINTMENTS

· Blood may need to be drawn at each visit for continuing evaluation.
· You can expect to have regular follow-up appointments with your doctor.

CAUTION

· Read the label each time before giving this medicine.
· Wash and dry your hands before handling drugs.
· Do not give more or less of this medicine than is ordered by your doctor.
· Stay with your child until he has taken the medicine.
· Do not give this medication to anyone other than the person it was prescribed for.
· STORE ALL MEDICINE OUT OF CHILDREN'S REACH. Store in locked cupboard if possible.
· When medicine is no longer needed, flush it down the toilet.
· If too much of this medicine is accidentally taken call your doctor IMMEDIATELY (doctor's phone: _____), the Poison Control Center (phone: _____), or the Emergency Room (phone: _____).
· Do not use this medicine after the expiration date.

If you have any questions, please call _____.

Index